THE CRAFT OF LIFE COURSE RESEARCH

The Craft of Life Course Research

edited by
Glen H. Elder, Jr.
Janet Z. Giele

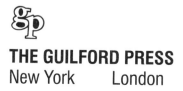

THE GUILFORD PRESS
New York   London

© 2009 The Guilford Press
A Division of Guilford Publications, Inc.
72 Spring Street, New York, NY 10012
www.guilford.com

Printed in the United States of America

This book is printed on acid-free paper.

Last digit is print number: 9 8 7 6 5 4 3 2 1

Library of Congress Cataloging-in-Publication Data

The craft of life course research / edited by Glen H. Elder, Janet Z. Giele.
    p. cm.
  Includes bibliographical references and index.
  ISBN 978-1-60623-320-7 (pbk. : alk. paper) — ISBN 978-1-60623-321-4
(hardcover : alk. paper)
    1. Life cycle, Human—Research—Methodology.   I. Elder, Glen H.
II. Giele, Janet Zollinger.
  HQ799.95.C73 2009
  305.2—dc22

                       2009021253

Preface

This book is intended to show how experienced investigators do life course research. Just as craftsmen introduce newcomers to a field by showing them how expert work is done, this book is meant to impart to other scholars and students in neighboring fields some of the newest and best research methods for studying the life course by showing how leading practitioners do their work. Accordingly, we invited distinguished specialists on the life course to contribute chapters that draw upon their own research, thereby providing a view of each project "from the inside." The book begins with an introductory chapter on life course research as an evolving field. The three main sections of the book then demonstrate several ways to collect different kinds of data, how to measure dynamic processes, and how to investigate the micro and macro explanatory factors that have an impact on the course of lives.

In our opening section on methods of data collection, each chapter walks the reader through a particular research process, such as designing a longitudinal study of the life course, collecting life record data, using ethnography to investigate hidden behavior in families, and posing research questions to fit a specific longitudinal data set. In Chapter 2 Robert M. Hauser describes nearly four decades of involvement in the Wisconsin Longitudinal Study (WLS) and tells how the project evolved from a statewide investigation of high school seniors' aspirations to a long-term study of their lives. The WLS is now one of the premier data archives in the world for the study of life course patterns and aging. In Chapter 3, on collecting and interpreting life records, Dennis P. Hogan and Carrie E. Spearin outline a variety of sources, such as tax records, membership lists, street directories, and court documents, that can enrich and supplement other longitudinal data. Ethnographic observation over time is the form of data collection taken up by Linda M. Burton, Diane Purvin, and Raymond Garrett-Peters in their account of the

Three-City Study of mothers on welfare (Chapter 4). Over time, the trust that is established between ethnographers and respondents allows many important, but previously hidden, experiences to be revealed, such as past or ongoing physical and sexual abuse. The last chapter (Chapter 5) in this section on data collection moves to another level, where Glen H. Elder, Jr., and Miles G. Taylor explore how to make the most of longitudinal data that are already available. Using such classic examples as the Terman Study of gifted children begun in the 1920s, they demonstrate how new questions can guide recoding and the addition of relevant new data through follow-up of the original participants.

Part II of the book takes up a central concept of aging and life course development, namely, the conceptualization and measurement of dynamic processes by which earlier events and transitions shape and influence later experience. Each chapter in Part II represents a marked advance in clarifying and measuring the processes by which earlier life events and transitions influence subsequent states. In Chapter 6, on cumulative processes, Angela M. O'Rand discusses the concept of cumulative advantage and disadvantage, and notes the underlying similarity between conceptual models and strategies for measurement of social inequality and accumulation of stress. It turns out that education is a pivotal factor for improving the likelihood of both upward mobility and better health. Life transitions often entail stress, and David M. Almeida and Jen D. Wong (Chapter 7) show how the microstudy of daily stress illuminates transition experiences and their health implications. They observe a remarkable consistency in studies of stress—that it appears to be higher for younger people than for older people, perhaps because later life transitions are more expectable, and individuals learn adaptive strategies that can reduce stress as they grow older. In Chapter 8, on trajectories, Linda K. George asserts that the central focus of life course research is *intraindividual* change, and that the measurement challenge is to identify which factors of timing, duration, sequence, or turning points result in a given trajectory. Along with giving examples of thematic and investigator-designed classifications of trajectories, she carefully explicates the difference between two major quantitative methods—hierarchical linear modeling and latent class analysis (both of which are actually illustrated in this book in the chapters on stress and crime). Finally, in Chapter 9, Elaine Eggleston Doherty, John H. Laub, and Robert J. Sampson demonstrate the use of group-based trajectories in life course studies by identifying several major life patterns that characterize delinquents. For example, the trajectories of incarceration vary according to the age of males when they began offending, with the highest curve for those institutionally raised youth who typically began offending by the age of 7.

The chapters in Part III of the book focus on explanatory factors that range from micro- to macrostructural and contextual influences that affect life course outcomes. At the *intrapersonal level*, Michael J. Shanahan and Jason D. Boardman (Chapter 10) show that genes are expressed "across the life span" and consequently require a life course framework to investigate interactions and correlations between genetic and environmental influences. For example, they report the results of a longitudinal study, which indicate that a genetic risk factor (*DRD2*, a dopamine receptor) is associated with lower rates of school completion in boys, but if the child comes from a higher socioeconomic status, the influence of this risk factor is greatly reduced. In Chapter 11, on life stories, Janet Z. Giele shows that qualitative themes expressed in life histories reveal marked differences at the *personal level* in self-concept, motivation, relational, and adaptive style. Among college-educated white and black women, these differences are strongly associated with being a career woman or a homemaker. At the *interpersonal level*, Phyllis Moen and Elaine Hernandez (Chapter 12) draw upon extensive research on linked lives to outline ways of thinking about and measuring the impact of "social convoys" of family and friends on major life transitions and trajectories. Important life transitions, such as when to retire, are very often affected by the needs of a spouse or an aging parent. In the closing chapter (Chapter 13), Hans-Peter Blossfeld systematically reviews cross-national research on life course phenomena at the *societal level* through the use of comparative methods to assess differences in major social institutions as a source of life course variation across European countries. He finds, for example, that characteristic national patterns in fertility behavior, educational attainment, and women's employment are associated with societal differences in family, market, education, and social welfare institutions.

As editors, we first joined forces some years ago to undertake our first volume on methodological issues in life course studies, *Methods of Life Course Research* (Giele & Elder, 1998b). The thinking and collaboration that brought us together began over two decades ago, when our research interests converged through professional friendship, mutual involvement in life course studies, and participation in interdisciplinary committees. In that first volume, as in this book, we invited leading practitioners of life course studies to prepare a chapter that revealed the process of doing such work, with abundant references to their own research.

After a decade of notable expansion in the variety of available longitudinal data and the life course studies being conducted, it is instructive to note how this second book is different from the first. The field of life course studies has matured. There appears to be more consensus on methods of data collection and on analytical strategies, and the chapters in this book reflect such changes. Longitudinal survey research and panel studies are the principal ways to chart changes in the life course over time, with other methods, such as linkages to life records, ethnographic observation, or archival enrichments, as important supplements. Likewise, there appears to be a methodological convergence on measurement of cumulative processes by the use of growth curves and latent classification of trajectories. In regard to explanatory strategies, there also appears to be progress in identifying multiple levels for causal analysis (intrapersonal, personal, interpersonal, and societal), both within and across levels. All in all, this book, which represents the current work of outstanding life course researchers, is testimony to major advances in the methods by which investigators actually do life course research.

In the course of this project, we have been assisted in countless ways. Most of all, we are indebted to C. Deborah Laughton, our editor at The Guilford Press. She embraced our plan, helped us work through the book's structure, and generously guided and supported us with wise counsel and enthusiasm. Terry Poythress at the Carolina Population Center (University of North Carolina at Chapel Hill) played a key role in assisting us with communications, coordination of activities, and other technical matters as we brought our book manuscript to press. This included the painstaking task of building a unified set of references. Her expertise kept us moving along, and we thank her profusely for all she has done to ensure a successful outcome. It has been a great pleasure to work with our distinguished list of authors as they sought to identify and present some of the most significant developments in their domain to a broad audience. We appreciate their patience and dedication in working through multiple revisions.

As editors, we are grateful for the support of institutions that have helped us to sustain our work on life course projects. A Senior Scholar Award to Glen Elder from the Spencer Foundation provided both time and essential resources in the development of the book manuscript. He especially appreciates many years of financial support from the National Institutes of Health and the National Science Foundation for longitudinal studies of lives and families in changing environments. His life course studies began at the Institute of Human Development at the University of California at Berkeley in the early 1960s, and both directors and staff encouraged and supported the continuation of this work. In addition, he wishes to thank the MacArthur Foundation and the U.S. Army Research Institute for generous research support. In Chapel Hill, his home for many years, the Carolina Population Center, the Center for Developmental Science, and the Institute on Aging have made the University of North Carolina a rewarding place to conduct longitudinal studies of the life course, human development, and aging.

For Janet Giele, an interest in life course research grew as she studied the changing lives of women. Beginning with comparison of the lives of 19th-cenury temperance and suffrage leaders, she turned to analyzing survey data from 20th-century cohorts of women graduates of Wellesley, Oberlin, and Spelman. Her foray into qualitative analysis of life stories began with a Radcliffe Institute fellowship and additional funding from the Murray Research Center and Brandeis University. Her research on women's lives has received support over the years from the Ford Foundation, the Social Science Research Council, the University of Michigan, the Lilly Endowment, the Rockefeller Foundation, the German Institute for Economic Research, and the German Marshall Fund. She is especially grateful for the collaboration and stimulation of colleagues and students at Brandeis and the Heller School, particularly the former Policy Center on Aging, the former Family and Children's Policy Center, and the Department of Women's and Gender Studies.

Contents

CHAPTER 1

Life Course Studies

An Evolving Field

Glen H. Elder, Jr.
Janet Z. Giele

Lives are influenced by a changing society, though little is known about how this occurs. Immigration posed such a challenge to W. I. Thomas and Florian Znaniecki (1918–1920) in their landmark study, *The Polish Peasant in Europe and America*. They provided an ethnographic–historical account of life in the old country of Poland, and of eventual settlement in urban environments of Northern Europe and America. But they did not have the methods or resources to follow immigrants to communities in the New World and to study the personal effects of this social transition. Decades later in World War II, research teams (Stouffer, Suchman, DeVinney, Star, & Williams, 1949) used cross-sectional surveys to assess the impact of wartime experience on soldiers morale. However, they could not identify sources of changing morale, because they did not observe the soldiers over time. Today *The Polish Peasant in Europe and America* and *The American Soldier* are recognized as pioneering classics of early social science, and the study of people's lives has flourished, moving well beyond these limitations for addressing questions at hand.

Ever since the 1950s, there have been extraordinary advances in studying lives over time, and they extend across disciplines in the social, behavioral, and biological sciences. The times called for new thinking about people's lives, society, and their relationship, now identified with life course concepts (Elder, Johnson, & Crosnoe, 2003). Aging populations contributed to this perspective by focusing attention on relations

1

between the early and later years. Most noteworthy among data collection methods is the explosive growth of longitudinal studies that follow people into new situations and across their lives. In a special issue of *Science* (Butz & Torrey, 2006), this research design has been described as the "Hubble telescope" of the social sciences and as one of the most important methodological innovations in the field (Phelps, Furstenberg, & Colby, 2002; Menard, 2008). Sequential surveys of a sample or birth cohort generate data that enable scientific observers to "look back in time and record the antecedents of current events and transitions" (Butz & Torrey, 2006, p. 1898). With this perspective, longitudinal studies have brought a greater appreciation of temporality, process, and contextual change to the study of people's lives.

This introductory chapter provides an overview of major methodological issues in life course projects by showing how all share in a new paradigm on the life course. The paradigm emerged out of the convergence of theoretical and empirical strands of research that link social change, social structure, and individual behavior. We make explicit the paradigm's core principles, especially as it has come to be understood in sociology, and describe how it developed out of empirical discoveries after 1960. We turn next to new directions in life course studies and include the methodological developments reported in this book.

Emergence of the Life Course Paradigm

How new models emerge from a time of contrary practices is often puzzling. A prime example involves the sudden appearance of "major longitudinal studies" of the life course after years of survey research. Most social research between World War II and 1960 was based on cross-sectional surveys that offered snapshots of a person's life. Studies also investigated the effects of social structure on individual behavior at a point in time, even though both factors are known to change. And, too often, people were depicted as if they lived in what Nisbet (1969) has called the "timeless realm of the abstract." In short, social research of the 1950s in the United States neglected change in people and environments, an observation that also applies to greater Europe.

This scientific climate began to change in the 1960s, when a number of developments favored longitudinal studies and a contextual life course perspective. They include the rise of new scientific questions that take advantage of the medical/life histories of people, and the perceived relevance of longitudinal designs for their study. More questions focused on the etiology of health and illness, owing in part to the postwar establishment of the National Institutes of Health (NIH) in the United States, with emphasis on pathways to health and disability. For example, the Framingham Heart Study was launched in 1948, with over 5,000 men and women from Framingham (Massachusetts) between the ages of 30 and 62. Based on funds from the National Heart, Lung and Blood Institute of the NIH, this pioneering longitudinal and intergenerational study has been extended to the Framingham grandchildren. Similar changes in research questions in Great Britain are evident in government support for national longitudinal cohorts. Medical Research Councils in the United Kingdom have played a major role in managing and promoting national longitudinal cohorts, from 1948 to 2001 (see Ferri, Bynner, & Wadsworth, 2003, pp. 313–324).

The model for such research designs may well have been influenced by the prewar writings and initiatives of social psychologists and developmentalists in the United States. During the mid-1920s, W. I. Thomas, a social psychologist, asserted that priority should be given to the "longitudinal approach" to lives, that studies should investigate "many types of individuals with regard to their experiences and various past periods of life in different situations " (in Volkart, 1951, p. 93). Thomas appears to have had in mind a study that followed children from their earliest years to young adulthood. The first decade of life would set in motion the pathways of later life. The impact of Thomas's recommendation is unknown, although he knew that a small group of psychologists at the Institute of Human Development at Berkeley was involved in launching such studies of children with birth years at opposite ends of the 1920s (Elder, 1999). The resulting projects focused on child development, but the study participants were eventually followed through the Depression and War years to their middle years and old age (Eichorn, Clausen, Haan, Honzik, & Mussen, 1981).

Research Questions, Designs, and Contextualization

New scientific questions about the etiology of health and illness, and the proliferation of longitudinal studies were necessary but clearly not sufficient as catalysts for the development of life course models in the 1970s. For example, the Framingham Heart Study made excellent use of its longitudinal data, but the investigators did not chart the social pathways of the study members or the timing of events. The Berkeley longitudinal studies focused on issues of behavioral continuity from early childhood to the middle years. The investigators devoted no attention to the routes—whether college, the workforce, or military service—that young boys and girls followed into adulthood. The historical time and place of these studies were not part of the research. This neglect of life contexts was not unique to these studies. Lewis Terman's (1925) sample of talented Californians (born 1903–1920) entered college and the workforce during the 1930s, and over 40% of the men served in World War II (Holahan & Sears, 1995). But neither of these historical periods was of interest to the investigators; they also paid little attention to the life course of the study members.

The essential influence to consider is the rise of "contextualiza-tion," which had its beginning in the late 1950s. Social history began to flourish at this time, with emphasis on the lives of people, their families and communities, instead of Kings and Queens (Thernstrom, 1964). In the field of historical demography, manuscript census files have been used to generate individual-based data files. Steven Ruggles (2002) at the University of Minnesota has pioneered the development of public use microsample files of federal census reports, extending all the way back to 1850. In preparation of the files, his team has provided data in a standardized format that enables intercensal comparisons. Each census file is based on at least a 1% sample of the national population. The files enable investigations of life course patterns over historical time in population subgroups defined by race and ethnicity, immigrant status, and age and sex. Though individuals cannot be tracked across succes-sive censuses, Hogan and Goldsheider (2003, p. 684) point out that indi-vidual persons in households can be used to track the aggregate life course in carefully defined birth cohorts over time.

In the 1970s, life course specialists began to collaborate with social historians on historical studies of the life course, as in the Essex County–1880 study in Massachusetts (Hareven, 1978). Historians launched social histories of the life course, with a focus on adolescence (e.g., Modell, 1989) and on decline in the textile industry, expressed through the lives and families of workers (Hareven, 1982). A good many developmentalists also shifted their interests in the direction of study-ing children's lives and families in context (Eccles & Midgely, 1989). Schools, neighborhoods, and communities were investigated as child-hood contexts with potential effects on development.

Perhaps influenced by a new awareness of the connection between life patterns and social change, significant theoretical work emerged in the 1960s on this link, highlighted by Norman Ryder's seminal essay, "The Cohort as a Concept in the Study of Social Change" (1965). He stressed the notion of life stage in his account of cohort differences in the life course. As each birth cohort encounters a historical event, it "is distinctively marked by the career stage it occupies" (p. 846). In the early 1970s, Matilda Riley and her colleagues wrote about the dual functions of age (Riley, Johnson, & Foner, 1972). Age distinctions order social roles, and they also order people according to birth cohort (the year of birth). Children's life chances are influenced by the economy's health at the time of their birth. For example, Americans born at opposite ends of the 1920s (1920–1921 vs. 1928–1929) experienced different life chances through the Depression and war years (Elder, 1999). Boys in the older cohort, unlike the younger cohort, were not wholly dependent on their families during hard times, but they were recruited to military duty early in World War II, whereas the younger cohorts of males were too young to be drafted for service in this war.

In the field of sociology, investigators applied newly formed interests in the life course to the recasting of unused data archives (see Elder & Taylor, Chapter 5, this volume). For example, Robert Sampson and John Laub (1993) injected new vitality and purpose into Sheldon and Eleanor Glueck's archive (1950) of data on 1,000 men who had grown up in a low-income area of Boston, 1924–1932. This study employed a matched control design with 500 young males who had a delinquent record and 500 who did not. The authors recoded the available data to measure life pathways and adaptations up to the young adult years. In a subsequent volume, Laub and Sampson (2003) analyzed crime and death statistics on the men, and succeeded in collecting new interviews from a small number of them in late life. Divergent life lines emerged from the shared origins of this disadvantaged sample.

To set up these studies, the authors used an age-graded theory of informal social control that has since been modified to include historical context and human agency. The meaning of age in lives, developed initially and most extensively by Bernice Neugarten (1996) in the 1950s and 1960s, was used in constructing an age-grade perspective. This included the social definitions of age status, normative divisions of the life course (e.g., adolescence and young adulthood), and age norms, as expressed in expectations regarding the timing of life transitions. "According to theory, age expectations define appropriate times for major life events and transitions. In moving through the age structure, individuals are made cognizant of being early, on time, or late in role performance" (Elder, 1975, p. 175). A second aspect of this theory involves ties to significant others and the constraints of role relationships. Both social embeddedness through relationships and age became primary components of a developing life course perspective. For Sampson and Laub (1993), age as birth year located their study members in history as young men during World War II, and a large percentage entered the military at that time.

Life Course versus Child Psychology/Life Span Studies

In theory, a longitudinal life course perspective refers to multiple levels—from aggregate, institutionalized pathways to the lived experience of people working out their life course. Life course studies (see Elder & Shanahan, 2006) tend to relate the lived experience of individuals to their developmental processes. Life span developmental psychology, established at the end of the 1960s by Paul Baltes and Warner Schaie, also claims this field of investigation with a commitment to the study of contextual effects (Nesselroade & Baltes, 1974). However, there is an important difference between the two perspectives.

Developmental psychology models, including some in the life span field, frequently focus on individual development in a "typical life course" (see Hetherington & Baltes, 1988). This might be the typical pathway from early childhood into adolescence or into adulthood. From this perspective, life course variation is not recognized as a potential source of behavioral change (but see Heckhausen, 1999). By contrast, such variation is of primary interest to the life course specialist, along with variation by cohorts and historical context. This interest is being expressed among investigators of child development studies that have been continued into the young adult and middle-age years (see Magnusson, 1988). We hope that the future will bring more fruitful cross-fertilization in the years to come.

Longitudinal Data Collection

Longitudinal projects launched in the contextual world of the 1960s and 1970s accelerated the application and advance of life course research, often by adopting conceptual distinctions, such as the timing of a change in status (a transition) and duration in a state, trajectories, and turning points. In this regard, Hogan and Goldscheider (2003) refer to the formative early 1970s, a time when demographic study became heavily dependent on secondary data files based on national samples, such as the Panel Study of Income Dynamics and the National Longitudinal Surveys:

> These studies served multiple purposes, with a design that was driven by the broad community of researchers (by means of national advisory panels). Once the life course perspective was adopted by a few leading demographers on these advisory panels, it quickly became the standard by which national surveys was judged. Thus, data necessary for life course research were quickly available to all demographers. (p. 682)

In fact, all users have benefited from this change. Mayer (2009) refers to the widespread dissemination across the social sciences of "a longitudinal life course perspective," and that longitudinal data collections have increased in dramatic fashion and have become the current "gold-standard" of quantitative social science.

Empirical applications of these studies include the National Longitudinal Study of Mature Women (Moen, Dempster-McClain, & Williams, 1992), the National Longitudinal Surveys (NLS; Pavalko & Smith, 1999), and the Panel Study of Income Dynamics (PSID; Duncan & Morgan, 1985). Economists played an important role on the advisory committees of the NLS and the PSID. The PSID became a model for longitudinal studies in other countries, ranging from the United Kingdom and Germany to Canada and Sweden, among others. The British National Cohort studies (1946, 1958, 1970, and 2001) represent an impressive standard of longitudinal data collection for the study of changes in society and in lives (see Ferri et al., 2003). Finally, the well-known Stockholm Longitudinal Study was established by developmentalist David Magnusson (1988).

In addition to prospective studies, a retrospective method for collecting life history data in a reliable form, with an age–event matrix, began to take shape in the late 1960s (see Brückner & Mayer, 1998; Scott & Alwin, 1998). This matrix facilitates accurate memory through comparison of events in a particular year, and events across the life span. The method represents a giant advance over the retrospective interview dating back to the early years of the 20th century. It maximizes accuracy in self-reports (except for emotional responses, subjective accounts). Also, the retrospective method enables researchers to conduct life course studies in places that lack prospective data archives, such as Germany after World War II. Overall, the impressive array of prospective and retrospective studies has launched generations of potential investigators into a study of human lives and development across the life course. These studies have encouraged research on pathways through a sequence of life stages and increased the need for models of lifelong development and aging.

Advances in life course models and sequential data collection have placed a premium on essential techniques of data analysis, such as event–history models for age-graded life events (Mayer & Tuma, 1990; Blossfeld, Gotsch, & Rohwer, 2007); trajectory analysis with latent growth curve and latent class models (Laub & Sampson, 2003); and the analysis of multiple levels with hierarchical linear models, as in studies of neighborhood- and family-level effects on children (Singer & Willett, 2003). Each of these techniques of analysis deserves more detailed elaboration, and we do so in George's masterly account of trajectory research in Chapter 8 (this volume) and in Doherty, Laub, and Sampson's (Chapter 9, this volume) account of group-based trajectory analysis. More longitudinal life course studies are combining both quantitative and qualitative data.

Elements of the Life Course Paradigm

As coeditors of this volume, we bring different intellectual and research histories to this introductory chapter, but we also acknowledge a convergence in what we consider the common elements of the life course paradigm. Elder first encountered longitudinal studies in the early 1960s, when he arrived at the Institute of Human Development to work with sociologist John Clausen, then director of the Institute. His task was to design interview codes for the Oakland Longitudinal Study members, born in 1920–1921. Though Elder approached this research project with an interest in the effects of social structure on people, life records in the data archive directed his attention to the challenge of studying lives in a changing world. The data revealed much change in lives and relationships across the 1930s. A good many study members could say that they had been well off at one time but were now "quite poor."

These observations focused Elder's attention on ways of thinking about social change, life transitions, and trajectories as modes of behavioral continuity and change. Transitions, such as entry into first grade and graduation, are part of a life trajectory that gives them meaning. The multiple pathways of individuals and their developmental implications became key elements of the life course in Elder's *Children of the Great Depression*, published in 1974, followed by an enlarged 25th anniversary edition in 1999. This edition compared the Oakland young people up to the middle years with Berkeley study members, who were much younger during the Depression era (born 1928–1929). This younger life stage placed the Berkeley children at greater risk of economic hardship, especially the boys. The two birth cohorts of young men were also compared on experiences during World War II.

From the time of Giele's graduate studies at Harvard under Parsons, Homans, Inkeles, and Stouffer, she has been most keenly interested in the question of how social system requirements become articulated with individual motives and goals through links between individuals and the social structure. She asks not only how the environment shapes the person but also how, in turn, people intentionally try to change their own situation, as well as the larger society. She began her research career with a doctoral dissertation on the 19th-century American women's movement that contrasted the lives of women's temperance and suffrage leaders. Later, she turned her research to a comparison of the lives of women college alumnae from different eras to pinpoint the differences in the life course that preceded the rise of the new women's movement and steady growth of married women's labor force participation.

This work generated questions about innovations in women's lives— how they change their roles and initiate efforts to change the larger institutions of work and family. Life course change and feminist activity are bidirectional in Giele's research, a perspective shaped by her studies of Wellesley College graduates and other college alumnae groups in the 1970s and 1980s. She discovered a shift toward multiple roles among women born since 1930. Additional comparisons of data from Germany and the United States identified changes in jobs, family life, and education that had begun in the 1940s and 1950s, and contributed to the rise of feminism in the 1970s.

Emergence of the Fourfold Paradigm

From the accumulated findings of his work on children of the Depression, Elder (1994, 1998a) identified four paradigmatic factors that affect the diverse ways the life course and human development are influenced: *historical and geographical location*, *social ties* to others, *human agency* in the construction of one's life course, and *variations in timing* of events and social roles. Each factor applies to the full life span, consistent with the principle of life span development—that human development and aging are lifelong processes. This principle of aging as a continuous dynamic (see Riley et al., 1972) reflects a general shift from "age-specific" studies to research that extends across long segments of life. Human development and aging cannot be explained fully by restricting analysis to a specific life stage in question. According to this perspective, the early years of childhood are relevant to understanding social adaptations in later life, not just in the adolescent years and young adulthood.

Historical and Geographical Context

The biographies of people are located in specific communities and historical times. To address these matters, investigators began to draw upon the insights of a deeper knowledge of the meanings of age. Ryder (1965) and Riley et al. (1972), among others, developed the historical meaning of age as birth year. People born in a certain year are members of a birth cohort, with a particular historical experience and range of life opportunities that depend on geographic location. The life course principle of historical time and place is derived from this research.

Social Embeddedness

The principle of *social ties* to others is derived from a role change and relationship-based approach to lives. Lives change as relationships and social roles change. The concept of life cycle focused this perspective on intergenerational relationships and change—as a reproductive sequence

high school to new
—long lasting friends

of parenthood stages over the life course, from the birth of children through their departure to their own childbearing. This process is commonly known as a "family cycle" (Hill & Foote, 1970). Typically, the stages are not defined by age, and they follow a prescribed sequence of marriage, childbearing, and survival to old age, an increasingly atypical pattern in contemporary society. Nevertheless, the life cycle processes of intergenerational relations and reproduction depict an important functional domain of linked lives. Social ties to significant others establish forms of socialization and control in channeling individual actions and decisions.

Agency and Personal Control

The "principle of agency" refers to the process by which people select themselves into roles and situations. In doing so, they construct their own life course within given constraints. People are planful and make choices that give them a chance to control their lives (Clausen, 1993). Elements of agency have been prominent in life history research (Thomas & Znaniecki, 1918–1920) and are central to life course studies that relate individuals to broader social contexts.

The inclusion of people and social structures in models of the life course establishes the potential for what might be termed "loose coupling" between the age-graded life course and lives as lived by individuals. "Age-grades and loose coupling exemplify two sides of the life course—its social regulation and the actor's behavior within conventional boundaries, and even outside of them" (Elder & O'Rand, 1995, p. 457).

Timing

Here the question of interest is *when* an event or transition occurs in a person's life, whether early or late relative to other people and normative expectations. Neugarten (1996), a social psychologist, broke new ground by developing the normative and subjective meanings of age in the late 1950s. Social or normative expectations determine in part whether a role transition, such as marriage or promotion to supervisor, is early or late. The principle of timing is based on this research literature.

To Giele, these four principles appear to be a variant that can be independently derived from Talcott Parsons's (1966) four-function model of the social system (the familiar AGIL in reverse—Latent pattern maintenance, Integration, Goal attainment, and Adaptation) as applied to social change and the life course (see Figure 1.1). In her book, *Two Paths to Women's Equality*, Giele (1995, pp. 18–23) used four elements—cultural background, social membership, individual goal orientation, and strategic adaptation—to describe the ways in which the historical women's temperance and suffrage movements carried the life course change of leaders into the broader social structure. In her recent work on variations in men's and women's roles, she has used the same schema to characterize differences between traditional homemakers and married women with careers (Giele, 2004, 2008).

How is it that basic elements of the Elder and Giele paradigms correspond with each other? Elder's core principles of the life course are filtered through the individual, whereas the corresponding dimensions identified by Giele are focused on relations between the individual and the surrounding social structure. Linking the two frameworks is useful for tracing the interplay of person and setting, and of dynamic change

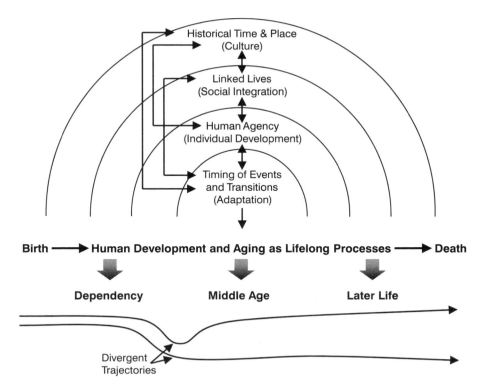

FIGURE 1.1. Elements of the life course paradigm.

by the individual in a context of social leads and lags, as spelled out in the following paragraphs. Moreover, in linking the life course paradigm with a more general theory of action (which has long been a major project of leading theorists), the life course approach is greatly expanded, and explanations and models of analysis can be integrated and applied across an ever-wider set of problems and disciplines (Giele, 2002b).

Historical Time and Place (Cultural Background)

This principle underscores the multiple layers of human experience; the social hierarchies, cultural and spatial variations; and the social/biological attributes of individuals. Children who grew up in the Great Depression encountered hardship at different times in their lives, and their experiences may have varied across urban and rural places as well. Indeed, all historical events are likely to have different meanings across geographic areas and individual life stages. In the case of early feminist leaders, their regional and historical backgrounds set them apart from the general population of women. To establish a new order, they developed an ideology that would promote new cultural patterns.

One of the most dramatic illustrations of historical and spatial change in a birth cohort comes from a longitudinal study that followed 12th-grade students (1983–1985) from 15 regions of the former Soviet Union up to 1999 and beyond (Titma & Tuma, 1995). Called Paths of a Generation, the study assessed the life aspirations, achievements and cultural backgrounds of young people before the Soviet Union disintegrated circa 1990, then traced their lives into a period of exceptional change and instability. One region retained the command economy of the old Soviet Union (Belarus), whereas others adopted a market economy (e.g., Estonia) or returned to a more primitive rural exchange system (e.g., Tajikistan).

The socioeconomic lives of young men and women tended to resemble the changes of their respective regions of the old Soviet Union. For example, the Estonian cohort ranked at the top on prosperity, whereas downward trajectories were common among youth from Belarus. Despite such regional variations and economic instability, the future of this cohort to date was written in large part by members' personal accomplishments, self-appraisals, and goals during high school. Academic success and high aspirations were more predictive of high occupational status and income than family background. The young men who had become entrepreneurs with hired personnel were most distinguished by their ambition in high school and positive appraisal of personal skills in managing people.

Linked Lives (Social Integration)

The life of a person is interwoven with the lives of significant others. In the Great Depression, economic hardship changed decision making, the division of labor, and emotional ties among deprived families in ways that were not experienced by the nondeprived children. This difference forced boys and girls from hard-pressed families into assuming household responsibilities. In Giele's study of feminist leaders, family, religious and educational networks played an important role in channeling the women toward the role of reformer, an influence that differed for women who focused on charitable work rather than on changing the laws. Such relationships can be thought of as a context for development and aging. Antonucci and Aikyama (1995) refer to this moving social network as a "social convoy."

New relationships can lead to a change in the composition of friends, as in the case of marriage. Wellman, Wong, Tindall, and Nazer (1997) report that a new marriage typically leads to a turnover in the friends of the husband. Similarly, Sampson and Laub (1993) found that the marriage of young men with a history of crime leads to a turnover in their friends and a decline in the likelihood of more criminal activities. By contrast, shared military experience tends to establish enduring social ties that extend beyond the temporal boundaries of a war. Among veterans of World War II and the Korean conflict, exposure to combat and loss of comrades increased the likelihood of enduring social ties through visits, letters, and phone calls (Elder & Clipp, 1988).

Human Agency (Individual Goal Orientation)

Elements of human agency and structural constraints are central to any effort to relate individual lives to broader social contexts. People's motives to satisfy personal needs result in decision making that organizes their lives around goals within the options and pressures of their situations. Thus Giele (2008) found that feminist leaders who had experienced some personal loss were more likely to be interested in temperance and charitable work. However, women who had been denied higher education, opportunities for work, and/or a political voice because they were women tended to support the suffrage movement.

In the Great Depression, girls from economically deprived families grew up seeking traditional homemaker roles, whereas nondeprived girls were likely to obtain more education and gratification from the combination of paid work and family life. Although some girls with deprived backgrounds moved beyond homemaking to education and employment, the future of girls from more privileged backgrounds depended on their intellectual ability and resourcefulness.

Social constraints restrict and channel the expression of agency. Consider, for example, a planful view of one's future in the 1930s to 1940s (Shanahan & Elder, 2002). Events beyond one's control were prominent in these decades, and an uncontrollable environment was characteristic of the lives of older men in the Stanford–Terman study, who were born between 1903 and 1911. Most had completed college before the Stock Market Crash; consequently, they entered a labor market that soon became stagnant in the economic crisis of the 1930s. Their dismal chances in the labor market kept them in school, acquiring advanced degrees. Nevertheless, a significant number of these men eventually rose to positions of high accomplishment. By contrast, younger men (born between 1911 and 1920) remained in some form of schooling throughout the 1930s, long enough to find attractive jobs as the economy improved because of World War II.

Timing of Lives (Strategic Adaptation)

To accomplish their ends, people and groups (e.g., families) coordinate responses to the timing of external events, such as loss of employment, to undertake actions that use available resources most effectively. In this manner, the timing of life events can be understood as both passive and active adaptations for attaining individual and collective goals. How and when a person acquires wealth or education, enters a new job, or starts a family illustrates potential strategies. Among early feminists, a number of women were interested in temperance early in their careers, then graduated to the suffrage movement, a pattern that was reflected in feminism as a whole. Temperance became the most popular women's reform movement in 1890, whereas suffrage soon dominated the succeeding decades.

In the dependency years, a girl's relatively early transition (e.g., physical maturation) can significantly increase developmental risks, such as a premature exposure to older boys and sexual pressures. In the field of criminology, studies show that the earlier the age at first arrest, the greater the risk of subsequent incarceration. In the well-known Dunedin Longitudinal Study, Moffitt, Caspi, Harrington, and Milne (2002) followed the males up to their 26th year, an age that still proceeds the median age at first marriage in New Zealand. In a comparison of two groups on age at onset of antisocial behavior (childhood vs. adolescence), investigators found that the childhood group displayed the most elevated pattern of psychopathic personality traits, violent and drug-related crime, problems of mental health, substance abuse, and economic–work problems.

Figure 1.1 depicts all of these principles and theoretical elements coming together through the funnel of life course timing to influence life trajectories. Whatever a person's cultural heritage and social location, friendships and networks, or personal motivation, they are experienced through the individual's adaptations to concrete situations and events. As we show later in this volume, historical time and social timing give structure to the life course.

New Directions and Challenges in the 21st Century

As the preceding pages indicate, a great many advances in theory and method have distinguished the evolving field of life course studies over the past half-century. Especially noteworthy from a methodology standpoint is the spectacular growth of longitudinal studies, both prospective and retrospective. In thinking back to the 1950s, when the social survey reigned supreme, no one could have imagined how prominent this longitudinal design would become in social science research by the 21st century, and in promotion of a new field of study and thinking known as the life course.

The small cluster of pioneering longitudinal studies, launched before World War II, began to pose challenging questions by linking childhood to the adult years and late life as study participants grew up and entered their middle years. Child-based models were also challenged theoretically by the question of how to think about the organization of human lives and their development over the life span. Because these longitudinal studies found subjects in changing environments, investigators confronted the question of how to think about the relation of development to an ever-changing society (Elder, 1998b). What theories would be helpful in connecting lives to changing contexts? The answer at the time called for fresh thinking in the direction of the life course paradigm, because longitudinal studies at that time paid virtually no attention to the pathways of lives, or to their historical context and place.

But the influence process did not merely flow from longitudinal studies to theoretical orientations on the life course. As life course concepts began to take the form of a theoretical perspective, this framework played a role in shaping decisions made by senior social scientists concerning the design of survey instruments for national longitudinal studies in the United States (the National Longitudinal Survey, etc.) and perhaps elsewhere. Hogan and Goldscheider (2003) tell this important story, and we have drawn extensively from their essay in representing the evolving perspective on the life course, with its trajectories and transitions (Elder, 1985b; Mortimer & Shanahan, 2003). Life course dynamics evolve over a lengthy period of time, within a trajectory of work or marriage, and over a short span of time, such as leaving one job and entering another.

By following a birth cohort of young people into adulthood and the middle years, longitudinal studies have collected data from lengthy sequences of survey waves. Given sequenced data on key outcomes, such as emotional health, the measurement and analysis task has centered on trajectories, with emphases on both level and rate of change. A case in point is the Monitoring the Future sample, which has followed seniors out of high school and into adult pursuits. The longitudinal component of this sample has more than 10 data waves on topics such as work values. For example, Johnson (2002) used latent growth curve analysis to identify work–value trajectories of stability and change from adolescence to the young adult years. She found a pronounced growth of realism toward jobs as study participants progressed toward the later years of young adulthood. In this volume, George (Chapter 8) and Doherty et al. (Chapter 9) discuss the strengths and limitations of individual- and group-based analyses of life course trajectories.

Up to the present, a small number of longitudinal samples have followed their study participants across multiple stages of the life course. This has led to research that links socioeconomic disadvantage to cardiovascular disease in later life (Kuh & Ben-Schlomo, 1997/2004; O'Rand & Hamil-Luker, 2005) and to mortality (Hayward & Gorman, 2004). These studies and others add compelling empirical documentation to the principle that human development and aging are lifelong processes. But even in this fruitful research domain, few longitudinal studies have actually investigated the interplay between developmental/aging processes and the socially patterned life course (see Mayer, 2009).

Longitudinal studies that extend across most of the life span remain exceedingly rare. This limitation may change as studies add follow-ups, but analysts are also using available data to extend the scope of their inquiry, for example, by pairing strategically related longitudinal samples for each half of the life course. Brown (2008), for example, has paired the National Longitudinal Survey of Youth sample (late adolescence to mid-40s) with the Health and Retirement Survey (ages 50+) to investigate the wealth and health trajectories of African Americans and European Americans. Birth cohorts in the two studies are not identical; thus, potential historical effects require some caution, but this strategy at least enables the investigator to apply the insights gained from young adult experience to an understanding of late-life trajectories.

With these issues in mind, we turn briefly to four themes that identify new directions for theoretical work and method on the life course: (1) the contextualization of lives, (2) analogies to cumulative advantage–disadvantage, (3) stress and the life course, and (4) the life course as social interventions.

Placing Human Lives in Context

The analytic task of placing lives in context refers to an extended temporal process in long-term longitudinal studies. With the extension of active longitudinal studies, lengthy prospective histories can link changing times to lives. The longest running study, the Terman Project, illustrates the potential of such research. This project followed a sample of Californians from birth in the first decade of the 20th century to 1992. Over 40% of the men served in World War II (Elder, Shanahan, & Clipp, 1997), and their overseas duty increased the risk of poor health in late life.

Today with the availability of geocodes and coordinates to map households in national data sets, investigators have the information to locate people in context. These data and spatial techniques of analysis enable researchers to take major steps toward contextualizing lives in neighborhoods. Crowder and South (2008, p. 792) note that in the field of migration "prior work tends to treat neighborhoods as isolated islands, largely divorced from their broader social, geographic, and economic context." The authors based their project on the view that neighborhoods are "embedded in a larger mosaic of urban communities" and conclude that the "conditions of nearby neighborhoods influence the behaviors of individuals in a given neighborhood" (p. 809). Likewise, Sampson, Morenoff, and Earls (1999) observed that studies of spatial dynamics indicate that the crime rate and collective efficacy of youth in neighborhoods affect these outcomes among youth in adjacent neighborhoods.

Beyond Cumulative Advantage and Disadvantage

The concept of cumulative advantage and disadvantage that is used to measure inequality has some analogues in the domains of education, health, and stress. In a seminal essay, published in 1960, Howard Becker proposed a theoretical account of a process by which people become committed to a line of action through their acquired ties to others and their social control. In life course terminology, the process involves duration dependence. The concept of "duration" refers to the waiting times between changes in a person's status. The duration of a person's job indicates the stability of employment, and duration of residence in a particular neighborhood indicates a person's residential stability. Strong local ties discourage residential change.

This perspective provides a useful way of thinking about the cumulative dynamic of social ties—enduring, weak, or broken. Change in social ties can affect health and well-being. In *Crime in the Making* (1993), Sampson and Laub proposed an age-graded theory of informal social control in which the individual with weak conventional ties is especially vulnerable to the temptations of crime and deviance. With a longitudinal sample of 500 delinquent males from low-income areas of Boston (birth year, 1924–1932), they found that young men who desisted from a life of crime were most likely to have entered new sets of conventional relationships during the transition to adulthood, primarily in jobs, marriage, and military service (Laub & Sampson, 2003). As turning points in the life course, these transitions pulled men away from deviant friends, while involving them in strong, competing relationships.

At present, little is known about the cumulative dynamic of social relationships, even though it is a vital component of health, broadly considered, and of cumulative advantage and disadvantage (see O'Rand, Chapter 6, this volume). In their analysis of social convoys, Moen and Hernandez (Chapter 12, this volume) emphasize the obvious but often neglected point that all individual lives are linked lives. They show that much is lost in understanding dual-career couples when only one career is studied in terms of work that spills over into marital life. Consistent with their recommendations, data collection from multiple respondents (e.g., partners, siblings) has become more common during the past decade, and one of the best illustrations comes from Hauser's discussion of the Wisconsin Longitudinal Study (Chapter 2, this volume) in which data were collected from not only the primary respondents but also family members and others. Nevertheless, much unfinished business remains in terms of network studies of family and/or close friends over the life course.

Stress and the Life Course

Up to the 1990s, studies of stress and the life course were largely carried out in splendid isolation, with researchers barely acknowledging each other. Today this separation is hard to imagine: Stressors affect people's lives, and life transitions often entail stressful adaptations. Even by the mid-1990s, sociologists noted a continuing neglect of life course models and methodology in "studies of stressful life events and judged research on stress and well-being to be still largely uninformed by knowledge of how lives are socially organized and regulated by age norms, demographic patterns, and social structures" (Elder, George, & Shanahan, 1996, p. 248; also see Pearlin & Skaff, 1996). However, much change has occurred since then. Indeed, Leonard Pearlin, a leading sociologist in the study of stress, spoke about the affinities between stress and life course models in his Matilda White Riley lecture at the 2008 American Sociological Association meeting. These affinities are well expressed in *The Handbook of the Life Course* (Mortimer & Shanahan, 2003) and by Almeida and Wong in this volume (Chapter 7) in their discussion of life transitions and daily stress. More generally, dynamics of the stress process have become essential elements of the sequence of events and adaptations that link the early life course to health and illness in late life.

This research model addresses the "black box" characterization of longitudinal studies on the antecedents of health and illness, in which the mediational mechanisms and contexts are ignored. In the field of epidemiology, Kuh and Ben-Shlomo (1997/2004) also regard the life course approach as a notable advance beyond such limitations, with emphasis on the etiology of chronic disease. As they make clear in an anthology of this empirical work, a temporal and multilevel life course approach generates "knowledge of how past events have shaped the risk of subsequent exposure, the responsiveness of physiological systems, and behavioural patterns" (p. 459). The life course perspective gained prominence in epidemiology during the 1990s, when an increasing body of longitudinal evidence documented the link between childhood adversities and the risk of disease in later life. Life course epidemiology emerged from this research as a recognized field of epidemiological inquiry.

The Life Course as Social Intervention

The status passage of young people into and through the young adult years is marked in distinctive ways by departures from multiple social roles and entry into new roles, such as leaving home and establishing an independent residence. Within the framework of life course analysis, this period of role transitions provides an opportunity for youth and for social institutions to change the course of young lives toward a better future. In their study of this transition among delinquent Boston youth (born 1924–1932) from low-income areas, Sampson and Laub (1993) refer to these transitions as *turning points*. Stable employment, marriage, and military service altered the life trajectories of a significant proportion of these young people. In 21st-century America, the all-volunteer military provides potential access to higher education for disadvantaged youth (Segal & Segal, 2004), and a variety of social interventions aim to promote a more constructive direction in the lives of these young people.

An example of the life course as a social intervention comes from the Miami Youth Development Project (Kurtines et al., 2008), a community outreach program that has been in operation through alternative schools in the Miami–Dade County System for nearly two decades. A key component of this community program is known as the Changing Lives Project, which offers, through alternative schools, counseling services that employ a participatory learning and transformative approach to empower troubled youth. The counselors address the presenting problems through psychoeducational and individual counseling, as well as group sessions on topics such as substance abuse, anger management, and troubled families. Approximately 250 students participate in these counseling sessions each year. The overall strategy, then, consistent with the life course perspective, focuses on developmental gains that assist youth in changing circumstances that adversely affect their lives. In this manner, these young people become agents of their own life courses.

These are only a few of the new directions and challenges we have observed in life course research up to 2009. A much broader sample is provided by the chapters of this book.

Plan of the Book

We begin with a focus on data collection (Part I), led by Hauser's description of the Wisconsin Longitudinal Study (WLS) and its development over four decades (Chapter 2). This is an appropriate beginning, given the important role of longitudinal research in the evolution of life course studies. The WLS was launched before the crystallization of life course models that eventually shaped its theoretical framework on aging. As the project became a longer-term longitudinal study, it gradually assembled life stories of members of its Wisconsin cohort. Across the life stages of this cohort, data collection foci and practices tended to reflect the intellectual currents of the time. For example, the role of biology in life course development and aging did not become a major research theme until the late 1990s, with the advance of data collection technology. The WLS has since collected biomarker data and buccal saliva samples for genotyping.

Hogan and Spearin (Chapter 3) detail the process of gaining access to marriage, divorce, birth, and crime records, and the research opportunities that are experienced by merging these records with a primary data archive. Sometimes a "discovery" research strategy is needed to understand life experience; a method that calls for ethnographic study. In Chapter 4, Burton, Purvin, and Garrett-Peters show that this method of data collection is well suited to uncovering hidden behaviors in lives that typically are not detected in quantitative studies. Research questions typically guide the collection of data and the use of data archives, but as Elder and Taylor note in Chapter 5, longitudinal studies tend to outlive their original questions. As a result, investigators must ask new questions of old data and maximize the goodness of fit. To achieve a better fit, life records may be merged with the data at hand. As a whole, these chapters bring to mind the advantage of mixed methods of data collection in research on lives.

Data collection can be thought of as the foundation of life course research, providing appropriate data to address investigators' questions. Though much is known about methods of data collection, this is not the case in the formulation of thoughtful research questions. Robert Merton (1959, p. ix) has noted that posing research questions might seem to present no difficulty "and yet, the experience of scientists is summed up in the adage that it is often more difficult to find and to formulate a problem than to solve it." As readers, you may bring research questions to these chapters on data collection and find better ways of formulating them, or even develop different questions. This is the process of matching research questions and data.

The varieties of data collection surveyed in Part I provide empirical documentation of changing lives across the life span and historical times, with related challenges for conceptualization, measurement, and analysis. These challenges involve ways of thinking about changing lives, personalities, and contexts, along with the development of useful measures and techniques of analysis. Three concepts and their measurements are especially prominent in current studies of life course dynamics: cumulative processes of advantage and disadvantage, life transitions, and life course trajectories. All three represent new directions as the focal point of chapters in Part II.

Changing lives and personalities pose questions concerning relevant mechanisms, such as the cumulation of advantages or adversities. For many years, cross-sectional studies documented an association between socioeconomic status and health, with no attention to the potential cumulative dynamic of this effect into the later years. However, the rapid growth of long-term longitudinal studies has shifted research efforts to the cumulative process of socioeconomic disparities in health and well-being. O'Rand (Chapter 6) provides a guided tour of this line of work, its accomplishments, and unfinished business. Stress is a likely mechanism in this process. Almeida and Wong (Chapter 7) survey empirical evidence on the daily stresses of life transitions and provide a "backstage" introduction to the measurement and analysis of relevant stressors.

The concepts of trajectory and transition represent the long and the short perspective on life course change and continuity. Life course dynamics, for example, a trajectory of education or work, occur over a lengthy period of time, and they also evolve within a short time span marked by specific events, such as leaving or entering a job. Transitions are always embedded within a trajectory, such as job changes in a work career. In Chapter 8, George distinguishes between social and developmental trajectories, and notes that not all trajectories evolve from a sequence of transitions based on categorical data. Some are measured by continuous data, as in the case of sequential reports of emotional distress.

A life trajectory is often regarded as either an independent or a dependent variable. However, both types of trajectories are frequently measured and analyzed in the same study. To introduce the reader to the measurement of trajectories (using the methods of latent growth curve and latent class analysis), George has sequenced selected studies according to the number of trajectories they employ and their function. Doherty, Laub, and Sampson (Chapter 9) supplement the breadth of George's survey by focusing on group-based trajectories, as applied to a central problem in the field of criminology—age variations in the desistance from crime. Why do some men stop their criminal ways at the end of adolescence, while others continue this life a decade or more into adulthood? The authors used latent class analysis to identify an optimal number of groups of men defined by similar desistance patterns. In measurement and analysis, trajectories identify diverse life course patterns.

Variations in the life course reflect a broad set of influences. In Part III, we examine four influences and their particular strategies for investigating explanatory factors—genetic dispositions, differences in personality and behavioral adaptation, interdependent lives, and institutional–cultural variations by country. Over the years, studies have shown that exposure to a particular event does not affect all members of a population in the same way. As Shanahan and Boardman indicate in Chapter 10, this is so, in part, because people bring differing genetic tendencies to the event. Unlike most work in this field, the authors argue that genetic influences must be investigated across the life course, not just at a particular point in time. Gene expression takes place over time and is subject to modification through environmental changes. The interplay of genes and environment provides an opportunity to investigate genetic dispositions in the self-selection of people into life transitions and pathways (Caspi, 2004). Selection is a vital process of life course development, though we still know very little about it.

A recurring puzzle in longitudinal studies of the life course centers on the lives of people who do not follow the "continuity or conventional script" from social origin to their destination in later life. Contrary to predictions based on social origin, some people do much better than expected in life, whereas others do much worse. What are the personal qualities and experiences that help to explain these different life paths? In many cases, the investigator draws upon survey data, collected at different points in life, to address this question. But such data typically fail to provide an understanding of motives, goals, and strategies of people who followed these different life paths.

Giele (Chapter 11) faced this limitation in understanding motives in the feminine role by turning to the life story method to achieve a deeper understanding of women's lives. This method used retrospective interviews with open-ended questions to obtain an explanation for why college-educated mothers of similar age, both white and black, had become homemakers or career women. Distinctive themes differentiated the women by role outcome. She discovered their personal views of life and accounts of how things had evolved in their lives. An important part of this view concerns the people to whom they are linked, as Moen and Hernandez show in (Chapter 12). Giele concludes by reviewing the theoretical and methodological principles of the life story method, as applied in her own studies of differences in women's lives by race and gender.

Though most life course projects focus on the lives of individuals, Moen and Hernandez (Chapter 12) persuasively show how incomplete such research can be in understanding the transitions and trajectories of people's lives. The social convoys of life include family, friends, and coworkers, among others. The successes and failures of children in establishing their adult lives beyond the family of origin have enduring consequences for the lives of parents, as do the problems of the older generation in the later years of life. Moen and Hernandez highlight such interdependencies within and across the generations.

Most longitudinal studies are based on samples from a single society, but the phenomenal diffusion of such studies across developmental societies during the past half-century offers hosts of new possibilities for cross-national research, as surveyed in Blossfeld's pioneering chapter. In the early days of cohort studies of the life course, analysts became increasingly aware of the perils of assuming that one could generalize findings based on a single cohort to an entire population. Since then, studies have shown that life patterns vary across successive cohorts. Likewise, Blossfeld emphasizes the strategic values of cross-national comparisons of life course longitudinal analyses for the purpose of determining the generalization boundaries for empirical findings. The same social institution, such as education or the family, often assumes different forms and functions across societies. For example, Blossfeld's comparative research shows that the contingent lives of couples (see Moen and Hernandez, Chapter 12) assumes different forms in relation to the partners' resources by region of Europe and country. In the Mediterranean countries, the family system is malecentric and few wives are gainfully employed.

The new directions for life course studies that are so prominent across the chapters of this volume represent major challenges that promise to stretch our minds, talents, and external resources. Among other things, we are urged to study people over their lives and times, and to do so in multiple societies; to collect life record data on social networks or linked lives over time; and to bring biology into the study of health and the life course. This is an exciting time for life course research, and we hope this book proves to be useful to our readers.

PART I

METHODS OF DATA COLLECTION

One of the key methodological contributions to the growth of life course research has been the advance in survey technology that began with post–World War II surveys and panel studies (Giele & Elder, 1998b). Using these methods, Stouffer et al. (1949) reported in *The American Soldier* the effects of combat experience on later attitudes, and Lazarsfeld et al. (1944) examined in *The People's Choice* how people made up their minds, over the course of several months, on the way they would vote in a presidential campaign. In the ensuing half-century, the techniques for tracking changes in individual behavior and attitudes over time have progressed remarkably. There is growing consensus that representative longitudinal surveys are the most comprehensive and accurate way of capturing changes not only in behavior of a population over time but also in the lives of individuals. As Mayer (2009) says in a comprehensive review of life course research since 2000, the longitudinal survey or panel study with repeated administration of questions to the same persons is now considered the "gold standard" for high-quality life course data. The basic data from longitudinal surveys are then supplemented by more intensive studies of specific age groups who report either retrospectively on past experiences or prospectively about successive current events, transitions, and feelings. The result is that longitudinal survey methodology has become institutionalized. There is consensus among researchers that the data can be trusted. The means for administering and analyzing the surveys have been standardized, and there are mechanisms in place that make the data accessible for a wide range of research purposes.

There is also recognition that since the 1960s large public invest-ments have been made in projects, such as the Panel Study of Income Dynamics (originally the Five Thousand Family Study) and the National Longitudinal Surveys on labor market experience. Therefore, it behooves researchers, when possible, not simply to collect their own new data on a particular problem but to use what is already available. Publicly acces-sible websites now make it possible to download and reanalyze data with one's own purposes and hypotheses in mind.

Fortunately, Chapter 2 by Robert M. Hauser gives us an inside view of the development of one of the key ongoing longitudinal studies of the last 50 years. His chapter, "The Wisconsin Longitudinal Study: Design-ing a Study of the Life Course," describes the initial impetus for launch-ing the survey in 1958 to study the aspirations of Wisconsin high school seniors. These students born in 1938–1939 are now 70 years old. It is possible to chart how their lives have unfolded with respect to family life, education, employment, and health. The project began with a focus on the precursors of upward social mobility and the effects of childhood circumstances on health and well-being. But over time, as the original cohort has grown older, uses of the study have shifted to a focus on healthy aging, differential access to health services, and the precursors of high cognitive functioning as compared with cognitive decline. The chapter provides a fascinating inside view, through Hauser's eyes, of how the study evolved. The chapter also suggests the many possibilities for other investigators to use these data to answer their own questions. A comprehensive description of the questions, samples, and mechanisms for downloading and analyzing data are all available through the Wis-consin Longitudinal Studies public website.

At the same time that large national repeated surveys have become the standard for achieving representativeness, it has also become clear that not all relevant and significant information can be captured by quantitative survey methods. Several other kinds of data are needed for validating the results, uncovering important influences not included in a survey, or incorporating relevant archival material. Three other chap-ters in Part I describe ways of collecting these different but important kinds of life course data.

Chapter 3, "Collecting and Interpreting Life Records," by Dennis P. Hogan and Carrie E. Spearin, takes us to the largely unnoticed trove of written public records that can be used to reveal the health, marital, employment, and civil status of individuals. Of potential interest are tax records, membership lists, and court documents, which are not provided by the individual directly but can be used to reconstruct the history of populations and the life course of persons. Such reconstruction can be done for a population in a specific historical period. Written records can also be used to put together a running description of a person's life at several points in time and to serve as a valuable alternative or supplement to repeated surveys or a person's self-reports. However, making use of such data requires imagination to be able to picture in one's mind's eye what records might have been left behind and where they might be found. Hogan and Spearin list some of the possibilities: high school and college yearbooks, employment records, marriage licenses, health records, insurance data, and tax records.

Chapter 4, "Longitudinal Ethnography: Uncovering Domestic Abuse in Women's Lives" by Linda M. Burton, Diane Purvin, and Raymond Garrett-Peters, alerts the reader to the vast unknown territory of individual behavior that goes unmentioned both in surveys and public records. This is particularly true of any kind of embarrassing, deviant, or illegal activity. The authors claim that by using ethnographic methods based on close observation over time, these hidden behaviors will gradually come out, and the ethnographers themselves will become confidants. They illustrate these principles with unforgettable and troubling accounts of domestic abuse, both physical and sexual, from participants in the Three-City Study of mothers who had been dependent on public welfare. Especially valuable for the practitioners of life course research are the recommendations about the ethical dilemmas that face the ethnographers when they must decide how to maintain trust, yet also sustain their professional integrity. Such questions arise when the researchers are confronted with the demands of confidentiality, along with the professional obligation to report abuse to the authorities, or when they are torn between giving help and maintaining professional distance.

In Chapter 5, "Linking Research Questions to Data Archives," Glen H. Elder, Jr. and Miles G. Taylor further expand the range of alternatives for collecting longitudinal data. They present three major strategies for linking longitudinal data to new research questions. The first is a *recasting* process, in which the investigator records and restructures existing data to maximize the fit between the available information and the question, as has been done with the Terman data on gifted children and the Gluecks' data on juvenile delinquents. The second strategy is *merging* of supplemental files with existing longitudinal archives that might contain health, death, or military records. A third approach is a *follow-up study* of the original members of a longitudinal sample for the purpose of supplementing information on a particular topic. Several follow-up studies are given as examples. One, Elder's own work on the Terman data, which examined experiences of men in the military during World War II, found links between age of entry, length of service, and measures of later health and well-being. Another example is the remarkable success of Moen, Dempster-McClain, and Williams (1989, 1992) in tracing respondents of a 1956 study and discovering 20 years later that respondents who died early had smaller social networks at the time of the first study than those who were still alive.

CHAPTER 2

The Wisconsin Longitudinal Study

Designing a Study of the Life Course

Robert M. Hauser

The Wisconsin Longitudinal Study (WLS) is just over 50 years old, and it has become the most enduring study of its scope and size in the United States and perhaps in the world. What began in the late 1950s as a state-inspired survey of what happens to Wisconsin youth after high school has become a biosocial study of health, cognition, and well-being in the retirement years, as well as a vehicle for studies of intergenerational social and economic stratification. A lone investigator at the University of Wisconsin–Madison has been replaced by a loosely coordinated team of several dozen researchers that spans the nation. A once-private and distinctly modest data resource has evolved into a complex combination of survey operations and administrative record links with a Web-based system for public distribution of massive data files, extensive documentation, powerful search and extraction tools, and hundreds of publications (see *www.ssc.wisc.edu/wlsresearch*).

The importance of the WLS as a resource for studies of the life course depends on the extensive data that have been collected from 1957 onward—or even earlier in some cases—and on the investments made by the National Institute on Aging in the study since the early 1990s (Sewell, Hauser, Springer, & Hauser, 2004). The WLS can contribute to basic knowledge about social, behavioral, and biological processes in three fundamental ways. The first is by providing new information about the consequences of childhood and adolescent conditions and experiences. The second major contribution of the WLS is to provide new information about the extent to which early life conditions affect later life outcomes, above and beyond the known effects of the conditions and experiences of adulthood. Finally, because of its rich, complete, and contemporaneous records of careers and family events, the WLS provides unique opportunities to analyze the characteristics of whole-life trajectories that may affect the quality and length of later life.

Today's research and policy environments are far different from those of the late 1950s. On the one hand, both the feasibility and the scientific value of longitudinal studies of the life course are well established. Such studies have become the backbone of observational research in psychology, sociology, and economics. In the realms of human development and health, by dint of the well-known Barker hypothesis (Barker, 2001; Kuh & Ben-Shlomo, 1997/2004), life course research now extends back into the womb, and a national study of child development aims to follow health and development that ranges from couples' childbearing intentions to their offspring at age 21. In each decade since the 1970s, the National Center for Education Statistics has followed a cohort of youth from secondary school to the end of the school years. The Bureau of Labor Statistics has fielded three waves of longitudinal studies of adolescent youth since the late 1960s. The National Institute on Aging (NIA) supports longitudinal studies of aging in the United States—including the WLS—and in many foreign nations, but its premier data resource, the Health and Retirement Study, now provides continuous longitudinal coverage of the U.S. population age 50 and above.

In current and future work, the WLS will be used to explore the implications of the changing social, political, economic, and technological contexts of the early 21st century for the well-being of a large cohort of men and women transitioning to old age. Among the most important social and economic changes are the deinstitutionalization and individualization of retirement; that is, retirement is no longer a well-defined economic status—simply a matter of leaving the labor market—but a distinct and expected, yet highly variable, stage of the life course in which time spent in paid work tends to decline and may be replaced by unemployment, leisure, or disability.

Over the past 20 years, both the government and employers have shifted more of the responsibility associated with planning and managing the retirement years toward individuals. The capacity of individuals to make good choices about their investments, medical care, insurance, and other domains of increased uncertainty and personal responsibility will be an important determinant of both financial and health-related well-being in old age. Moreover, technological advances—ranging from the expansion of the Internet to the development of life-extending medical technologies—also offer older adults an unprecedented number of options about health insurance, choice of health care providers, and types of medical treatments. The contexts in which people are making these choices will play a significant role in shaping the quality of those choices, and ultimately, in older Americans' quality of life.

Among other questions, WLS data will be used to ask, "In what psychological, cognitive, social, and health contexts do WLS graduates plan for then actually manage health and financial arrangements in the retirement years?" In short, what kinds of resources and constraints frame the process of their decision making? Because decisions about the retirement years are increasingly in the hands of individuals, it is critical that we adequately understand the contexts that shape peoples' lives. How do these provisions affect the lives of their survivors in the event of their death? A second key question is, "What are the earlier life factors, both individual and contextual, that lead to better outcomes in the postretirement years?" How is the quality of later life affected by childhood circumstances and their repercussions across the life course? Are there lagged effects of early life conditions, or of job and familial trajectories across the life course, or are circumstances in the later years connected to childhood only through intervening circumstances? We expect that analyses of the cumulated WLS survey and biomarker data, along with rich administrative and public data, will resolve old questions and open new areas of interdisciplinary inquiry about health, aging, and the life course.

I wish I could write that the evolution of the WLS followed a well-established plan, or at least an aspiration, that from the outset the WLS was intended to track the entire life course of thousands of Wisconsin youth and to become a resource for a research team in Madison and hundreds of other researchers across the globe. But in the late 1950s there was no such intention, nor were there appropriate theoretical or methodological templates for such an endeavor. Rather, the study has been like Topsy: "It just grew." To be less flippant, the evolution of the WLS has paralleled that of the human life course; it began and has changed as a consequence of its initial location in time and place, social and intellectual connections, individual initiatives, and adaptation across time to external events (Giele & Elder, 1998a). In this chapter, with its focus on development of the WLS, I draw repeatedly on this parallel, but more important, I try to highlight some of the decisions—regarding content, design, and method—that have shaped the project.

The WLS: Its Origin and Research Context

The WLS began with a 1957 survey of the educational plans of all high school seniors in public, private, and parochial schools of Wisconsin.

Not only was there a rising demand for college and university education in the late 1950s, but also economic and technological competition with the Soviet Union was a major public issue. Many states, including Wisconsin, were then consolidating and upgrading their postsecondary educational institutions. At that time, most of the units of the present University of Wisconsin System were state and county teachers' colleges. J. Kenneth Little, Professor in the School of Education at the University of Wisconsin, conducted the statewide survey with the cooperation of the Wisconsin State Superintendent of Schools, and it was used to plan the expansion and consolidation of public higher education in the State (Little, 1958, 1959).

In 1962, William H. Sewell, one of the academic leaders who brought the behavioral and social sciences into the National Institutes of Health (NIH) (Sewell, 1988), learned that the 1957 survey schedules and punch cards were sitting unused in the University administration building. Sewell had long been interested in the formation and consequences of youthful aspirations, but he had lacked access to an appropriate population for study. At that time, social scientists had little real evidence about the extent of social and economic mobility between generations in the United States. Only in 1962 was the first large, national study of social mobility in America conducted (Blau & Duncan, 1967). Researchers could do little more than speculate about the processes of selection and socialization that accounted for social stability or social movement.

Sewell selected for further study a random sample of one-third of the graduates, comprising 10,317 cases. He then added information on the measured mental ability of each student from files of the Wisconsin State Testing Service, which, since 1929, had conducted a testing program covering all high school students in the state (Froehlich, 1941; Henmon & Holt, 1931; Henmon & Nelson, 1946, 1954). Although Sewell's collection of the test score data followed naturally from his interest in postsecondary educational entry and completion, that measure has proved to be one of two key variables that have sustained the value of the WLS data. Moreover, the files of the Wisconsin State Testing Service have subsequently provided test scores for other participants in the study, including siblings of the graduates and spouses of the graduates and siblings.

Sewell developed a number of indexes based on information from the survey—including the socioeconomic status of the student's family, the student's attitudes toward higher education, educational and occupational plans, and perceived influence of significant others on educational plans—and then added these to each student's card. Finally, using secondary sources, he constructed relevant measures of school, neighborhood, and community contexts. These included the socioeconomic composition of each senior class (Sewell & Armer, 1966a, 1966b, 1972), the percentage of its members who planned on going to college, the size of the school, the size and degree of urbanization of the community of residence, and the distance of the student's place of residence from the nearest public or private college or university (Anderson, Bowman, & Tinto, 1972). However, the second key variable in the WLS was a 4-year average of parents' incomes from 1957 to 1960 that Sewell was able to obtain from files of the Wisconsin Department of Revenue; unlike many other longitudinal studies, up to the present day, he obtained a direct and highly reliable measure of economic standing in adolescence. Thus began a research program that is in its sixth decade and that now focuses on the lifelong antecedents of health and aging.

In the early years, WLS research focused mainly on the ways in which adolescent achievements and aspirations formed and then influenced postsecondary schooling and occupational careers. This work led to the so-called "Wisconsin model of status attainment" (see Figure 2.1), which became a template for subsequent research on the life course—and for critical attention to the social-psychological theory of status attainment (Sewell, Haller, & Ohlendorf, 1970; Sewell, Haller, & Portes, 1969; Sewell et al., 2004).

The essential ideas of the model are as follows: Social background affects school performance. These two sets of variables affect social influences—the expectations and modeling behaviors of significant others. Social influences largely determine educational and occupational aspirations, thus carrying much of the influence of social background and school performance. Aspirations in turn have large effects on postsecondary schooling and occupational careers, and they carry much of the effect of social influences, school performance, and social background.

The key theoretical idea of the model is the importance of social-psychological processes in mediating the connections between positions in the social structure across generations. This idea now seems simple, because it is widely accepted among social scientists. The model is also simple in a second, more important sense, that it is a modified causal chain. Not every earlier variable affects every later variable in the scheme. Of 15 possible paths from antecedent variables in Figure 2.1, only the seven paths marked with an asterisk (*) carry large effects.

It is well known that the Wisconsin model is a social-psychological elaboration of the Blau–Duncan (1967) model of intergenerational occupational stratification, but the marriage of that model with the social psychological theories of Sewell and his colleagues was neither accidental nor inevitable (Sewell & Hauser, 1992). It grew out of the

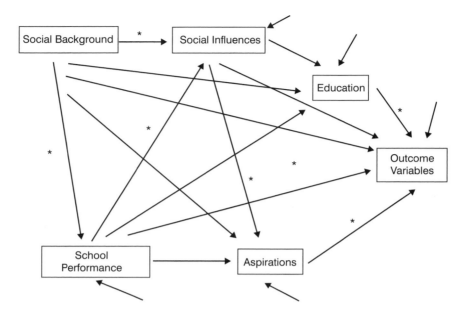

FIGURE 2.1. The Wisconsin model.

close personal and intellectual relationship between William Sewell and
Otis Dudley Duncan. Sewell had been hired in 1937, fresh out of the
University of Minnesota, by Otis Durant Duncan, who was then chair
of the Department of Sociology at the Oklahoma State University in
Stillwater. Sewell and the elder Duncan were neighbors in Stillwater.
Otis Durant's son Dudley was first babysitter for Sewell's children, then
academic advisee, and, by the 1960s, scientific advisor to Sewell.

The distinctive scientific contributions of the Wisconsin project lie
not merely in proposing the model but in testing it by means of careful—
and repeated—measurement of key variables across the entire adult
lives of the vast majority of participants in the study. These two features
of the study work hand in hand, for repeated measurements are costly
to obtain, requiring either sample retention or proxy reports (from well-
informed others), and their analytic use requires sophisticated statistical modeling. The Wisconsin model serves to illustrate these points,
though other analytic work in the WLS might also have been chosen.

It is patently clear that to follow occupational and economic achievement across the life course, one needs repeated measurement. Thus,
the Wisconsin model has repeatedly been estimated and validated as
the cohort has aged, starting with the original and modified versions
of Sewell and colleagues (1969, 1970), continuing with the addition of

earnings as an outcome variable (Sewell & Hauser, 1972, 1975), adding occupational standing at midlife (Sewell, Hauser, & Wolf, 1980), and culminating in a model of occupational achievement from school-leaving to the preretirement years (Hauser, Warren, Huang, & Carter, 2000).

However, in research that followed introduction of the model, both that based on WLS data, and in the hundreds of replications and extensions that followed (Sewell et al., 2004), the central social-psychological argument—that the process followed a modified causal chain—was forgotten, and researchers simply estimated recursive models in observable variables. This practice began as early as the second paper on the model (Sewell et al., 1970), in which additional paths were added to the model, based on the size and significance of simple regression estimates from observed variables.

I joined the WLS project in the summer of 1969. Otis Dudley Duncan, who had been my advisor at the University of Michigan, had suggested me to William Sewell as a possible collaborator. I arrived at Madison only after the two formative status attainment papers had been completed, and my early work with Sewell mined the same vein— running recursive models in observable variables (Sewell & Hauser, 1972, 1975). However, I also began collaborating with David L. Featherman to undertake a modified version of the Blau–Duncan study (Featherman & Hauser, 1975, 1978; Hauser & Featherman, 1977). Largely because of economist Samuel Bowles's (1972) critique of measurement in the Blau–Duncan survey, Featherman and I commissioned follow-up surveys of small samples of black and white men, in which we obtained repeated measurements of key socioeconomic variables. This led to a series of papers in which we estimated Blau–Duncan-type models with correction for measurement error, and we learned that these corrections had substantial effects—though not as anticipated by Bowles (Bielby & Hauser, 1977; Bielby, Hauser, & Featherman, 1977). Among other findings, we learned that—after taking account of response error—the process of socioeconomic attainment appeared to be more similar among blacks and whites than we had previously believed.

With this work in mind, I began to wonder whether it would be possible to estimate the Wisconsin model with corrections for errors in variables, and whether such estimates would sustain or invalidate the social-psychological theory that motivated the model. To carry out this agenda, we needed repeated measures of all of the variables in the model. Thus, in the 1975 telephone survey of graduates, our first direct contact with them since high school graduation, we not only ascertained information about military experiences, careers, family formation, and social participation across the previous 18 years, but we also remeasured social background characteristics, educational and occupational aspirations, educational attainments, and early occupations.

Working with Shu-Ling Tsai, a brilliant student from Taiwan, Sewell and I were able to estimate error-corrected models using Jöreskog and Sörbom's (1996) LISREL (Linear Structural Relations) program (Hauser, Tsai, & Sewell, 1983). Back in 1980, this was a very tedious process; we worked on the paper for 2½ years, and estimating a single variant of our model took days on the computers of that era. Now, it takes only a few seconds to estimate those models on an ordinary desktop or portable personal computer.[1]

The main finding from this study was that the original, parsimonious version of the Wisconsin model was correct, that the theoretically specified relationships were even stronger than initial estimates suggested, and that the unexpected relationships, later added to the model, were negligible. Unfortunately, the main lesson from this analysis has not been widely heeded, and almost all researchers continue to estimate models of social stratification "on the cheap," declaring as plain truth whatever comes out of simple regressions in observable variables.

One other example of the value of correcting for measurement error is the series of random effect models of sibling resemblance, largely based on data from the WLS, in which response error biases "within-family" but not "between-family" regressions. Hauser and Mossel (1985, 1988) provide a primer in the design and estimation of such models.

An even more striking example is provided by stratification research that compares models of aspiration and attainment between black and white youth in the United States. Across more than 30 years, the standard finding has been that the estimated coefficients of such models are much smaller for blacks than for whites, leading researchers to conclude that the corresponding processes are different in the two populations and directing them toward competing "structural" explanations of attainment differences (Kerckhoff, 1976, 1989; Porter, 1974; Portes & Wilson, 1976). For many years, these ideas could not be tested directly, because there were no longitudinal data with repeated measurements of key variables: social background, academic achievement, aspirations, and attainments. Such data are at last available from the National Educational Longitudinal Study of 1988 (NELS88). Megan Andrew and I find that, when appropriate corrections are made for response error in all of the relevant variables, there are essentially no differences in educational attainment processes among black, Hispanic, and white non-Hispanic youth (Andrew & Hauser, 2008).

The 1950s were a lively period in American sociology and social psychology. They were also a period of growing affluence, during which adolescence was redefined by the emergence of youth culture. Thus, Little and Sewell were by no means alone in focusing on adolescent circumstances and aspirations as the stepping-stone to adult lives. Other influential studies of American youth included James Coleman's *The Adolescent Society* (1961) and Albert J. Reiss, Jr.'s studies of Nashville youth (Reiss & Rhodes, 1961; Rhodes, Reiss, & Duncan, 1965). Sociologists of that time—and later times—were also captivated by Ralph Turner's provocative thesis contrasting "sponsored" mobility in British school systems with "contest" mobility in the United States (Turner, 1960, 1964). The Wisconsin study had been preceded by careful and insightful, but small and selective, longitudinal studies that had long been in progress, such as the studies of exceptionally able youth initiated by Lewis Terman (1925; Burks, Jensen, & Terman, 1959; Oden, 1968; Terman & Oden, 1959a, 1959b) and the two small studies of youth in California communities that were made famous by Glen Elder (1974) and John Clausen (1991, 1993).

In addition, the WLS was soon followed by large, national longitudinal studies of youth, the first of which was the ill-fated Project TALENT of 1960 (Flanagan et al., 1964, 1966). Three highly successful school-based national longitudinal studies of youth followed—the National Longitudinal Study of the High School Class of 1972, High School and Beyond (the class of 1982), and the National Educational Longitudinal Study (the class of 1992). However, none of these larger studies continued for more than 15 years. In my judgment, it is tragic that the division of labor among federal agencies has precluded a level of cooperation and integration that could have extended these studies across working life and into the retirement years. The National Longitudinal Studies of Labor Market Experience began with cohorts of 14- to 24-year-old women and men in the late 1960s, but the male sample was soon abandoned because of high attrition rates. Only with the aging of the cohorts in the 1979 National Longitudinal Study of Youth—who are only 43–50 years old in 2008—is there likely to be a national longitudinal study of women and men that compares favorably with the WLS both in size and coverage of the life course.

From Adolescence to the Life Course

Over the years, the WLS has collected data in many different ways—and has always protected it carefully regardless of its source. Table 2.1 provides a succinct overview of data available to the WLS or under development. After the 1957 survey of graduates, the next two waves of survey data were collected from the graduates and their parents in 1964 and 1975. In 1964, Sewell and his colleagues sent a very brief mail survey to parents of WLS graduates in the belief that 7 years after high school

TABLE 2.1. Survey and Administrative Record Data in the Wisconsin Longitudinal Study

Sources of survey data

- 1957 Senior Survey of Graduates
- 1964 Postcard Survey of Parents
- 1975 Telephone Survey of Graduates
- 1977 Telephone Survey of Siblings
- 1993 Telephone/Mail Survey of Graduates
- 1994 Telephone/Mail Survey of Siblings
- 2003–2007 Telephone/Mail Surveys of Graduates, Siblings, Spouses, and Widows
- 2007 Mail Survey about Medicare Part D enrollment
- 2009–2010 Personal Home Interviews and Assessments (in development)

Available public or administrative record data

- Henmon–Nelson Mental Ability (9th and 11th grades for graduates, other years for siblings and spouses)
- Rank in high school class
- High school yearbooks (including senior-year photos and extracurricular activities)
- Parents' adjusted gross income, 1957–1960
- Male graduates' earnings, 1957–1971
- College characteristics
- Employer characteristics, 1975
- National Death Index–Plus (and Social Security Death Index)
- Elementary and high school resources (from Wisconsin state archives)
- Wisconsin health insurance plans
- Local health resources (Area Resource File and Interstudy data)
- Medicare enrollment and claim data (at present, only for older siblings)
- Wisconsin Worker's Compensation records

Biomarkers

- DNA samples (graduates in 2007, siblings in 2008)

Administrative record data in process

- Wisconsin State Tumor Registry
- Geocoded addresses across the life course

graduation, youths would be unlikely to respond to such queries, whereas parents always like to talk about their children. The questionnaire—just one side of a folded postcard—asked about educational attainment, marital status, military service, and occupation of the graduate, and—in the case of women—the occupation of the graduate's husband. After five waves of mailing and a telephone reminder, the response rate was 87%. This rate of coverage in a large-scale study across a 7-year interval was unprecedented at the time, and it demonstrated feasibility for the large national studies that followed.

In 1975, after demonstrating the feasibility of tracing virtually all graduates for 18 years after high school graduation (Clarridge, Sheehy, & Hauser, 1977), the WLS carried out 1-hour telephone interviews with the graduates, in which more than 90% of the survivors participated. Taken together, the 1964 and 1975 waves of the WLS provide a full record of social background, high school curriculum, youthful aspirations and social influences, schooling, military service, family formation, labor market experiences, and social participation. Early survey data were supplemented by earnings of parents from state tax records; mental ability test scores and rank in high school class; and characteristics of high schools and colleges, employers, industries, and communities of residence. Data on the occupational careers of male graduates were supplemented by Social Security earnings histories from 1957 to 1971 (Sewell & Hauser, 1975).

We have continued to come up with new ways of learning more about the early lives of the graduates. Recently, state archival data on high school district resources from 1954 to 1957, and from elementary schools in the early childhood of the cohort, have been added. A creative and energetic graduate student, Sheri Meland, became interested in the long-term effects of facial attractiveness. She thought of the WLS as a source of appropriate data and was able to collect, scan, rate, and scale senior high school yearbook photos for thousands of WLS graduates by borrowing yearbooks from schools and libraries—beginning with the larger schools in urban areas. Meland (2002) developed visually anchored scales of facial attractiveness and a computer-based protocol for applying the scales to individual photographs. The success of this effort has led to studies of the Duchenne smile (Freese, Meland, & Irwin, 2007) and—by extension of the scaling method to facial mass—to a study of the long-term consequences of adolescent obesity (Reither, Hauser, & Swallen, 2009). The high school yearbooks also filled another gap in the early history of the WLS cohort by providing a comprehensive record of extracurricular activities in high school.

With all of these resources in mind, we decided to obtain yearbooks for all of the WLS graduates. Early in 2007, we designed a multipurpose contact with the graduates. We distributed reports of findings from the most recent (2004–2005) surveys, along with a short questionnaire about experience with the Medicare Part D prescription drug benefit, and, in addition, we enclosed a personalized letter asking whether we could borrow a high school yearbook from each student for whom we had not already borrowed and scanned one. The response was exceptional, and we now have coverage of 86% of the original graduates, whether or not they participated in later rounds of the study.

Linking Lives through Data Collection

In the 1975 telephone survey, the combination of two circumstances led us to obtain a roster of living siblings and to choose a focal sibling at random for each graduate (plus all twins). First, I was strongly impressed by the work that Otis Dudley Duncan (1968) and Christopher Jencks and colleagues (1972; Hauser & Dickinson, 1974) had done with survey data on the resemblance of siblings in cognitive ability and socioeconomic attainment. They had each made the most of the fragmentary data available at the time, and much as I admired their methods and models, I hoped that it might be possible to create a complete set of sibling resemblance data with the WLS. Second, in the early 1970s, I had witnessed many complaints that so-called "status attainment research" was excessively individualistic, that it did not take a relational approach to social stratification or consider the networks and social structures in which individual lives were embedded. While I strongly disagreed with such arguments, I also concluded that we would do well to situate the lives of graduates firmly in their social contexts.

With this in mind, we proceeded on four fronts. First, we asked each graduate to name his or her three best, same-gender friends from their high school graduating class. Using this definition, about half the graduates have a named peer in the sample (of which many are reciprocated choices). We chose not to ask women about men or vice versa, because—at that time—women tended to date older men, and men to date younger women. Similarly, to maximize the chances of matches within the sample, we limited choices to each graduate's own high school. Second, we obtained a roster of all children born to graduates that was organized by age and gender. We chose a focal child at random from this roster and asked the graduate about his or her hopes and expectations for that child. Third, we asked about the current social and economic characteristics of spouses and about their social origins. Fourth, as noted earlier, we obtained a roster of siblings that included age, gender, first name, and highest level of completed schooling. Then, we chose a focal sibling at random (or the graduate's twin) and asked about the occupation and the full name and address of that focal sibling. Our uses of these linked data are described below.

Figure 2.2 suggests a way of looking at the WLS study design in terms of the set of role–relationships about which the study provides information. Although the WLS data originally centered on the 1957 graduates, we now find it useful to think of them as focal points in sets of relationships with parents, spouses, adult children, and siblings, as well as relationships with the localities and social institutions through which they have passed—high school, military service, college, and employers.

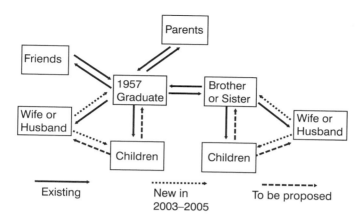

FIGURE 2.2. Some social links in the Wisconsin Longitudinal Study. Arrows go from source to subject of reports.

Available WLS files include survey and administrative data records for graduates, linked with those of friends and siblings. Parents were the initial post–high school informants about graduates, but a great deal of our information about parents has come from administrative records or from graduates and siblings. Data have first been obtained from spouses (and widows) in the 2004–2006 wave of the study, and we hope to add (adult) children eventually.

Going back to the files of the Wisconsin Testing Service, we were able to locate adolescent cognitive ability test scores for 6,619 of the focal siblings of graduates (75%). In 1977, with support from the Spencer Foundation, we interviewed a highly stratified sample of 2,100 of these randomly selected siblings—controlling the number of female–female, male–male, female–male, and male–female pairs, among other variables. These relational data proved so useful that we have included all selected siblings in the two subsequent waves of the study. Briefly, our work with the sibling data has shown that resemblance between siblings is greater with respect to ability than educational attainment, and greater with respect to educational attainment than later occupational and economic success. Moreover, the economic resemblance of siblings gradually declines as they grow older (Hauser, 1984, 1988; Hauser & Mossel, 1985, 1988; Hauser & Sewell, 1986; Hauser, Sheridan, & Warren, 1999; Hauser & Wong, 1989; Warren, Sheridan, & Hauser, 2002).

The 1980s were difficult years for the WLS. Until then, the project had been supported very well by the National Institute of Mental Health (NIMH) by dint of its focus on the antecedents and consequences of aspirations. However, the Reagan administration had no use for such studies, and we were summarily told that NIMH would no longer consider WLS proposals for support. The project managed to survive through a combination of local resources and small grants from the National Science Foundation, and in the absence of data-collection activities I was able to focus more on analytic issues, including the development of statistical models of repeated measurements and of sibling resemblance.

New Focus on Aging, Retirement, and Health

By the early 1990s, we realized that the years of work and child rearing were ending and that, if the WLS were to continue, it ought to focus on health, well-being, and retirement. We immediately regretted that we had failed to ascertain even the most rudimentary information about health in the previous round of the study. All the same, we decided to change the direction of the project and began to work with staff of the NIA.

In 1993–1994, the WLS conducted four major surveys with NIA support: telephone and mail surveys of graduates, and nearly identical telephone and mail surveys of an expanded random sample of focal siblings. Measurements included marital status, child rearing, education, labor force participation, jobs and occupations, social participation, and future aspirations and plans among graduates and siblings. The content of earlier follow-ups was expanded to include psychological well-being, mental and physical health, wealth, household economic transfers, and social comparison and exchange relationships with parents, siblings, and children.

In 1993–1994, the 1-hour telephone interview covered life history data, family rosters, and job histories, which have many skips or branches. The mail instrument also added measures of well-being, social contact, exchanges, and health, including an extensive account of menopausal experience. The sibling mail survey was modified to obtain additional measures of physical health and health-related behaviors, richer accounts of menopausal experiences, and more information about relationships between the focal sibling and other family members—including indicators of childhood abuse.

By 2001, when we were planning proposals for a new round of surveys, it was evident that the project would not survive if its content were limited to the interests of sociologists, economists, and psychologists, as traditionally conceived. This was the beginning of the era of biosocial surveys, and science of the life course was moving rapidly toward a truly interdisciplinary mix of traditional social science, epidemiology, neuroscience, medicine, and genetics. A series of excellent panel reports from the National Research Council (2000, 2001, 2006a, 2006b, 2008) charts this movement and provides guidance to researchers. The existing group of WLS investigators was ill-equipped to move in this direction, so we reached out for new collaborators.

New surveys of WLS participants were carried out, beginning late in 2003, when graduates were 63 and 64 years old. As in the 1993–1994 round of the study, WLS graduates and the sample of their brothers and sisters were first interviewed by telephone for about 1 hour, and more than 80% of survivors participated. Telephone interviews were followed by mail-out, mail-back surveys, which were longer than those in 1993–1994—more than 50 pages in some forms. I was at first overwhelmed by the number of items my colleagues offered for this instrument. However, in a chance meeting with Don Dillman (1991, 2000), an expert in mail and other self-administered surveys, I was assured that there is no documented relationship between response rates and the length of a well-designed instrument. In fact, 89% of persons interviewed by telephone completed the mail survey.

In the 1993–1994 round of the WLS, we sent mail instruments only to those participants who had completed a telephone interview, on the assumption that mailing to telephone refusers was hopeless. However, we learned that many of the telephone refusers in 2004–2006 had said they would fill out a questionnaire if one were sent to them. We initially took this as a form of polite refusal, then decided to learn whether it was true. We sent mail instruments to a random pilot sample of telephone refusers and 40% responded, so we did the same for all telephone refusers. In the full sample, 40% of those who did not complete the telephone survey did complete the mailout, which we modified to update basic demographic information that had been included only in the telephone protocol. In fact, despite survey attrition and deaths across the decade, we obtained a larger number of completed mailouts in 2004–2006 than we did in 1993–1994.

The telephone interview schedules build in supplementary sections for (1) graduates or siblings who are widowed and (2) those who have a physically or mentally disabled child or have experienced the death of a child. Permission was obtained from almost all WLS participants to record the telephone interviews for studies of respondent cognition and interaction with interviewers. To prepare the way for studies of joint survivorship and (eventual) widowhood, and to cross-validate reports from graduates and their siblings, shorter (30-minute) interviews have been carried out with spouses and with approximately 900 widows or widowers of graduates and siblings. These interviews focus mainly on health and family relationships.

Collection of Biomarkers

None of these efforts satisfied our interest in obtaining biomarkers—other than those such as height and weight—that could be ascertained by self-report. For several years, WLS staff had attended an annual, NIA-sponsored workshop on biomarkers hosted by the University of Chicago and Northwestern University. In 2006, we learned of a new DNA collection protocol, DNA/Genotek, that was noninvasive and could be collected by mail, and that yielded a very large sample of DNA in a solution that would be stable for years at room temperature. For example, our initial set of assays, now underway to identify 95 SNPs (single-nucleotide polymorphisms), will use less than one-tenth of each of our samples.

Each participant first receives a mailing that contains a report of recent findings. A follow-up telephone call ascertains the willingness of the participant to donate DNA, and the next mailing includes the DNA/Genotek kit, a consent form, and a return mailer. The kit is rather like an oversized contact lens case. The participant spits into the lower half up to a designated level. This is sometimes difficult for older persons, and the instructions suggest sucking a sugar cube and washing the mouth with water before filling the container with saliva. The upper half of the kit is sealed with a preservative that is released when the kit is closed.

Almost 70% of graduates who participated fully in the 2004–2006 survey protocol completed DNA donation in the spring of 2007, a total of 4,500 cases. This rate appears high—especially for a mailout operation—and it is comparable to response rates in some other biomarker data-collection operations (but see Rylander-Rudqvist, Hakansson, Tybring, & Wolk, 2006). However, it does not meet our standards, and WLS staff expect to increase participation during forthcoming home interviews. One of the reasons we are not satisfied with the current level of DNA donation is that we identified a very strong response differential by self-reported current health status. Respondents who classified themselves as in fair or poor health were far less likely to donate DNA than those who said they were in excellent health.

As of spring 2009, WLS is undertaking a major new challenge, interviewing graduates and siblings personally in their own homes. WLS staff have planned this change of mode for two major reasons, because (1) hearing and comprehension problems may make it more difficult to carry out telephone interviews when the graduates are around 70 years of age, and (2) it will be possible to extend the content of the study to include functional and more intensive cognitive assessments, to collect additional biomarkers, and to obtain waivers for collection of Medicare and personal health records. This is challenging for at least two reasons.

First, the cost of home interviews is far greater than that of telephone interviews. Survey costs will be about 50% greater to survey only the surviving graduates in 2009–2010 than the cost to survey graduates, siblings, spouses, and widows in 2004–2006. Second, because the sample is geographically dispersed, and travel costs are a large share of all survey costs, we will no longer be able to change instrumentation on the fly, without affecting the integrity of the samples; that is, all of the protocols, subsampling designs, and alternate forms have to be fixed before we enter the field.

Many new purposes will be served merely by repeating measurements that we have ascertained previously, for example, health, economic resources, preparation for the end of life, and psychological characteristics (e.g., cognitive performance, personality, well-being, depression, and anxiety). However, we also have extensive plans for new measurements that, we hope, will illuminate the ways the WLS cohort ages in a social environment where individual decision-making is increasingly the norm. These include anthropometric and functional assessments; more intensive cognitive assessments; measurements of health and financial literacy, and Internet skills; experimental trials of impulsive and risk-averse preferences; waivers for access to Medicare and other medical records; and experience with the deaths of family members.

In 1975, WLS concepts and measures resembled those of the Current Population Survey (CPS) and the 1973 Occupational Changes in a Generation Survey (OCG; Featherman & Hauser, 1975, 1978; Hauser & Featherman, 1977). In 1992, continuity was balanced with comparability to other well-designed surveys (e.g., the Health and Retirement Study [HRS], the National Survey of Families and Households [NSFH], NIH surveys of work and psychological functioning [Kohn & Schooler, 1983], and the National Opinion Research Center [NORC] General Social Survey [GSS; Davis & Smith, 1992]). The WLS design was also coordinated with members of the MacArthur Foundation Research Network on Successful Midlife Development, with Michael Marmot's Whitehall II study (Marmot et al., 1991), and with Michael Wadsworth's (1991) longitudinal cohort study of births in Great Britain in 1946.

Interview data from siblings and spouses are a special strength of the WLS. They provide unique data—self-reporting variables that cannot be obtained from proxies, cross-validating information about graduates and their families and complementing accounts of interhousehold (and intergenerational) exchanges. Analytically, the relational data permit construction of multilevel models of family and individual effects on life course outcomes.

The WLS has linked graduates and siblings to the National Death Index–Plus (NDI-Plus) using Social Security numbers, names, and birth dates as identifiers to obtain cause(s) of death and to confirm date and place of death (Bilgrad, 1990; National Center for Health Statistics, 1994, 1999). Similar searches have been undertaken for parents of the graduates and for siblings. However, the data for parents are of limited value because many parents died before the baseline year of the NDI-Plus (1979; cited in Bilgrad, 1990), and many of the mothers of graduates who never worked outside the home did not have Social Security numbers. It has recently become possible to purchase regular updates of the Social Security Death Index (SSDI), and this has enabled us to identify deaths among graduates and siblings on a timely basis and to focus searches for records of cause of death in NDI-Plus.

Since the 1970s, each phase of WLS survey operations—from tracing through coding—has been carried out in a series of 10 replicate subsamples within each major component of the design (graduates, siblings, and spouses). This had four advantages. First, it smoothed the flow of easy and of difficult cases, thereby evening out the workload. This accommodated the inevitable entry of new and inexperienced interviewers into the field operations, and it prevented the accumulation of a large backlog of hard-to-interview cases near the end of the field period. Second, it permitted us to estimate final response rates and costs early in the survey operation, and to fix problems in the instruments without systematically biasing responses in the entire sample. Third, it gave us the opportunity to vary content systematically, both by using alternate forms for similar content, and by adding and dropping content in known, random fractions of the samples. Finally, it gave us the capacity to terminate survey operations at any of several thresholds, without lowering the response rate among cases that had been entered into the field. In fact, because the University interrupted field operations with a building renovation project in the early 1990s that increased our fixed costs, we eliminated telephone interviews with the last two replicates of siblings who had not been interviewed in 1977—without affecting the response rate in other replicates.

In development of the 2004–2006 round of the WLS, project staff decided that it would be desirable to record all of the telephone interviews. The original reason for our investigation of recording technology was that two of the collaborators, Nora Cate Schaeffer and Douglas Maynard, wanted to obtain high-quality recordings of about 1,000 randomly selected interviews that could be used for intensive analysis of respondent–interviewer interaction in an older population. A second reason, which applied to parts of all interviews, was that some of the more attractive protocols for cognitive assessment could not be administered reliably unless the responses were recorded; furthermore, recordings could be used to validate appropriate administration of the assessments.

We asked all respondents at the beginning whether we could record the interview. If they agreed, the interview was recorded, and respondents were asked at the end of the interview whether we could retain the recording for research purposes. If the respondent declined to be recorded at the beginning of the interview, the recording equipment was turned off, but the respondent was asked again, at the beginning of the cognitive assessments, to give us permission to record just that portion of the interview.

Aside from the future value of the recordings in research, which includes an improved ability to edit the raw survey data, they also have proved most useful in the process of instrument development in the WLS. For example, it was efficient for researchers to listen to each instance of a pretest telephone module (e.g., a family roster or employment history) to detect and to solve problems in the logic and content of the instrument, and to identify problems in interviewing that could then be addressed in training sessions. There has been just one major disadvantage to the recorded interviews: Despite improving the quality of the survey data files, their existence has also permitted and encouraged endless data editing, perhaps beyond the point of diminishing returns.

The Wisconsin Study in 2000: Social Composition and Differential Nonresponse

Among Americans aged 60–64 in March 2000, 66.7% were non-Hispanic white women and men who completed at least 12 years of schooling; thus, they resembled the Wisconsin cohort. The WLS is unusually valuable in its representation of women, as well as men. Also, because the WLS is the first of the large longitudinal studies of American adolescents, it provides the first large-scale opportunity to study the life course from late adolescence through the mid-60s in the context of a full record of ability, aspiration, and achievement. The WLS graduates and their siblings have lived through major social changes: rising affluence, suburban growth, the decline of old ethnic cleavages, the Cold War, and changing gender roles. Moreover, the WLS cohort, born mainly in 1939, precedes by a few years the baby boom generation that has taxed social institutions and resources at each stage of life; thus, the study can provide early indications of trends and problems that will become important as the larger group passes through its early 60s. The WLS overlaps the youngest cohorts that entered the HRS in 1992, and this provides continuing opportunities to check the scope of our findings. Unlike the WLS, HRS is nationally representative, but it does not cover the lives of participants from adolescence to old age.

The WLS data also have obvious limitations. Some strata of American society are not represented. Everyone in the graduate sample completed high school. It is estimated that about 75% of Wisconsin youth graduated from high schools in the late 1950s; about 7% of siblings and 12% of spouses in the WLS did not graduate. There are only a handful of African American, Hispanic, or Asian persons in the WLS, and there is no way to generalize from the WLS to the unique conditions of these population groups. Given the minuscule proportion of minorities in Wisconsin when the WLS began, there is no way to remedy this omission. About 19% of the WLS sample is of farm origin; this is consistent with national estimates for cohorts of the late 1930s. In 1964, 1975, and 1992, 70% of the sample lived in Wisconsin, but 30% lived elsewhere in the United States or abroad. Fifty-seven percent of WLS graduates resided in Wisconsin at every contact. WLS graduates are homogeneous in age, but the ages of selected siblings vary widely, mainly within the range of 10 years older to 10 years younger than the graduates.

From Sewell's 1964 parent survey onward, the WLS has done exceptionally well at maintaining a high overall level of survey participation. We cannot offer any definitive explanation of this success. Among the reasons we can offer informally are the regional location of the sample in the northern Midwest, the educational level of the sample, and our efforts to identify participants with their state, their high school class, and their state university. But we have no evidence to support any of these ideas.

All the same, there are problems with differential response in the WLS. I have already noted the sharp differential in DNA donation by self-reported general health status. Another, pervasive problem is differential response by cognitive ability. Up through the 1975–1977 wave of the WLS, we were unable to detect any notable response differentials relative to variables that were available for all participants. One WLS investigator, Marsha Seltzer, showed me that in the 1993–1994 surveys, and especially the mail component, there was a regular gradient in response by adolescent cognitive ability, with a sharp fall-off among the bottom 10%. We surmised that the cognitive demands of a lengthy interview, and those required to read and respond to hundreds of survey items, were just too great for participants with limited cognitive skills.

Further investigation demonstrated that in the WLS, the well-established survey response differentials by gender and socioeconomic status, favoring women and those of high status, were present in the 1993–1994 data but were entirely explained when adolescent test scores and rank in high school class were controlled (Hauser, 2005); that is, it appears that there is a normative, as well as a cognitive, effect on survey response. Not only are cognitive skills a limiting factor, but also women—who obtain better grades than men by dint of more normative behavior—are more likely to respond, because that normative orientation persists across the life course.

To compensate at least in part for these differentials in the 2004–2006 round of the WLS, we encouraged participants to complete telephone interviews in more than one session if they grew tired and, likewise, to take their time in filling out the mail instruments. In my judgment, the take-home lesson here is that for both methodological and theoretical reasons, longitudinal surveys should obtain at least a brief cognitive assessment at an early stage and use it to monitor survey response in subsequent waves. Contrary to earlier opinion, such assessments can be administered by telephone, as well as in person, and almost all research participants agree to and enjoy completing a brief assessment.

Study Documentation

When the WLS began, data documentation was primitive. A huge typed codebook with marginal distributions was supplemented only by the meticulous handwritten notes of William Sewell's exceptional research assistant and coauthor Vimal P. Shah. Around 1970, my wife Tess Hauser established two permanent series of internal documents to record project research activities. Computer Operation Requests (CORs) were prepared before a programmer would undertake any new tabulations or estimates, and WLS memos recorded substantive decisions, operations, findings, and methodological notes. Now, all documents are created electronically, and the early entries in each series have been scanned. As interactive computing has evolved, it is no longer practical to create a record of every computing operation, but final operations are documented fully, including computer code and intermediate data files. The goal of these efforts has always been the same, namely, that any research carried out in the WLS project should be reproducible by others, even if all of the present staff and faculty were to disappear from the scene.

The Scope of the WLS

There is every reason to expect that the WLS will continue to be an important resource for research on aging and the life course for decades to come. In this regard it is both a blessing and a curse that the sample is composed almost entirely of non-Hispanic whites who have completed high school. Based on recent U.S. life tables, there is good reason to expect that more than half the women graduates in the WLS and more than a third of male graduates will live until at least 2022, when they will be 83 and 84 years old. Thus, the current round of the WLS has reached not an end but a beginning.

As the WLS has become a full-fledged study of aging, it serves a very broad agenda of research and policy interests. Anonymous public data and documentation from the WLS have long been available to qualified researchers (*www.ssc.wisc.edu/wlsresearch*). Sensitive data are accessible through the secure data enclave in the Center for Demography of Health and Aging at the University of Wisconsin–Madison. The research agenda ranges from the effects of childhood circumstances and work life on late adult health and well-being, to the effects of children's prospects on the life course of their parents, to differential access to health care services, to the behavioral precursors of high cognitive functioning and cognitive decline. No smaller agenda will justify the long-term investment that investigators, students, funding agencies, and an exceptionally generous cohort of research participants have made in the WLS.

Acknowledgments

The research reported herein was supported by the National Institute on Aging (Grant No. R01 AG-9775 and P01 AG-21079) and by the William Vilas Estate Trust. I thank my colleagues—students, staff, and faculty—on the WLS over the decades, especially those from whom I have gleaned parts of this text, but most of all, the many thousands of research participants whose generosity and trust has made the WLS possible. The opinions expressed herein are my own.

Note

1. LISREL code to estimate the two key versions of our model is available from the author.

CHAPTER 3

Collecting and Interpreting Life Records

Dennis P. Hogan
Carrie E. Spearin

Life records provide unique information for the study of the life course of individuals and descriptions of cohorts of individuals over time. Historical life records, such as population registers, enable researchers to reconstruct the lives of past populations to examine historical change. Contemporary life records, collected from a variety of sources, can be used to reconstruct the recent past lives of individuals when retrospective reports are likely to be unreliable or inaccurate. Life records can also reveal the subsequent life course of individuals after a one-time study or a prospective panel ends.

In this chapter, we discuss life records that provide information about an individual and are not based on the individual's own report to the survey researcher. Although not always the case, such life records often involve official records of statuses or events occurring in the lives of individuals. Sometimes these records result from individuals' reports to data-collection agencies (e.g., tax records), but they can also include records of observed activities (e.g., traffic violations or court appearances) or the official record of some individual action (e.g., getting a driver's license or marriage license). Life records need not be legal documents. Life records can include ecclesiastical records, membership lists of voluntary or political associations, social registers, or credit histories. Table 3.1 illustrates a few of the many possible types of life records that can be of potential use to life course researchers.

TABLE 3.1. Some Types of Life Records

- Vital registers (birth, death, marriage, divorce certificates)
- Population registers and censuses
- Migration and residential records (immigration declarations, residential directories)
- Licenses (vehicle licenses, licenses to driver, business and professional licenses)
- Ecclesiastical records (church membership, baptisms, marriages, burials)
- School records
- Employment records
- Military service records
- Health records (physician, hospital, pharmacy, insurance and government reimbursement)
- Financial filings (insurance claims, credit applications and reports, property transfers, tax forms)
- News reports (newspapers, magazines, directories)

As used in this chapter, a "life record" is any written or electronic record that is entered at the time of an event or observation and archived afterward by someone other than the individuals themselves. We take life course research using life records to be a special form of the use of archival records, in which the purpose is to track individuals over a significant number of years of their lives.

In this chapter, we discuss three major uses of life records: the reconstruction of the population and individuals during some historical time period; augmented description of present life, with records of current behaviors (without interview); and use of life records as supplements to individuals' self-reports about their lives. After indicating the extent to which these life records have been used in life course studies, we discuss assessing life records in terms of quality, accuracy, and limitation. Whereas linking life records provides detailed information on individuals for researchers, it also poses some significant ethical concerns. We end the chapter with a discussion of the ethical considerations we must bear in mind when linking life records from numerous sources.

The Reconstruction of Past Lives from Records

Historical life records have proven useful in examining changes in fertility and mortality over time. Gutmann and Fliess (1993) created a continuous population register of individuals in Gillespie County, Texas, during the 19th century by linking 19th-century manuscript censuses, civil (marriage, births, deaths) and ecclesiastical vital registration systems (baptism, marriage, funerals), and tax assessments. However, relatively few population reconstitution studies for the United States cover the first half of the 20th century, because manuscript census data from that era are closed to researchers to protect the privacy of individuals and households.

Historical life records from Europe are often much richer in detail than those found in the United States. For example, Alter and Oris (2001) used population reconstitution to assess how individual and family behaviors affected mortality and the transition from high to low mortality in the commune of Sart, Belgium, during the 18th century. Using periodic census data to identify individuals in families, these registers of individuals within households were continuously updated in a population in which commune authorities recorded every instance of birth, death, and migration in a household. An unusual feature of this study was that all death notations recorded the cause of death, allowing the researchers to study mortality changes due to the control of infectious diseases.

A common cornerstone of historical life course studies is the population census or some other complete listing of the population in an area, such as a tax list or church membership records. Birth and death registers are essential for identifying the individuals present in the population during any given historical year. Population censuses and population registers capture the mobility of the population in terms of migrants to and from the community. Such continuous information is essential, because it allows for the definition of populations at risk of experiencing key events during any specified year. This information provides the denominators for rates of events.

Although historical studies have often used life record data to study temporal changes in the life course of individuals, the data more commonly are aggregated so that the behaviors of groups of people (by social class, ethnicity) may be examined across different birth cohorts or specific historical periods. These analyses can include life course topics such as the age patterning of events that mark the passage from youth to adult life or the relationship between ascribed and achieved characteristics that influence economic opportunities, choices, experiences, and transitions over the life course.

As illustrated earlier, a wide range of life records is available to researchers interested in almost any social topic or historical period. However, this list is far from exhaustive. Researchers have made use of religious records (church membership, marriages, annulments) and place records (burial plots, ownership of businesses and properties), as well as personal diaries and newspapers, or other media sources, to examine the life course.

Reconstruction of Past Lives: An Example from Casalecchio di Reno

Overall, historical life records provide researchers with a unique opportunity to reconstruct the lives of individuals from the past. Typically, these studies focus on smaller communities with relatively few members for good reason. Such communities have been selected for study because they have intact historical archives, with data on individuals linked to households, making it simpler to keep track of individuals over time. Community studies are also a popular method to study the life course of persons in contemporary populations.

Although data from smaller communities may be less overwhelming to analyze than those from larger communities, states, or nations, the process is nonetheless complicated, complex, and time consuming. Although paper archives can be scanned and computerized, changed spellings of names, inconsistent information across data sources, and the disappearance and reappearance of individuals at different times during the period of study all necessitate the intensive involvement of researchers in accurately linking records of persons over time.

Kertzer and Hogan (1989) used life records to reconstruct the life paths of individuals in the Italian town of Casalecchio di Reno. This town, a rural community outside of Bologna, exemplifies the shift from an agricultural economy, with large complex households engaged in sharecropping in 1861, to a predominantly industrial economy, with nuclear family households by 1921. It was a period of declining papal and church control, and the ascendancy of the secular government of the new nation of Italy.

This changing political and economic landscape (the political economy) led to dramatic changes in the ways families were organized as units of production and consumption (the family economy). In 1861, families were bound to sharecropping contracts by elite landholders. Because all potential agricultural land was farmed and new methods of agricultural production had not yet arrived, the major way that landowners increased production was to maximize the number of laborers farming their land. They could enforce this strategy by canceling the annual contract of any sharecropping household that supplied insufficient labor, forcing the peasants off of the land and into economically desperate lives as landless agricultural wage laborers (*braccianti*). The *braccianti* found jobs as individual laborers, and their households were not units of economic production. Following the agricultural crisis of 1883–1896, the number of *braccianti* increased dramatically, supplying labor for the industries that developed in the early 20th century.

There are hundreds of Italian communities that exemplify this period of transformation. Why did Kertzer and Hogan (1989) study Casalecchio di Reno? The answer is in the archival life records that were available. The Casalecchio town hall was one of the few government buildings in Italy whose records were not destroyed by the Allied bombing campaign of World War II. An additional critical feature is that Casalecchio archival sources were meticulously maintained, with individual records stored in the folders of the households in which the people lived. This greatly simplified the matching of individual records over time, because, for most cases, the entire Casalecchio database did not have to be searched for matches on each of the 32,916 names that were recorded in one of the archives.

The census of 1861 was the basis for the newly established population register, through which the unified Italian government began to establish a secularized citizenry. The register continued for 60 years. In 1920 the socialists scored an electoral victory in Bologna. Fascists attacked the Bologna city hall, deposing the municipal government. Fascist violence and the socialist response spread fear and disorder throughout the province of Bologna. In 1922, the Fascist government of Mussolini deposed the Casalecchio socialist town government. Thus, the Casalecchio population register system effectively ended with the census in 1921.

Kertzer and Hogan (1989) were able to draw on manuscript census records; annual tax records that recorded heads of household, household size, and social class; baptismal records and the appearance of new infants in the population register; records of civil and church marriages; and migration records. These databases identified 19,052 different persons living in Casalecchio sometime during the period of study. The wealth of individual records included, for example, 20,290 instances of migration, 2,490 marriages, and 2,007 conscription records of young men. Household information included 3,868 different household heads, 7,769 different household configurations, 22,342 instances of coresidence in households, and 18,882 annual household tax records. All of the information for this study was coded in terms of events that occurred, and needed to be recorded, retrieved, and analyzed using methods appropriate to the analysis of life history events (Karweit & Kertzer, 1998).

With this information, Kertzer and Hogan (1989) were able to match individual personal records, along with records of the households in which the person lived, across all sources of information annually from 1861 to 1921. This dynamic data set allowed for a thorough investigation of social class transformation among families, declining rates of mortality, changing patterns of migration, and the conflict between civil and religious authorities during a period of rapid economic change and political turmoil. Because the Casalecchio database included information on the ways that individual life courses were structured by the political economy and the exigencies of family life, the researchers were able to examine whether all members of the population responded in the same way to the dramatic social changes going on, and whether these differed across birth cohorts, or within cohorts by social class. Although the Casalecchio life records were unusually rich, the study illustrates the vast potential of life records for life course research.

The Construction of Contemporary Lives with Records

Even though the use of birth, death, and marriage records in studying life histories is not a new technique, these data do serve as a powerful source for estimating and projecting national estimates of trends in vital rates, both in the past and the present. In a recent study, Elo, Turra, Kestenbaum, and Ferguson (2004) used vital records, along with Medicare data, to estimate both age and sex specific death rates for a range of Hispanic subgroups in the United States. This combination of records allowed for corrections in data errors and provided researchers with additional means of determining Hispanic origins. Mortality rate estimates for Asian American subgroups have also been inferred with the use of similar data, with an additional source provided by Social Security records (Lauderdale & Kestenbaum, 2002).

Individual driving records and accident reports have been used by researchers to address a multiplicity of unique research questions. For example, Elliott, Shope, Raghunthan, and Waller (2006) used state driving records to examine the link between gender, substance use, and environmental factors, and the incidence of high-risk driving. Accident records are also being used in a study on aviation accidents and alcohol use. This research project links data from three sources: state driving records, crash investigation reports from the National Transportation Safety Board, and medical examiners' records of fatally injured pilots. These pooled data allow researchers to examine how alcohol involvement in aviation crashes, combined with pilots' histories of driving while impaired (DWI), is linked to both fatal and nonfatal aviation crashes.

The population registers maintained by the Scandinavian nations have proved to be a rich source for life course studies based on life records. For example, to determine the effect of high-quality and affordable day care availability on women's transition to motherhood, researchers have used Norwegian birth records. Utilizing the birth records in conjunction with geographic information, Rindfuss, Swicegood, and Rosenfeld (2007) found that the proximity of child care facilities had a positive effect on fertility in Norway.

Life records can also uncover acute changes in life patterns that result from key historical events. Using monthly birth records, Rodgers, St. John, and Coleman (2005) examined the potential influence of the 1995 Oklahoma City bombing on fertility patterns throughout Oklahoma. They found a direct increased fertility response in residents closest to this disaster.

Construction of Work Careers:
An Example Using Government Records

A fresh approach to studying advances of workers in the low-wage labor market is use of program data from the Longitudinal Employer–Household Dynamics (LEHD) study. The motivation for constructing this dataset was to reduce respondent burden from yet another government survey of the labor force. Respondents were sampled using workers' unemployment insurance (UI) wage record data. The quarterly employers' UI reports were matched using Social Security numbers to provide information on the course of individual occupational change and wages from 1993 to 2001. An advantage is that the UI data provide a sample of individuals in their workplaces. These data were then matched to personal household-level information, as well as information on establishments and firms in the business register (Andersson, Holzer, & Lane, 2005). These comprehensive records were used to analyze the situations and trajectories of workers in low-wage jobs and to identify career tracks that led low-wage workers into better paying jobs. The data were also used to identify the types of firms in which low-income jobs were concentrated, and to determine whether low-wage workers could change their economic situations by moving from one kind of firm to another with a more promising occupational profile. Researchers found that almost half of those with persistent low earnings were able to improve their economic situations over time (Andersson et al., 2005).

Life Records as Supplements to Self-Reports

The most common and direct way that researchers now collect life histories is by means of longitudinal survey interviews. Data collected from the same individuals at different times over the life course can provide researchers with unique opportunities to examine cohort changes over time, as well as the effects of age-specific historical context. Researchers can also identify how these patterns differ among individuals by social class, ethnic origins, and individual differences.

However, a more dynamic approach to examining longer stretches of an individual's life is to use mixed methods that draw on both survey interviews and life records. When information gained from these longitudinal surveys can be matched with factual records, researchers are able to compare the "true" pasts of individuals and biographical

interpretation of their past life experiences. These mixed sources of longitudinal information typically have an advantage over studies that use
life records as the sole basis for identifying respondents (e.g., population reconstitution studies), because they typically are representative of
a broader range of people's social characteristics and diverse life course
experiences. For the analysis of social contexts (quality of community,
schools, and labor markets), these data are also superior because they
contain large samples of persons from many different locations.

One noteworthy example of this is a longitudinal study of Detroit-
area married couples who experienced the birth of a child in 1962
(a sample of couples based on official birth certificates). This study
matched information on the reported dates of first marriage and first
birth to official records of marriages and births to obtain a correct measurement of which couples were pregnant with their first child at the
time of their marriage. They found that many of the couples reported
their marriage dates to be earlier by 1 year, so that it appeared that
their first births were conceived within marriage. This is an example
of how respondents' accounts of life events can be made more accurate
through the use of life records. Longitudinal follow-ups through survey
interviews tracked the effects of pregnancy prior to marriage on the
long-term economic well-being and the marital relationships of these
couples (Freedman & Thornton, 1979).

Laub and Sampson (2003) used an archive that tracked the juvenile and adult crime careers of a cohort of young persons to study desistance from a life of crime and the relationship of criminal life histories
to employment, family transitions, and other features of the life course.
Numerous researchers had collected the data they used over the course
of decades, permitting an unusually complete look at the entire life
course of an adolescent cohort. The study collected information from
a variety of sources, including interviews with adolescents identified as
delinquents, parents and social workers, police and probation officers,
and juvenile and adult arrest records and court records. Maintenance of
this rich life record archive allowed these researchers to apply new ideas
and methods to the study of the life course of these young persons.

Another example, the National Maternal and Infant Health Survey
(1988), used birth and perinatal mortality records to sample women
whose pregnancies reached term. This was done to investigate the origins and impact of pregnancy loss and very low birthweight infants on
the lives of the infants and their mothers in the short term. Much of this
information was provided through interviews with the mothers at about
9 months and 30 months after the birth. This study contacted the offices
of medical doctors and hospitals to obtain recorded health information on the infants and mothers. Because of high nonresponse and the

low quality of much of the reported patient information, these medical records were of limited use. However, the birth registry and survey data provided rich information that Hogan and Park (2000) used to study the effects of pregnancy and birth experiences, nutrition and medical care, and program participation on the developmental trajectories of the children.

To study life course outcomes such as psychosocial adjustment and academic and occupational pathways, researchers have matched individual student files to school-level data and survey interviews. Information provided by schools on students' Individualized Education Plans can be used to identify students with disabilities and investigate the success of special supports and programs designed to help them do well academically (Wells, Sandefur, & Hogan, 2004). Grades, obtained from student files, are used to measure academic outcomes and to study their relationship to parental involvement and family composition. Beyond grade point averages, student files often contain classroom assignments and sizes, standardized test scores, and basic levels of academic engagement, along with broader, school-level data, such as school size and rankings. Such data can give researchers a comprehensive understanding of the school environment.

Recently, historical military records have been scrutinized in terms of their usefulness for accurately measuring height, as height has been used as an indicator of improving or declining standards of living (Guthrie & Jenkins, 2005; Komlos, 2004). Researchers studying the Vietnam era often utilized military records to determine war-zone stressors and the likelihood of posttraumatic stress disorder. It is likely that such records of deployment and action on the battlefield will continue to be relevant as effects on the life course of veterans of the wars in Iraq and Afghanistan become apparent.

Linking Responses and Records: An Example from the Wisconsin Longitudinal Study

Throughout the life course, data on individuals are collected from a variety of sources. If these sources' potential is maximized, this trace evidence, often in the form of written or electronic records, allows researchers to reconstruct important events in the lives of individuals. An excellent example is the Wisconsin Longitudinal Study (WLS) that began with interviews of high school students in 1957. These same students were then followed and reinterviewed over time (1964 [parents], 1975, 1992, and 2004). This study also accessed Wisconsin state tax records to obtain family income information when the adolescents in the initial study lived at home. Later, federal Social Security Administration data on incomes were attached to individual records as the adolescents reached the adult years (see Hauser, Chapter 2, this volume).

The life history information available in the WLS is exceptionally complete, and the availability of life records has enriched the scope and accuracy of information about the subjects' life courses. It is a unique study because of its full inclusion of young women at a time when most studies of social stratification were restricted to males. In perhaps its most unusual use of life records, the WLS had project personnel examine yearbook pictures of the high school seniors to measure physical attractiveness and relative body mass. The yearbooks were also used to record school activities in which the students participated.

WLS participants were asked to provide identifying information (names and locations) of schools they attended and places of employment. Postsecondary schools were classified according to their selectivity, academic specialization, programs offered, and other factors likely to be important in assessing the impact of colleges on the life course. Researchers have been able to build on this life course information by using other official records relevant to the specific schools and occupations of the respondents. Furthermore, a unique aspect of these data is that additional life records were linked not to individuals but to specific characteristics of individuals at various points in their life course. For example, Leicht, Hogan, and Wendt (2006) matched indicators of college selectivity and quality to the respondent records through the specific survey information about the schools attended. They also attached Dictionary of Occupational Title information and career pathway information based on census data on reported occupations to identify which persons by age 52 were working at jobs associated with career pathways that maximized occupational prestige and income. Finally, the researchers were able to take advantage of the county of residence information of members of the senior class of 1957 to determine how young and midlife men and women were able to capitalize on new employment opportunities associated with the growth of technological and service sectors of the economy, and to minimize their exposure to risk from the shrinking manufacturing sector. As this example shows, individual life histories, when combined with individual and group identity life records, can provide an exceptionally rich resource for life course studies.

Assessing the Quality and Limitations of Life Records

When utilizing life records, researchers must consider several issues related to their accuracy. Historical studies using census and annual records from population registers, and official certificates of births, deaths, and migration, typically base the cohort on an initial census of the population, with subsequent events in the population at risk being recorded from an event register (birth, death, marriage records). To the extent that studies cover more than a few years' time, it is essential that the initial population count be adjusted to include new entrants to the population through birth or in-migration and to subtract those who have died or are out-migrants. The cohorts in this population need to be "aged" in the database, so that in any given year the survivors of the previous year are recorded as being 1 year older. In this way, investigators can correctly calculate age- and sex-specific birth, death, marriage, and migration rates each year, and study changes in these rates over time.

When more than one census represents the population, this initial census of the population should be compared to the reconstituted population to determine whether population counts by age and sex match across the two sources of data. If they do not, the extent of errors in closure can be calculated, and particular sources of disparity in records identified. In the Casalecchio study, census data on households were available for 1861, 1865, 1871, 1881, 1911, and 1921. In these years, households and individuals recorded on the census forms were compared to the population register. This comparison indicated that the extent to which the enumerated persons in the censuses were not included in the population register population was 1.3% in 1871, 1.9% in 1881, 3.4% in 1911, and 2.5% in 1921. Examinations of these missing persons from the continuous population register database indicated that about 75% were servants, apprentices, foundlings, or other nonkin living in the households. Records for these individuals were added to corrected population registers.

A similar issue in the use of life records is whether the records for the resident population in an area are complete at a given point in time. One example of such incompleteness in life records is the failure to include persons who are not "officially" part of the actual population (e.g., undocumented immigrants in the United States). This difference can be especially critical for the calculation of rates, because the "unofficial" residents may have children, marry in churches, or die, and these events are recorded in registers. In Casalecchio, soldiers were typically regarded as outsiders who were not members of the population. Traders, merchants, or landholders who lived in Casalecchio only for short or intermittent periods typically were also not recorded as residents. But events in their lives do sometimes appear in the event archives.

Beginning in the last decades of the 18th century, major new transportation routes permitted much greater interaction between the residents of Casalecchio and Bologna. Bicycles, a major method of transportation, allowed workers living in one place to travel weekly or daily to work in another place. The commuter rail made daily transit between workplaces and homes a practicality. Thus, it was possible to use government and church archives in Bologna to supplement local archival information to complete the life histories of the Casalecchio population.

What is important to the researcher studying the occurrence rates of events in life records is that the count of events in a population be consistent with the population at risk for these events, with both numerators and denominators of rates referring to the same people. Often the most problematic event involves out-migration from an area, yet for most population recording systems, in-migration rather than out-migration is recorded. In Casalecchio it was relatively easy to identify in-migrants, because they appeared either in the censuses or in the population register. It was more difficult to determine why some household members "disappeared" from the household register; in the Italian population register, out-migration could only be recorded when the new community to which migrants moved informed individuals' communities of origin.

Another critical issue in the use of life records is the correct matching of individual records of events over time. This can be especially difficult in places whose residents have many common names (e.g., John Smith). A related problem occurs when the surname used may vary (as in many nations of Latin America in which the father's family name is the primary surname, and the mother's maiden name is sometimes used as a secondary surname). The use of nicknames also can be an issue (e.g., in the case of a person whose formal birth certificate name is "Margaret" but the name she uses as an adult in official documents is "Peggy"). Finally, alternative spellings of a name can also raise confusion (e.g., Meghan or Megan). In surveys, however, information from respondents can help to pinpoint the location and date of the record, making mismatch less likely. There are a variety of procedures available to match individuals across types of life records and periods, but most require some combination of names that sound similar, have some common written elements, are identical in report of sex, and are a match or near-match on age. This issue of accurate matching across records is most serious for studies that analyze the lives of individuals, since mismatches increase the apparent rate of change and create inexplicable flux in life patterns.

These problems are more vexing in studies that rely on different sources of life records, without any individual survey information. There is no substitute for direct access to archival records in the assembly of life histories with life records (Elder, Pavalko, & Clipp, 1993). The Casalecchio study made scrupulous use of the actual archives *in situ* to reconcile and to match a large proportion of the individuals and families in the community over 60 years. Even so, after the data were assembled and entered into computer files, further checks were necessary to deal with inconsistencies, impossible response codes, and missing data for particular items. Although some algorithms were used to fill in missing data, most corrections were done in a case-by-case inspection of the computerized records from the multiple archives that provided information. This process consumed more than 2,000 hours of researcher time. The ultimate product was a historical archive that was ideal for life course research during this exciting period of social and economic transition.

Additionally, there can be systematic differences across life record systems. These frequently arise when there are different official reasons for collecting and recording information. For example, the occupation of a woman reported on a census may refer to current occupation, but occupation information on the death certificate is usually reported by someone who is less knowledgeable and reports on the woman's "usual" occupation. Any attempt to calculate occupational differentials in mortality using these two sources of life records may be confounded by such differences in classification across types of life records.

There can also be differential recording of behaviors in official registries. In studies of delinquent behaviors of adolescents, official records may underrepresent the delinquent behaviors of whites or wealthier young people compared to the fuller documentation of illicit behaviors by minority or poor persons. These differences can occur when police treat one group of adolescents more informally and another group more formally. In general, these differences become more pronounced at each step of the legal process: Charges of delinquent behaviors brought by police typically are less biased than measures of delinquency from conviction records.

It is helpful to consider how researchers in the Casalecchio study dealt with these issues. The central data source was the population register. All other sources of data were matched to the information in the population registers. But this rich longitudinal data also was subject to a variety of errors. Newborn infants who died typically were not recorded in the household register. Household members were perhaps less well recorded among the *braccianti*, because these households were not bound by a formal labor contract. The inclusion of servants or other persons temporarily present in households might not be recorded in the register. Correction of the population register that was the core of the Casalecchio database relied on other sources of information.

A frequent source of discrepancy can arise when ecclesiastical and public records of the same events are recorded. In places without well-established birth or death recording systems, church records of baptisms and funerals may provide the most complete information. However, church records typically represent faithful adherents to that religion, potentially excluding many secular individuals, some of whom may be social innovators. In Casalecchio, this created a particular problem for the recording of marriages, because persons receiving civil marriage licenses were officially not permitted to marry in the church. Among sharecroppers, marriage licenses were essential to bind new brides to the household legally, but among the *braccianti*, they were less important.

In prospective longitudinal surveys (i.e., studies that begin with a sample survey, then follow respondents in periodic reinterviews) an important source of error is loss to follow-up (Scott & Alwin, 1998). In other cases, segments of life histories are missing because a respondent is absent from one of the periodic surveys. Retrospective longitudinal surveys (i.e., studies that begin with a sample survey that gathers information from respondents about their past lives) are not subject to these follow-up errors but they are more subject to recall errors and the misreporting of dates. Retrospective data also are inferior to prospective studies when the mortality of cohort members is salient. Retrospective life histories represent only persons who survive long enough to tell their stories; persons who have died are not represented (Scott & Alwin, 1998). The WLS matched death certificates to their panel members to be able to model attrition due to mortality. Such information is important, for example, in analyses of how the health of an individual at one point in time affects subsequent well-being.

Considerations for Analytic Strategies

These potential sources of error in life records are important for the study of turning points in the life course. Mismatches can lead to the exclusion of critical events that may represent turning points (because of failure to match records that link such events to individuals). Or errors in matching can make the events actually happening to different individuals seem to be a life course turning point for a single individual. These errors are particularly problematic in studies of the life course that investigate developmental trajectories or discontinuities over the life course.

Because some apparent changes over the life course may be the result of errors in coverage, matching, or reporting, it is incumbent on any researcher using life records to assess the implications of errors for research on the life course. Often it is not possible to correct the errors, but analysts typically can determine likely error structures and assess their implications for bias in analysis. The methods used by demographers to assess and adjust for errors in census and vital registration data may be especially helpful in this regard, because they not only maximize the use of available data but also rely on practiced-derived commonsense methods. Sometimes the best solution is to place sensible confidence intervals around estimates to indicate the soundness of any conclusions.

It is possible to use more and less stringent algorithms to match persons across life records. Statistical models can then be estimated using the two sets of matched records. For example, Hogan and colleagues investigated the effects of infant and child disability on mothers' work, marriage, and fertility histories (Park, Hogan, & Goldscheider, 2003). They matched data from the 1993 National Health Interview Survey (which records infant and child disability) with the mothers' employment and marriage histories, as reported in the 1995 National Survey of Family Growth, which was based on the same sampling frame. Mothers were matched with certainty between the data sets. But individual children needed to be matched according to their age and sex, as reported in the National Health Interview Survey, with children recorded in the mothers' fertility histories in the National Survey of Family Growth. Consistent matches could be obtained for greater numbers of cases when the requirements for the age match were relaxed (e.g., requiring that the "matched" child have the same age within a 3-, 6-, or 12-month interval). But less stringent matching criteria increased the possibility that children would be mismatched. Park et al. estimated their statistical models based on the different samples of children obtained with the various matching algorithms to demonstrate that their statistical results were largely unaffected by the matching criteria they utilized.

Many of the methods for handling errors in longitudinal life course data are applicable to the use of life records. Analysts must carefully consider whether to replace missing data estimates using maximum likelihood and Bayesian methods. An alternative is to evaluate segments of the life courses of individuals for which complete records are available. Missing events can be treated as censored data in survival analysis. This strategy is only effective when the censoring events are unrelated to the outcomes of interest, something that often is not a valid assumption in life course research.

It is useful to use the Casalecchio study again to illustrate the many ways in which data from life records can be used to address critical questions about the life course of individuals, the family economy, and social change. Census data provided periodic snapshots of changes in the types of households (relationship of individuals to household heads). The infant mortality rate was calculated from the number of births each year divided by the population register number of infants born that year. Because of the small number of births and deaths each year, 5-year moving averages were calculated to identify the particular years (rather than broad time periods) in which the most dramatic changes in the infant mortality rate occurred. Kertzer and Hogan (1989) were able to document the sharp declines in infant mortality that occurred from 1885 onward, linking this to local government efforts to improve sanitation and to increased breast-feeding (by requiring employers to provide places and times for mothers working in factories to breast-feed). They were able to use the number of deaths recorded each year (by the social class of the households of the dead persons) and the number of person-years lived in each social class to demonstrate that nearly all of the mortality declines occurred among the *braccianti*.

Kertzer and Hogan (1989) used longitudinal data on individuals who had moved to Casalecchio, whether they had emigrated, and in what year they immigrated for an event history analysis of how the rate of emigration differed by a variety of social and economic characteristics. This demonstrated that the rate of emigration was exceptionally low among persons who moved to join kin in established households or moved to Casalecchio with their households, and quite high among non-kin residents of households (e.g., soldiers, itinerant workers, apprentices and servants). They used information on date of marriage from the civil and church archives, and dates of births recorded in the birth registers to estimate the annual proportion of brides who were pregnant at the time of marriage. With these data they were able to document that pregnancy of the bride was increasingly common after 1900, because many sharecropping grooms married *braccianti* women they had made pregnant. Kertzer and Hogan used the information on the households in which individuals lived and the others who resided in those households to show that relatively few widows of household heads were left destitute after the death of their spouses.

Ethical Considerations

Although issues related to accuracy of life records are greatly reduced in populations in which a national identity number is available (the Social Security number in the United States is becoming such a number), or in which modern population registers are utilized (e.g., in the Scandinavian nations), this same ability to "link" individual records can pose significant ethical concerns. There has been a meteoric rise in the sources of government and privately compiled life records. Government life records (for birth, death, marriage, divorce) are now computerized and typically include enough identifying information to link records. The ease of linking records electronically opens up entirely new avenues for the use of multiple life records to study intimate details of persons' lives.

Information from the Social Security Administration can be used to improve accuracy of income streams, the history of disability status, and income transfers. Medicare claims files can be linked to national surveys on the health of the elderly to obtain improved information about the type and cost of care received. In a similar manner, Medicare files and death certificates can be linked to elderly respondents in health surveys to study rates and causes of death, and to provide information on end-of-life care. The availability of comprehensive credit histories by name, address, and Social Security number enables investigators to follow the trajectory of spending, types of expenditures, and financial stress of individuals and households. All of these examples illustrate how official records enable prospective survey panels to be extended, even when the respondents themselves or their spouses can no longer be interviewed.

This expansion of available life records for research can be problematic even when the matched information is from legal records for which there is no assumption of privacy. When respondents participate in a survey, they consent in writing, based on the description of the survey instruments by study investigators. However, when matched with official records or credit records that are not known by the study participant to be available to the investigator, such mixed survey interview and life records studies can provide a far more comprehensive view of the life course of individuals than they intended in their informed consent. Such procedures might reveal sensitive, embarrassing, or even illegal activities. If survey respondents are not informed that the information they provide in the interview setting will be matched to life records, they are denied their right to informed consent. This means that study investigators who contemplate using life records at some point in future analyses should indicate this in the informed consent forms.

Another ethical issue in the use of life records in studies of the life course involves protecting the confidentiality and anonymity of the individuals' life histories. Typically, these data are released to investigators only after identifying information and detailed location data are removed. Sometimes the life record information is so sensitive that it can only be analyzed in a secure location at a government office or in the center collecting the survey data. An extreme example is that only census bureau employees or individuals who have special sworn status are permitted to work with LEHD data, and only after a Federal Bureau of Investigation (FBI) check. Investigators disclosing the identity of an individual or business in the LEHD can be fined up to $250,000 and/or sentenced to up to 5 years in jail (Andersson et al., 2005).

Institutional review boards (IRBs; panels that review research for ethical compliance) are becoming increasingly aware of these issues in the use of life records. At times, IRBs or research funding agencies (e.g., the NIH and the National Science Foundation) restrict the investigator from the comprehensive use of life records. As informed consent and data protection procedures are improved, these issues may pose less of a barrier to the use of life records.

Conclusion

This chapter has shown that life records can provide unique and valuable information for studies of the life course. Historical life records can be used to reconstruct the lives of individuals in past decades and centuries, providing an essential tool for understanding how long-term social transformations have affected the life course of individuals. Contemporary life records can provide insights into the current lives of large numbers of individuals when sample surveys are impractical or individual recall of life events is poor. This is important when there are many alternative pathways, when the incidence of significant life events of is low, or when frequent and short-term changes of status are common and easily forgotten. Life records can provide a useful (and often more accurate) supplement to the information that individuals provide in survey interviews, and they can be used to reveal the subsequent life course of individuals after a one-time study or a prospective panel ends.

Improved availability and methodologies for using life records have coincided with the growing interest of social scientists in the study of individual lives. Computer technologies have made more feasible the assembly and collation of life records for large numbers of individuals from a variety of archives. Software programs for matching individual records across sources and over time have greatly simplified these tasks. Although life records are subject to a variety of errors, the methods for assessing these errors have improved. Many studies of the life course, including classics such as Elder's (1974) *Children of the Great Depression* have been based on survey data. Indeed, the precursor to this volume, the *Methods of Life Course Research: Qualitative and Quantitative Approaches*, edited by Giele and Elder (1998b), primarily focuses on issues that arise in the use of survey data in life course research. While, of course, many of these same issues apply to studies that use life record data, life course researchers will benefit greatly by adding life records to their research toolbox. Studies that previously were not feasible become possible, and life records can provide a rich supplement to improve analyses that would otherwise be based solely on individual self-reports.

Identifying and accessing life records are two of the biggest challenges researchers must face in maximizing their potential for understanding the life course. In many ways, the use of life records in life course research requires scholars to return to the methodologies employed by social historians—visits to archives of historical documents, lengthy consultations with librarians specializing in government records, and attention to information used in biographies of individuals. But life course researchers, especially those interested in the lives of contemporaries, need to be attuned to all of the places that they themselves leave behind records—school transcripts; high school and college yearbooks; employment records; licenses (for marriage, divorce, birth, death); physician and hospital records; insurance data; credit card records of expenditures; wage, earnings, and tax statements; driving and accident records; memberships in churches, clubs, and organizations; and political groups. Indeed, we leave life records everywhere, every day.

The task for the life course researcher is to identify and obtain access to records that inform their particular research questions. Fortunately, many records are publicly available. Others might be accessible for research purposes under restrictive use agreements, especially if the results of the research are of benefit to the mission of the agencies that collect the data. Whereas there is no single word of advice for accessing extant life records, the best advice to researchers is to search widely, consult extensively, and be creative in negotiating access and funding. Once life records are accessed, the real challenges and pleasures attendant to life course research can begin.

Although there are numerous obstacles in the use of life records, the potential payoffs in rich life course information more than compensate for any problems. The use of life records is limited only by investigators' imaginations and their willingness to undertake the additional research involved. As the value of life records in combination with longitudinal survey data becomes increasingly clear, the matching of life records for the study of the life course will become the rule rather than the exception. This can only enrich and improve the scientific study of the life course.

CHAPTER 4

Longitudinal Ethnography
Uncovering Domestic Abuse
in Low-Income Women's Lives

Linda M. Burton
Diane Purvin
Raymond Garrett-Peters

Many family science and human development scholars argue that it is critically important to examine women's histories of physical and sexual abuse in studies of their life course. Yet, given the sensitivity of this topic and respondents' tendency to withhold troubling information about themselves, it is difficult to gather accurate and detailed information about the prevalence and nature of these experiences in women's lives (see Jouriles, McDonald, Norwood, & Ezell, 2001). For example, panel surveys of life course and family transitions, such as the National Survey of Families and Households and the Panel Study of Income Dynamics, either do not include questions about abuse or they employ less than ideal measures that result in significant underreporting of these experiences. Moreover, studies such as the National Violence Against Women surveys are designed specifically to identify the prevalence of abuse, but they do not gather information about processes (e.g., nuanced behaviors and styles of communication) involved in women's disclosures of abuse (Bachman & Saltzman, 1995; Finkelhor, 1994). Overall, most surveys rely on limited measures that fail to capture the full range of women's subjective experiences of abuse, or they neglect to consider abuse as a phenomenon affecting the entire life course of women and their families (Macmillan, 2001; Williams, 2003). Such problems in measurement and assessment impede our understanding of abuse prevalence and the ways it shapes the life course of women, particularly low-income women who face heightened vulnerabilities from its effects (Leone, Johnson, Cohan, & Lloyd, 2004; Sokoloff & Dupont, 2005).

Compared to surveys, ethnographic studies often find themselves "knee-deep" in data about women's physical and sexual abuse experiences. In many ethnographies, such issues typically emerge naturalistically as unanticipated themes during data collection. For instance, in ethnographic studies seeking to understand the life course of low-income women, researchers reported that although they did not specifically solicit information about abuse, it was a disturbingly common experience for their respondents, a fact of family life to be negotiated, along with the other, numerous challenges of poverty (Butler & Burton, 1990; Dodson, 1998; Fine & Weis, 1998; Musick, 1993). And, more recently, large-scale studies of welfare reform that include ethnographic components have reported the emergence of abuse issues as unanticipated yet significant factors influencing outcomes of interest (Cherlin, Burton, Hurt, & Purvin 2004; Scott, London, & Myers, 2002). These studies suggest that abuse, a highly influential force in low-income mothers' lives, is likely to go undetected in studies that neither address it directly nor employ sensitive enough methods to capture it naturalistically. In light of these findings, we ask the following questions: Could ethnography be one of the most useful and important methods for gathering accurate data about the prevalence of physical and sexual abuse in the life course of low-income women? What processes are involved when women reveal histories of physical and sexual abuse through ethnography?

In this chapter, we address these questions using longitudinal ethnographic data from *Welfare, Children, and Families: A Three-City Study* (hereafter, the Three-City Study). In this ethnography (described in greater detail later in this chapter) we sought to understand the life course experiences of 256 African American, Hispanic, and non-Hispanic white low-income mothers of young children in Boston, Chicago, and San Antonio over a 6-year period following the implementation of welfare reform. We begin this discussion with a brief overview of the features of ethnography that render it a viable life course method for gathering accurate and detailed data about physical and sexual abuse in women's lives. We then describe the processes involved in uncovering women's abuse experiences in the Three-City Study ethnography. In doing so, we illustrate the degree to which experiences of physical and sexual abuse permeate the lives of low-income mothers, and present methodological and ethical challenges to ethnographers. Our process of uncovering abuse in women's lives was characterized by distinctive respondent disclosure patterns evoked by certain trigger topics, recent crisis events in respondents' lives, and ethnographers' direct inquiries. The disclosure experiences also involved ethnographers' own emotional reactions and ethical responsibilities toward the respondents. The implications of these disclosure processes for research designs and methodological issues concerning life course research on low-income women also are discussed.

Ethnography and Revealing Experiences of Physical and Sexual Abuse

Very few people are completely revealing in what they do and say in the presence of others. This claim applies to passing interactants on a city sidewalk; close, lifelong friends; or even respondents answering a sociological survey. As social learning theorists would argue, all individuals are socialized to be mindful of some normative set of rules regarding thoughts, feelings, and behaviors gleaned through their participation in social life. Goffman (1959, 1963), with his emphasis on phenomena such as impression management, stigma, and passing, to name but a few, shed important light on this universal human tendency to guard the information we reveal to others. A main reason for this lack of disclosure is that people learn, both explicitly and implicitly, that their communication of information about self, others, thoughts, and actions can have consequences, both negative and positive (Blumer, 1955; Deutscher, 1966; Schwalbe, 1987). With this in mind, people often try to craft desired images of self, limit the kind and amount of information they share, and hide sensitive or discrediting information from others. And so, alcoholics may attempt to hide signs of inappropriate drinking; workers sometimes cover up evidence of laziness or mistakes to bosses; family members may reveal limited information about one another to outsiders; and women may hide or minimize experiences of sexual and physical abuse.

As social scientists intent on learning as much as possible from those we study, how are we to deal with this potential problem? And, more specifically, how can we gain access to important information, such as women's histories of being physically or sexually abused, especially when that data can better inform the understanding and interpretation of their life course circumstances? We argue that ethnographic research is an especially valuable means for gaining access to these types of sensitive data. The depth of information that emanates from longitudinal ethnography moves us closer than most data-collection methods to uncovering sensitive and hidden experiences that shape individuals' life course (Smith, Tessaro, & Earp, 1995). Ethnography allows for the discovery of such experiences in at least two ways. First, it enables researchers to collect a wide range of data by actually being there, over time, with those being studied to observe and question individuals under the conditions in which they usually act. Second, ethnographic research enables fieldworkers, through the development of trust and rapport with those studied, to elicit data on sensitive information in participants' lives—information that is less likely to be revealed in any single or limited number of encounters.

"Being There"

Ethnographic research, and fieldwork in particular, is a necessarily *social* research practice (see Gans, 1968; Gold, 1958; Jarvie, 1969; Stebbins, 1972; Vidich, 1955). Unlike other methods of social research, ethnographic fieldwork entails actually inserting oneself, to varying degrees, into the lives of the people being studied (see Clarke, 1975). In the course of doing research, ethnographers are inevitably enmeshed in social relationships with those studied by virtue of participating in the latter's activities. Asher and Fine (1991, p. 196), in their study of women married to alcoholics, underscore this feature of ethnographic research:

> Good field research inevitably involves the creation and cultivation of relationships. These relationships will, depending upon the goals of the research and the types of persons whom one is studying, take many forms, but in all cases there must be both a measure of personal caring and respect and an interpersonal distance that derives from the separate roles and social worlds of researcher and informant.

Any given ethnographic research project likewise comprises a series of social acts and relations, a history of cumulative acts that also entails the roles, identities, interactional pressures, and normative social obligations attendant to any set of social relationships (see Emerson & Pollner, 2001; Singer, Hertas, & Scott, 2000). Here, ethnography also stands out as social practice, precisely because of the need to cultivate and maintain relationships with those being studied, often over long periods of time (see Cassell & Wax, 1980; Clarke, 1975; Harrington, 2003).

As typically practiced, ethnographic study involves the close-up and detailed reporting of what people do and say in the flow of everyday activities. It is achieved through some mix of observation, participant observation, and formal and informal interviewing (see Agar, 1996; Spradley, 1980). Likewise, ethnographic research functions as a kind of ongoing, joint accomplishment with those individuals or groups studied, one in which fieldworkers are compelled to manage relationships, identities, and emotions as they attempt to maintain their good standing relative to the individuals and groups they are studying (see Kleinman, 1991; Kleinman & Copp, 1993). As a result, much of the epistemic and analytic power of ethnographic research comes from "having been there," from observing individuals or groups of people acting under conditions in which they usually act, and from describing a social world from the perspective of those who inhabit it (see Becker, 1996; Duneier, 2007).

It is in this sense of being there, and being there over extended periods of time, that ethnographic research serves as a useful way of getting at sensitive or potentially hidden behaviors. Part of this advantage derives from doing *sustained* ethnographic fieldwork that provides opportunities for collecting data as people go through their daily rounds across different settings and activities. Another particularly epistemological advantage comes from fieldworkers' actual participation in activities with research participants. Such participation (i.e., participant observation) provides opportunities to engage in close observation and questioning of social actors as they go about their lives, adapt to their particular circumstances, and provide understandings from the perspectives of those inhabiting distinct social worlds—worlds that typically are distinct from those of academic researchers (see, e.g., Burton 1990, 1997; Burton, Obeidallah, & Allison, 1996).

Rather than relying solely on what people tell them, for instance, in formal interviews, ethnographic fieldworkers are able to supplement, and, hence, to provide a check against these data in the course of doing participant observation and informal questioning. Thus, occasions can arise in which ethnographers experience contradictions between what people tell them and what they actually observe people doing or hear reported from others. The reasons for these contradictions, as discussed earlier, can be many: a desire to hide potentially embarrassing information; a fuzzy memory during formal interviewing; or even the phraseology of a particular interview question by an ethnographer. Regardless of the bases, by being there over time and participating in the social world being studied, fieldworkers gain opportunities to uncover new, contradictory, and potentially illuminating forms of data (see also Duneier, 2007).

Building Trust and Rapport

Ethnographic fieldwork also enables researchers to get at sensitive and hidden data in another way: by being there when research participants are ready to reveal previously concealed information on their own terms. Because many forms of sensitive data, such as experiences of physical and sexual abuse, are kept hidden by research participants, such data can be difficult to obtain, at least until researchers have earned some measure of trust (Dodson & Schmalzbauer, 2005; Wax, 1956). Sincere promises of confidentiality and anonymity can go some distance toward convincing participants to share sensitive data, but these measures are sometimes not enough. In settings in which those studied are concerned about revealing too much of themselves, not until a long-term, comfortable relationship has been established do research participants share information with ethnographers that could potentially have others see them in a less favorable light.

Part of this strength of ethnographic research to elicit sensitive data is a product of participants' felt obligations to reciprocate toward ethnographers in what has become over time a sustained relationship. Part of it derives from fieldworkers' willingness to serve as sympathetic listeners in the course of these cumulative interactions. Either way, central to such sustained relationships are feelings of trust and rapport that fieldworkers are able to establish and maintain with those they are studying. When trust and rapport are established, research participants often reveal sensitive information in the course of "altercasting" (Goffman, 1959; Weinstein & Deutschberger, 1963) fieldworkers into the role of therapeutic listener, someone to whom they can voice their fears and problems in confidence (see, e.g., Ortiz, 2004; Wax, 1956). This ability is made possible given an ethnographer's facility to listen without judgment and to make and keep promises of confidentiality—that is, to instill a sense of trust in the research participant. And for an ethnographer who comes to the research setting as an outsider, lack of involvement in the participant's immediate social world can make him or her all the more attractive (Kloos, 1969; Pollner & Emerson, 1983). In this context, ethnographers come to represent a special category of acquaintance or friend who, not bound up in the participant's network of close relationships, is not likely to spread gossip and create trouble.

Description of the Three-City Study

To illustrate the processes involved in how ethnography can facilitate uncovering physical and sexual abuse in the lives of low-income women we draw on data from the Three-City Study, a longitudinal, multisite, multimethod project designed to examine the impact of welfare reform on the lives of low-income African American, Latino, Hispanic, and non-Hispanic white families and their young children (for a detailed description of the research design of the ethnography, see Winston et al., 1999). Study participants resided in poor neighborhoods in Boston, Chicago, and San Antonio. In addition to longitudinal surveys of a random sample comprising 2,402 families, and an embedded developmental study of 700 families, the Three-City Study included an ethnography of 256 families and their children. These families were not in the survey sample but resided in the same neighborhoods as survey respondents.

Sample Description

Families were recruited into the ethnography between June 1999 and December 2000. Recruitment sites include formal child care settings (e.g., Head Start), the WIC (Women, Infants and Children) program, neighborhood community centers, local welfare offices, churches, and other public assistance agencies. Of the 256 families who participated in the ethnography, 212 families were selected if they included a child age 2–4 to ensure sample comparability with the survey and embedded developmental samples. To inform our understanding of how welfare reform was affecting families with disabilities, the other 44 ethnographic families were recruited specifically because they had a child age 0–8 years with a moderate or severe disability. At the time of enrollment in the ethnography, all families had household incomes at or below 200% of the federal poverty line (U.S. Department of Health and Human Services, 1999).

Table 4.1 describes demographic characteristics of the mothers in the ethnographic sample. The majority of mothers (42%) were of Latino or Hispanic ethnicity, with the largest groups being Mexican American, Puerto Rican, and Dominican, in that order. Over half of the mothers were age 29 or younger when they enrolled in the study and a majority had a high school diploma (GED), or had attended a trade school or college. Forty-nine percent of the mothers were receiving welfare (Temporary Assistance for Needy Families [TANF]) when they entered the study; one-third of these were also working. The 256 mothers identified a total of 685 children in their households, with most children under 4 years of age. Most mothers indicated that they were neither married nor cohabiting at the start of the study. However, longitudinal interviews and observations of the sample over time revealed that more respondents were in marital or cohabiting relationships than they had initially reported.

TABLE 4.1. Sample Characteristics: Three-City Study Ethnography Sample

Characteristic	N	%[a]
City		
Boston	71	28
Chicago	95	37
San Antonio	90	35
Ethnicity/race		
African American	98	38
Latino/Hispanic	108	42
Non-Hispanic white	50	20
Ages of primary caregivers		
15–19	21	8
20–24	67	26
25–29	62	24
30–34	36	14
35–39	35	14
40+	35	14
Education		
Less than high school	110	43
Completed high school or GED	67	26
College or trade school	79	31
TANF/work status		
TANF/working	40	16
TANF/not working	85	33
Non-TANF/working	64	25
Non-TANF/not working	67	26
Number of children primary caregiver is responsible for		
1 child	64	25
2 children	70	27
3 children	63	25
≥ 4 children	59	23
Children's ages		
< 2	190	28
2–4	174	25
5–9	205	30
10–14	88	13
15–18	28	4
Total	685	
Marital status/living arrangements[b]		
Not married, not cohabiting	142	56
Married, spouse in home	42	17
Married, spouse not in home/separated	24	10
Cohabiting (any marital status)	43	17

Note. N = 256.
[a]Percentages may not sum to 100 due to rounding.
[b]There are missing data for five cases in this category.

Ethnographic Methodology

To gather and to analyze ethnographic data on the mothers and their families a method of "structured discovery" was devised to systematize and to coordinate the efforts of the Three-City Study ethnography team (Burton, Skinner, & Matthews, 2005; Winston et al., 1999). An integrated and transparent process was developed for collecting, handling, and analyzing data that involved consistent input from over 215 ethnographers, qualitative data analysts, and research scientists who worked on the project over the course of 6 years. Interviews with and observations of the respondents focused on specific topics but allowed flexibility to capture unexpected findings and relationships among variables. The interviews covered a wide variety of topics, including intimate relationships; health and health care access; family economics; support networks; and neighborhood environments. Ethnographers also engaged in participant observation with respondents, which included attending family functions and outings; being party to extended conversations and witnessing relationship milestones (e.g., a couple's decision to cohabit) between mothers and their partners; and accompanying mothers and their children to the welfare office, hospital, day care, or workplace, noting both context and interactions in each situation. In 92% of the cases, ethnographers were racially matched with respondents and remained the families' ethnographers for the duration of the study. In most cases, interviews and participant observations were conducted in English, with the exception of 34 families who preferred Spanish. Ethnographers met with each family once or twice per month for 12–18 months, then every 6 months thereafter through 2003. Respondents were compensated with grocery or department store vouchers for each interview or participant observation.

Data Sources

The ethnography generated multiple sources of data that we used to identify processes in uncovering patterns of physical and sexual abuse within the sample. Ethnographers in each city wrote detailed fieldnotes about their interviews and participant observations with families, and all interviews were tape-recorded and transcribed. In addition, we consulted transcripts of principal investigators' group and individual discussions with ethnographers and qualitative data analysts about the families in this analysis. [During the data-collection process, we held monthly cross-site Thought-Provoking Questions (TPQ) conference calls with ethnographers and qualitative data analysts. The purpose of these conference calls was discussion of emergent themes in ethnographers' ongoing field observations and data analysts' synthesis of ethnographers' fieldnotes and transcribed interviews.] All sources of data were coded collaboratively [according to a general thematic coding scheme developed by the principal investigators] by ethnographers and qualitative data analysts for entry into a qualitative data management (QDM) software application, then summarized into detailed case profiles of each family. The QDM program and case profiles enabled counts across the entire sample, as well as detailed analyses of individual cases. When we use specific case examples in this chapter, the mothers and their family members have been assigned pseudonyms.

Uncovering Physical and Sexual Abuse: The Three-City Study Ethnographic Process

Although our ethnographic methods generated information on a variety of topics related to women's life course experiences, it is important to note that this ethnographic study *was not* explicitly designed to examine issues of domestic violence or sexual abuse in women's lives. Women's reports of abuse emerged naturalistically in the course of interactions with the ethnographers. When stories of abuse experiences began to surface early in the data-collection process in all three cities, the research team initiated a series of discussions about how to address these disclosures and observations. Principal investigators, senior ethnographers, data analysts, and family ethnographers met online and in conference calls to address a variety of ethical, empirical, and methodological dilemmas posed by "uncovering these experiences," and to develop procedures to protect the physical and emotional safety of both respondents and ethnographers.

During these discussions, those most directly involved in data collection (family ethnographers) emphasized the great degree to which they observed domestic violence and sexual abuse affecting respondent families. Informed by their concerns, the senior project staff requested that data collectors and analysts pay special attention to these issues, and attempt to document and understand their impact on women's and their families' lives, and their relationship to specific outcomes. As a result, the Three-City Study ethnography generated considerable interview and observational data on the patterns and effects of domestic violence and sexual abuse among low-income families over time and across generations. In efforts to analyze and disseminate these data, researchers affiliated with the study sought to place these findings in the context of prior research. Literature reviews conducted for this chapter, as well as for recently published articles (Cherlin et al., 2004; Purvin,

2003, 2007) and an article in press (Burton, Cherlin, Winn, Estacion, & Holder-Taylor, in press), indicate that issues of domestic violence and sexual abuse have not been adequately addressed in general studies of the lives of low-income women, and that gathering data on, measuring, and appropriately interpreting the incidence and processes of physical and sexual abuse among low-income women is complicated and difficult in practice.

The Prevalence of Abuse

Over the course of the study we determined that the prevalence of physical and sexual abuse experiences in mothers' lives was considerably higher than we had ever anticipated. Sexual abuse included mothers' reports of rape, molestation, parentally enforced child prostitution, and witnessing incest acts. Physical abuse comprised physical beatings, attacks with weapons, and witnessing consistent physical violence among parents, partners, and children. Drawing on existing studies that underscore the impact of witnessing sexual abuse and domestic violence on the life course (Feerick & Haugaard, 1999; Luster, Small, & Lower, 2002; Straus, 1992), and the severity of the exposure in our sample, we purposely included "witnessing experiences" in the sexual and physical abuse categories. Mothers' reports of witnessing sexual abuse or domestic violence of short duration or questionable intensity (e.g., "I saw my mother's boyfriend slap her one time") were not included in the analysis. However, witnessing experiences, such as the one recounted by Noel, a 34-year-old mother of five, were included:

> "My sister and I slept in the same bedroom in bunk beds. I slept on the top bunk and my sister on the bottom. Every night for as long as I can remember, my father would come to my sister's bed and force her to have sex with him. I lay there and listened quietly."

With respect to the incidence of physical violence, in most cases the violence was directed toward women and children by men, but in three instances women were perpetrators as well. For example, Serena, a 35-year-old mother, suspected her abusive partner of cheating on her and "followed him to the club with a gun." They argued, she pulled the gun on him, and in the struggle that ensued, Serena's partner was shot in the hand. Serena was charged with assault with a deadly weapon and received 2 years' probation.

Most mothers who reported sexual abuse also reported physical abuse, suggesting that sexual abuse often occurred in the context of physical violence. As Table 4.2 indicates, 36% of the mothers disclosed

TABLE 4.2. Percent Distribution of Physical and Sexual Abuse: Three-City Study Ethnography

History of physical and sexual abuse	% distribution[a]
None	35
Sexual abuse	3
Physical abuse	26
Sexual and physical abuse	36
Total %	100

Note. $N = 228$. Total ethnography sample $N = 256$ (28 cases were not included in this analysis because of insufficient data).
[a]Percentages do not sum to 100 due to rounding.

that they had been sexually and physically abused; 3% revealed that they had only been sexually abused (primarily in childhood), and 26% said they had only been physically abused (primarily in domestic violence situations as adults). In 35% of the cases, mothers reported that they had not been sexually or physically abused in their lifetimes. It is possible, of course, that some of these mothers may also have experienced abuse but were reluctant to mention it. Still, the extended duration of the fieldwork and the trust that developed between the ethnographers and respondents make it likely that our reports are more complete than many other studies.

Patterns of Disclosing Physical and Sexual Abuse

Overall, 64% ($N = 147$) of the mothers who participated in the ethnography disclosed that they had been sexually abused or had experienced physical abuse in childhood, adulthood, or both. What we found intriguing, and what we hope scholars who study life courses of women will find useful, are the ways in which the ethnographers uncovered mothers' histories of abuse.

Data on sexual abuse and domestic violence were gathered from mothers through a number of emergent approaches. For example, after several mothers revealed abuse experiences in early interviews with ethnographers, we developed specific questions in the interview protocol concerning lifetime sexual abuse and domestic violence experiences. Some mothers revealed their experiences to ethnographers in response to these questions, but most did so in response to questions about related topics (e.g., intimate relationships), others in the context of unrelated topics (e.g., discussions about housing), and still others as a function of experiencing recent episodes of abuse.

Three patterns of participant disclosure of abuse were apparent in the ethnographic data: *trigger topics disclosure, crisis or recent event disclosure,* and *ethnographer-prompted disclosure.* Of the mothers who disclosed a history of physical and/or sexual abuse to the ethnographers 71% demonstrated the trigger topics disclosure pattern; 19%, the crisis or recent event pattern; and 10%, ethnographer-prompted disclosure.

Trigger Topics Disclosure

The "trigger topics disclosure" pattern involved mothers unexpectedly revealing their sexual abuse and domestic violence histories to ethnographers when they were asked about not only related topics, such as health and intimate relationships, but also seemingly unrelated topics, such as transportation, family demographics, and intergenerational caregiving. For instance, general questions about health, particularly stress and coping, often triggered mothers' disclosures of sexual abuse and domestic violence experiences. The conversation between Sonya, a 37-year-old African American mother of three, and her ethnographer during a health interview is illustrative:

ETHNOGRAPHER: What would you say was the biggest source of stress for you in the past year?

SONYA: Dealing with a man [referring to her son's father, William]. They can really put you in a depressed stage. Here I am doing what I know is right with my kids, then this one person goin' try to come in and try to tell you another way, which, he just want to be the head of the household and treat you like you just nobody. And I couldn't go for that.... It was eating me up inside.

ETHNOGRAPHER: OK.... Let's talk more about William.

SONYA: He's crazy.... He was really jealous and just crazy. I had headaches daily when he was in the house. I was depressed, but I didn't take medication or nothing. My sister had told me to get rid of him. I was brainwashed though. He told me not to see my family because they didn't like him. I fell for it. He had me so stressed out. My pregnancy with Dante was hard, because I was sick.

ETHNOGRAPHER: You were sick?

SONYA: Yeah, he had been sleeping around and gave me gonorrhea. I'm still embarrassed talking about it. Sometimes I didn't want to sleep with him, but he'd rape me. I told him I was gonna' call the police and he said, "Go ahead. Ain't nobody gonna' arrest me for wanting to be with my woman."

In subsequent interviews, Sonya described in great detail the physical violence and sexual abuse she had experienced from other partners, as well as those experienced by her young daughter.

During Darlene's health interview, which was conducted by the ethnographer during her seventh monthly visit to Darlene's home, the ethnographer asked Darlene how she coped with stress. This 26-year-old Latina mother of four responded:

> "I used to keep a journal of my life, because, when I was younger, I was molested. And so was my sister, so you know, one of our things of therapy was, you know, to write down what we felt for the next time we [would see] our counselor, and I was just like, all right, you know, well, and then I just kept a habit of constantly writing...."

Darlene, like Sonya, went on, in several interviews thereafter, to provide explicit descriptions of her abuse experiences.

Liza, a 28-year-old mother of three, initially revealed her experiences with abuse when the ethnographer accompanied her to a doctor's appointment. At this appointment, Liza learned that her last Pap smear was abnormal. When asked about her sexual history, Liza noted that she was primarily intimate with her husband. The ethnographer seized the opportunity to ask her how she met her husband. Liza stated that this was a *funny* story. She nonchalantly recounted that she met her husband after having just ended a relationship with a man who *broke her nose*. This information was disclosed on the ethnographer's seventh visit with Liza.

Interview topics, such as work, transportation, residential mobility, and household composition, also triggered abuse disclosures from some respondents. For example, during the 23rd visit to the home of Delilah, a 40-year-old European American divorcée and mother of four children, the ethnographer conducted a follow-up interview concerning Delilah's past and current work experiences. Although she had failed to mention particulars about her work history in previous interviews, after 2 years of interviews, Delilah finally told the ethnographer that in the past she had worked at a bank as a switchboard operator until her former husband physically injured her. Delilah stated: "I went to work with a black eye. People at the bank noticed. When it happened a second time, I felt embarrassed coming to work, so I quit like cold turkey. And I really didn't like that idea 'cause, you know, it leaves you in a status of not good standing."

Residential history interviews also prompted disclosures of abuse. The following conversation between Estella, a 30-year-old Latina mother of three, and her ethnographer took place during a residential history interview. Estella had in fact mentioned to the ethnographer in a previous interview that as a child she had witnessed her mother being abused. The discussion of her former residences, however, prompted further disclosure:

ETHNOGRAPHER: So you remember that home, in that area.

ESTELLA: Umm, in that area.

ETHNOGRAPHER: You were like 7, 8 years old then?

ESTELLA: And, then I remember another one in [another city], right off of [street]. It was beautiful, too; it was called [name of development]. And I used to live there; we used to live out there. And, let's see how many more places I can remember.

ETHNOGRAPHER: But you don't have any one place in particular that would bring you memories.

ESTELLA: Yeah, there's one that's a sad memory, because I remember my mother being abused, between two men. One was her ex-husband and another was her boyfriend ... and another one where me and my sister were molested by my mother's ex-boyfriend. So it's like there's places that, you know, I remember that are bad, and then there's some places.

ETHNOGRAPHER: Different places or the same place?

ESTELLA: Right, different places, and I just remember places where they were happy places, where I can remember.

Gathering demographic information on marital histories also triggered abuse disclosures from mothers. Marital history interviews were generally conducted during the second monthly visit. Thus, when Marilyn, a 45-year-old European American mother of four, discussed her abuse experiences during a marital history interview, she became one of the study's earliest disclosers of abuse:

"So for 6 years I was married to him, well, not married to him. We got married for a year, and it didn't work out. We always fought, and then we renewed our vows for another year and that didn't work out. Sometime before she [Marilyn's daughter] was born he was very abusive.... [There is an extended silence before Marilyn continued on with her story.] He beat me up when I was pregnant with her. So I've been divorced since after she was born.... He physically and mentally abused me. He locked me in my apartment, in my bedroom. He told me if he wanted to, he could rape me. He said, 'Might as well get charged with something.' He gave me a couple of hits in the face, hit my head on the headboard, which was glass. I ended up with a contusion and went to the hospital for premature labor."

On the next visit to the home, the ethnographer learned that Marilyn's two youngest children had been sexually abused by her current boyfriend. In the 3 weeks that ensued, the police removed Les, Marilyn's cohabiting boyfriend, from the home for committing these crimes. Despite these very sensitive disclosures and unfolding events, Marilyn remained in the study for 6 years, until its completion.

Crisis Disclosure

The *crisis or recent event disclosure* pattern occurred when the ethnographer unexpectedly "walked in" on a domestic violence situation when visiting the participant, or when the participant experienced a sexual abuse or domestic violence episode a few days or weeks prior to the ethnographer's regularly scheduled visit. In both instances, the abuse situation was "fresh" in the minds of mothers, and they chose to discuss it with their ethnographers in great detail. In most of these cases, the ethnographers suspected abuse (as indicated in ethnographers' fieldnotes and in discussions with their supervisors and team members), but they did not feel that they could ask the participant about it directly until the crisis-prompted disclosure. For example, Janine, the ethnographer for Patrice, a 28-year-old European mother of two, describes the circumstances that led to Patrice's crisis-prompted disclosure:

"I arrived at Patrice's house 10 minutes before the interview only to find the streets covered with cops, patrol cars, and an ambulance. 'Oh my God,' I thought. 'What has happened?' They were taking one man out of Patrice's house. He appeared to be shot or stabbed. Patrice was on the porch screaming, her face bloody and cut. The kids were running around everywhere screaming and crying.... I feared that my worst suspicions about the prevalence of domestic violence in Patrice's life were about to be confirmed.... When I visited Patrice 3 weeks later the floodgate opened without me asking. I listened as she told me everything about the incident, and about other incidents of physical and sexual abuse she had experienced nonstop since childhood."

Ethnographer-Prompted Disclosure

The third pattern, *ethnographer-prompted disclosure,* reflects situations in which ethnographers directly asked mothers about their past and current experiences with sexual abuse or domestic violence. Ethnographers usually asked direct questions about these topics in an interview if they noticed a behavioral reaction from mothers when discussing their intimate relationships with their partners. One ethnographer's interview with Samantha, a 28-year-old European American mother of two, is illustrative:

> "When Samantha was telling me how she met Charles [her current husband], she said that her breakup from her daughter's father Byron was 'a whole big mess.' The expression on her face and the way she said it sent up a red flag for me, so I wanted to ask her more about it. I asked her whether, when she had split up with Byron, there was anything dangerous about it, or whether it was just upsetting in general. Samantha said, 'He was very violent, um, and then I found out he was cheatin' on me with a younger girl; at the time I was what, 20, 21, and he was about 23 goin' out with a 15-year-old, so...I just had it. He was very abusive, and I couldn't take it anymore anyways, so that just made me get the strength to say, 'Get out of my house.'"

The ethnographer asked whether Byron was abusive the whole time Samantha was with him. Samantha replied:

> "No, um, actually it didn't start until, um, the beginnin' of when I was pregnant. He didn't know I was pregnant; I didn't neither at the time, and then it stopped for awhile, and then after I had my daughter, it started up bad. 'Cause I didn't think, he didn't wanna be a family guy, you know, the responsibilities, so, and that's it. He hasn't seen my daughter since she was 2."

Samantha got two restraining orders on him after they broke up. After Samantha met Charles, about 7 months after she and Byron broke up, Byron would call up and threaten Samantha, and he would drive by her house. Later in this interview, and again in the intimate relationship interview, Samantha described in explicit detail the numerous bruises and injuries she received from Byron, and the effects of his abuse on her oldest daughter, who was exposed to it as an infant. Although Samantha initially described her current husband as not abusive, in an incident about a year after this, he became violent and she called the cops. I met with her about a week later, and she described to me what had happened in the course of explaining what had changed since our last meeting.

Timing of Disclosure

It is important to note that there was a range in the timing of disclosure, with approximately 12% of the mothers who revealed physical and sexual abuse experiences telling their stories to the ethnographers during visits or participant observations in the first 3 months of their involvement in the study. Twenty-nine percent disclosed physical and sexual abuse experiences during the 4- to 6-month visits with the ethnographers, 40% during the 7- to 9-month visits, and 19% after 10 to 24 visits. The variation in disclosure timing reflects a range of "turning points" between the mothers and the ethnographers. A turning point is the precise moment in time when the participant trusts the ethnographer enough to share intimate, highly sensitive, and often painful information, such as a history of sexual abuse.

Ethnographers' Reactions and Responsibilities to Participants

As the Three-City Study ethnographic data illustrate, the elements of ethnography that enable it to uncover experiences of physical and sexual abuse so effectively also present ethical and interpersonal challenges (see Becker-Blease & Freyd, 2006; Dodson & Schmalzbauer, 2005). Ethnographers, as we noted earlier, are very likely to find themselves in a privileged positions vis-à-vis their informants by virtue of their role as empathetic and supportive listeners who become, at least temporarily, trusted personal confidantes, yet are not bound up in participants' social networks. Although effective and ethical researchers prepare for and develop protocols to address such potential issues of blurred interpersonal boundaries and disclosure, physical and sexual abuse create unique dilemmas for researchers engaged in ethnographic data collection, analysis, and interpretation. In the Three-City Study ethnography two dilemmas are particularly noteworthy: vicarious trauma and safety.

Vicarious Trauma

Chief among Three-City Study ethnographers' reactions to participants' disclosure of abuse was secondary or vicarious trauma. Developed as a construct based in large part on the experiences of counselors working with victims and survivors of sexual assault and domestic abuse (Schauben & Frazier, 1995), "vicarious trauma" refers to the negative emotional and psychic impact on those "empathically engaged with clients' trauma material" (Pearlman & Saakvitne, 1995, p. 31). Because intensive qualitative interviews can be analogous to therapeutic interactions (Birch & Miller, 2000; Gale, 1992), ethnographers engaged in fieldwork with victims and survivors of traumas such as domestic and sexual abuse, particularly those who have not previously acknowledged or disclosed their experiences, are perhaps as likely as actual counselors to become recipients of such trauma disclosures. The potential for vicarious trauma in intensive qualitative research is just beginning to be addressed in the literature (Etherington, 2007).

Although the majority of sexual assault and domestic violence counselors do not become secondarily traumatized to an incapacitating degree, research suggests that significant numbers experience at least some formal symptoms of vicarious trauma (Bride, 2007; Schauben & Frazier, 1995). There is currently no information on the prevalence of vicarious trauma among researchers working with traumatized persons. However, the levels reported among counselors suggest that vicarious trauma is a potentially significant risk for ethnographers engaged in fieldwork with trauma victims or survivors. Recent work (see Etherington, 2007), as well as our experience on the Three-City Study ethnography, indicate that all research staff who engage intensively with narrative data on the trauma of physical and sexual abuse are potentially vulnerable to vicarious trauma. This includes data transcribers, coders, and analysts who may or may not have conducted direct data collection or fieldwork themselves. Within the Three-City Study team, our data analysts, who did not collect data but were coding it and writing family profiles, frequently had "melt downs," which included "having to pull off on the side of the road on the way home from work to have a good cry," "staying in bed all day because I just couldn't believe someone could do this to another person," or "sitting on the curb with two other ethnographers and just crying my eyes out because I didn't know what else to do."

Safety

An additional ethical and potentially methodological dilemma posed by the emergence of physical and sexual abuse in data collection is the problem of safety. Through their privileged positions of confidence, fieldworkers may become aware of threats to the physical safety of both informants and vulnerable others in the community, such as children. Such situations can potentially generate ethical quandaries over whether and how to break confidentiality and disclose threats of violence to outsiders, particularly in the context of mandatory reporting requirements in the event of child abuse or adult domestic violence. Additionally, the safety of fieldworkers themselves may be threatened when they are present in homes where there is the potential for violence, or if they are viewed as allies to persons who are the target of violence or abuse. Such incidents occurred numerous times in the Three-City Study ethnography. For example, one ethnographer observed a drug deal in a respondent's home and was threatened with murder. Another discovered that a respondent was being abused by her husband and was informed by the respondent's mother to "stay away and don't tell anyone what you saw or our family will fix you." Obviously, taking steps to protect the lives and well-being of those at potential risk is paramount, and any questions pertaining to the ethics of breaking confidentiality must be subsumed. Depending on the particular circumstances and the actions taken, the unfolding of such conditions in the course of data collection can create methodological dilemmas with respect to the nature of data collected, the relationship of the fieldworker to the informants and/or the setting, and implications for data analysis and interpretation.

Summary and Conclusion: Research Design and Methodological Recommendations in Uncovering Abuse

Using longitudinal ethnographic data from the Three-City Study we have described the aspects of ethnography that render it a viable life course methodology for gathering accurate and detailed data about physical and sexual abuse in women's lives. No method of data collection, of course, can ensure that people will disclose sensitive information or be truthful is sharing their life course experiences all the time. But good ethnographic research—which is based on close-up, careful, and detailed observation; participation in the flow of activities with those being studied; and development of trust-based relationships—makes disclosure all the more likely.

In describing the processes involved in uncovering women's abuse experiences in the Three-City Study ethnography we demonstrated the degree to which experiences of physical and sexual abuse permeate the lives of low-income mothers, and present methodological and ethical challenges to ethnographers. Our process of uncovering abuse in women's lives was characterized by distinctive respondent disclosure patterns evoked by certain trigger topics, recent crisis events, and ethnographers' direct inquiries. The disclosure processes also involved ethnographers' own experiences with vicarious trauma and safety issues.

Because physical and sexual abuse often emerge naturalistically in ethnography and are rarely a starting point of inquiry, many ethnographic studies that uncover these issues may not, at the onset, address the consequent ethical and methodological considerations in the study design or planning. Like other studies, the Three-City Study principal investigators did not include extensive preplanning to address specifically the potential for participants' various patterns of disclosure and ethnographers' vicarious trauma. However, based on previous field experiences of the ethnographic study's director and several of the research staff, fieldworkers did receive training to address potential safety issues related to abuse prior to entering the field. Despite this precaution, the extent, amount, and intensity of respondent experiences were significantly greater than anticipated. Because the premise of the Three-City Study ethnography was based on the concept of structured discovery (Burton et al., 2005; Winston et al., 1999), these issues became a focus of inquiry, and comprehensive protocols to address a variety of ethical and methodological concerns were instituted immediately. Based on our experiences, we offer the following suggestions for practices to researchers that may be helpful in the process of uncovering physical and sexual abuse in studies of women's life course:

• Individuals who directly gather data from respondents should be provided with extensive training and supervision concerning physical and sexual abuse, potential disclosure patterns, and vicarious trauma before, during, and after work in the field. That training also should be extended to those who are analyzing data, even if they do not have direct contact with respondents. Some researchers may be concerned that a training emphasis on abuse experiences would likely introduce bias in researchers' interactions with respondents and in data analysts' interpretations of the data. Our experiences suggest that it is better for individuals to have a comprehensive understanding of these issues, and that the potential for bias in data gathering and analysis is actually minimized when researchers are better informed about the realities of abuse in women's lives and how uncovering that abuse may impact them as researchers.

• It is critical that principal investigators and interviewer supervisors occasionally accompany interviewers and ethnographers into the field to assess potential dangers and provide "second opinions" on observed family behaviors that appear troublesome. Joint observations and field experiences provide an important level of support to interviewers and ethnographers, and can move the "onus" for verifying and reporting abuse from those who gather data about the families directly to those who direct the studies. We also developed protocols about mandatory reporting of abuse that we reviewed and revised as needed.

• Developing site-specific lists of contacts for referrals to shelters and other support agencies is imperative for any study. Principal investigators, and interviewer and ethnographer supervisors, should also establish good working relationships with referring agencies and keep abreast of agencies' capacities to accommodate the needs of respondents should referrals take place.

• Any study that has the potential for uncovering abuse experiences should include research team members with clinical expertise in abuse, and make them available to staff and supervisors across the study for consultation. Having a "quick response" strategy in place to address ethnographers', interviewers', and data analysts' experiences with violence in the field, or with vicarious trauma, is also imperative. We put together a reporting and safety committee on the Three-City Study that comprised clinical psychologists, social workers, and lawyers who were able to convene in person or via conference call within 24 hours to address ethnographers' issues concerning abuse. We also scheduled periodic, projectwide conference calls devoted to issues of abuse, as well as local site team meetings to ensure consistent peer support and debriefing.

To our knowledge, none of the published literature from ethnographies that have explored domestic and sexual abuse addresses these methodological and ethical challenges or describes how the research staff addressed them in either planning or practice. The literature does indicate that sexual and domestic abuse are very likely to continue to emerge as issues in any ethnographic or intensive qualitative research conducted with women and families in low-income communities (e.g., Dodson, 1998; Edin, 2000; Edin & Kefalas, 2005; Fine & Weis, 1998; Kurz, 1996; Scott et al., 2002). And the use of intensive qualitative methods in the study of poverty in sociology and policy studies is likely to increase (Newman & Massengill, 2006). Given this, and based on our experiences in the Three-City Study ethnography, we argue that it is incumbent upon researchers engaged in inquiry in low-income communities to take issues of physical and sexual abuse into account in study design and planning. Particularly when studies involve the collection, analysis, and interpretation of narrative life course data, it is critical to address the ethical and methodological challenges posed by the potential development of vicarious trauma and issues of safety among all levels of project staff and informants.

Acknowledgments

Writing and research for this chapter were supported by grants to Linda Burton from the National Science Foundation (No. SES-07-03968), the Administration on Children and Families (No. 90OJ2020) and core support to the Three-City Study from the National Institute of Child Health and Human Development through grant Nos. HD36093 and HD25936, as well as many other government agencies and private foundations. Most importantly, we thank the families who graciously participated in the research and who gave us access to their hidden life experiences.

CHAPTER 5

Linking Research Questions to Data Archives

Glen H. Elder, Jr.
Miles G. Taylor

The past half-century has witnessed a dramatic increase in the launching of longitudinal samples to study human lives. Many of the classic longitudinal studies that scholars use today (e.g., the Michigan Panel Study of Income Dynamics) were originally conceived as "short-term" projects for investigating behavior change from one year to the next. Fortunately for scholars, a good number of these projects were re-funded year after year, and now provide life record data spanning decades. More than ever, investigators usually find a number of longitudinal data archives that address specific research questions on the life course. Documentation of these studies has been transformed as well—from codebooks housed at a research institution where the specific study was based to PDF (portable document format) files that may be easily downloaded from publicly available data archives and "searched" with keyword commands.

With accessibility to longitudinal data at an all-time high, investigators now have the ability to choose from multiple archives. The problem they encounter is that these studies were not designed to address questions that are now relevant or timely to scholars in the field. This challenge is not a new one. It has been an obstacle since the very conception of longitudinal studies. Investigators faced the same problem more than a half-century ago, when they sought to link available data to new research questions. The technology has changed substantially since then, but the methodology and underlying thought processes are as relevant today as they ever were.

In this chapter, we address the challenge of how to make the most of readily available longitudinal data. We examine ways to breathe new life into existing longitudinal archives, so that they do not outlive their ability to address research questions that have evolved in life course research or that are relevant to contemporary policy issues. We do this by explicating three different strategies for linking existing longitudinal data to new research questions. For each strategy, we present one or more relevant examples from research to show the challenges and payoffs inherent in each. Some of the data archives, including that of the Terman study and the Gluecks' data archives, appear in multiple examples, underscoring the value of coupling research strategies to make the most of the data.

We begin with a discussion of the steps involved in making the decision to undertake one or more research strategy, featuring the iterative process of matching the research question to available data (Elder et al., 1993). Then we move on to discuss the three strategies for maximizing the usefulness of data that cannot address the research question in its present form. First, we discuss the "recasting process," in which a series of steps is taken to recode and restructure existing data to maximize the fit between data and the research question. In turn, the research question is also revised to enhance the fit. Second, we discuss ways in which supplementary data files can be merged with existing longitudinal archives to address new questions. For example, death, health, or military records may provide additional insight into life record data or provide outcome variables of interest that are not available in the original data. Finally, we discuss a third strategy, that of carrying out a follow-up study of the original members of a longitudinal sample for the purpose of gathering supplementary information on a particular topic, such as intergenerational relationships. This design may also be used to add a layer of detail or extend life record data that depict additional life stages.

With strategies of this kind, we aim to "make the best of what we have" (Hyman, 1972, p. 272), by ensuring that valuable longitudinal data are not overlooked or bypassed in the quest to answer contemporary research questions. Now, more than ever, scholars have options to make useful data applicable to contemporary research questions. In what follows we reintroduce scholars to examples from both classic and contemporary studies that have used one or more strategies.

Maximizing the Link

Making the most appropriate use of archival longitudinal data for current research questions involves achieving a satisfactory "match." This entails an iterative process between questions and available data or information. Throughout this section, we highlight the steps involved in this process. In addition, we use Dillon and Wink's (2007) recent work on religious practice and belief over the life course as an example in each step. Their work exemplifies the iterative process involved in achieving the best fit between research questions and data in life course research.

The first step in the matching process is to *locate an issue or problem and formulate one or more research questions that are answerable.* Merton (1959) noted that the task in scientific inquiry of identifying fundamental problems and framing them in such a way that they can be addressed is often more demanding than finding answers. Good research questions, in his mind, are "questions so formulated that the answers to them will confirm, amplify, or variously revise some part of what is currently taken as knowledge in the field" (p. x). The reasons for identifying a problem may vary, from questioning support for what Merton called existing "social facts" to clarifying a sociological or psychological idea that has become too narrow in its present form to address the facts to which it is applied. Regardless of what leads investigators to problems, they must then be translated into originating questions, statements of what we want to know. The next step is to formulate a rationale behind the question, why are we interested? Then, the question must be reformulated in a way that answers the question and satisfies the rationale for asking it in the first place.

The focus in this chapter is on finding ways to maximize the usefulness of existing longitudinal data. Thus, the original questions of investigators will likely not be the ones that motivated the data collection in the first place. Throughout this chapter we cite examples of investigators who used existing data based on other questions or topics to address their current sociological or life course questions. The importance of sound, specific, answerable research questions is the first step in recognizing where existing longitudinal archives can be of great use in addressing new lines of inquiry.

For example, Dillon and Wink (2007) were interested in the role of religion in the everyday lives of individuals and, more specifically, in how religious beliefs and behaviors change over the life course. As the authors note, the majority of sociological research on religion focuses on middle to late adulthood, with very little attention to childhood and adolescence, when beliefs and practices may be formulated. Also, early adulthood has been overlooked, although it is often noted as a time of transition into career, marriage, and parenthood. With the topic of religious involvement in mind, the researchers formulated a number of specific research questions. We focus here on one: "Does religious involvement change over the life course?" (p. 80).

The next step is to *identify one or more appropriate data sources* that appear to represent a good match for the question. No single data source is likely to offer everything a researcher wants, but a well-articulated question will enhance "goodness of fit" with the selected data set. In some cases a historical or biographical event is of interest, so the data must either sample individuals prospectively during the event or provide retrospective reports that enable us to link individuals to the past event. In other cases a developmental period may be the focus of inquiry, so relevant data would capture the time in question, either through observations of individuals over the entire period of interest or by staggering the ages of study members enough that statements about the entire period can be drawn with confidence.

Dillon and Wink (2007) observed that only a few longitudinal data archives in the world provide answers to research questions on change in religious involvement (p. 80). Few data sources track individuals from childhood to old age, and even fewer measure religious involvement. The authors report three potential data sources for this project: The Terman study at Stanford University (1922–1986), Valliant's (1977) study of male Harvard graduates, and the Berkeley Guidance–Oakland Growth Studies (1928/1929–1997/2000). Of these data sources, the Terman and Valliant data sets collected fewer prospective measures on religious involvement, and also offered less richness in their in-depth interviews on the topic of religious beliefs. Therefore, the authors chose to use the Berkeley–Oakland Studies (Dillon & Wink, 2007, p. 242).

At this point, *development of a research strategy* is helpful for refining the variables and data structure that are needed to address the research question adequately. If gender differences or racial/ethnic diversity are central to the research questions posed, then the data will have to include both men and women or have the necessary amount of racial or ethnic diversity to address such issues. This step includes an *inventory of what is and is not available in the data* source chosen. Listing measures by age tends to be helpful, because longitudinal surveys collect data on topics only in given waves or only particular data for certain groups (e.g., military service and labor force questions asked only of men). Part of this inventory may also include a *cursory analysis of the data* at hand, because codebooks do not always reveal important aspects of the data, such as frequency distributions for response categories or incomplete information on topics of interest to the proposed study.

In considering the Berkeley–Oakland data for questions on religious involvement and belief, Dillon and Wink (2007) found that in each wave of the data, all study members were asked detailed questions about religious beliefs, attitudes, and practices (p. 219). In the early waves, during the adolescence of study members, the parents were asked questions on religious behaviors and participation as well, thereby enabling the investigators to consider the role of religious upbringing in changes in religious involvement (p. 220). The study members were also asked a series of open-ended questions concerning religious activity, participation in religion-affiliated social groups, and religious attendance. Interviewers also collected data on other important aspects of individuals' lives, such as career, marriage, family, health, and so forth.

Through an examination of codebooks and open-ended questions, Dillon and Wink (2007) found a wealth of information on the topics listed earlier, although this information was scattered throughout the interviews in both quantitative and qualitative formats. Nonetheless, the data revealed that they could examine the concept of involvement in two important facets: *religiousness* (institutionalized or church-related beliefs and practices), and *spiritual seeking* (noninstitutionalized beliefs and practices). Furthermore, a cursory analysis of the data revealed that although the majority of study members grew up as mainline Protestants (63%), there was substantial variation in religious affiliation. Ten percent of the sample grew up with nonmainline Protestant affiliations (Mormon, Christian Scientist, etc.); 16% were Catholic; 5% came from mixed religious backgrounds; and 6% were nonreligious. This finding meant that the researchers could include differences in affiliation as part of their research question.

The final step in the process of adapting archival material for later use involves deciding whether the available data are adequate to address the research question at hand, or *whether some recasting, linking, or follow-up strategy is needed*. These strategies are undertaken when it is clear that although the data have strong potential to address part of the question at hand, some additional information is needed, whether in the form of a reorganization of the data itself (recasting) or in the addition of data to the original sample (supplementation and follow-up). In this decision-making process, some rewording of *the original research question* may be required to achieve the best fit with the data as they stand or once a strategy is undertaken to adapt the data.

Although Dillon and Wink (2007) had a rich data set that spanned the life course, they undertook two of the strategies discussed in this chapter to maximize the link between the research question and available data (recasting and follow-up). The first included recasting the data to create a *religious narrative* for each individual (p. 222). As mentioned previously, the data included a large amount of information on the lives of study members, but much of the information on religious involvement had to be pieced together in a manner that was consistent and reliable. Furthermore, the researchers conducted a follow-up of study members by adding a module of questions to the final wave in late adulthood (1997–2000) that focused on religious and spiritual beliefs, moral philosophy, the place of religion and the sacred in daily life, life after death, and any significant religious or spiritual experiences in addition to questions on religious attendance and overall involvement (p. 15). This module gave researchers the ability to ask rich, open-ended, and retrospective questions about the role of religion and spiritual belief and practice for study members as they looked back over their lives. The open-ended nature of the questions also allowed individuals to focus on what was most salient for them in terms of involvement.

In addressing the question, "Does religious involvement change over the life course?" Dillon and Wink (2007, p. 80) found that involvement does indeed change. They state that the shape of involvement is best described as a "shallow U-curve, with high levels of religiousness in adolescence and in early and late adulthood and a dip in religiousness in the middle years" (p. 81). Although this reduced involvement during midlife is not drastic, it likely coincides with children leaving the home and increased competition for time from work, community, and leisure activities.

In the sections that follow, we discuss strategies to make the most of longitudinal archives -—the processes of recasting, supplementation, and follow-up. For each strategy we present one or more examples from research to show the specific motivations, challenges, and benefits. The first strategy we discuss is recasting, a straightforward and useful way to reshape data not originally designed to answer life course questions, so that it can be used to address them.

Recasting: Recoding and Reshaping Data to Answer New Questions

"Recasting" refers to a restructuring or reshaping of the data to maximize its fit for a specific research question. It should be noted that recasting is more than just a recoding of data. Although some recoding may be involved, a new theoretical framework is generally applied to the data in a way that provides information for new research questions. As a rule, prospective longitudinal studies are carried out in a changing world, but information is seldom collected from study members on their historical experiences, except as inferred from their birth year and place. However, researchers need to know more about study members' journey through historical time and space. This information may be obtained by combining interview items that depict pieces of this journey, by coding open-ended questions that provide such information, or by using both measurement strategies.

Over his career, Elder has engaged in a number of projects that required making the best of available data to study lives in time and place. These endeavors have often led to the recasting of archival data, both qualitative and quantitative, to maximize the fit with the research question. In what follows, we present an example of recasting that resulted from the desire to answer questions on the mobilization experience during World War II, for which the data were not originally designed. The project focuses on military involvement and its role in the lives and health of men in the Terman data archive. We also return to the Terman data in the following sections as they provide an example of the use of multiple strategies to make the most of available data.

The Terman Men and World War II

The early 20th century witnessed a rise in research questions concerning the life span of individuals that coincided with advances in psychological, sociological, and human development theory. At the time, these questions far exceeded the reach of cross-sectional studies. As a result, a number of pioneering longitudinal studies on children and youth were extended into the early and later adult years. As mentioned in the previous section, most notable among these are the Terman study at Stanford University (see Minton, 1988a, 1988b), and multiple studies based at the University of California, Berkeley: the Berkeley Growth Study, the Berkeley Guidance Study (both with 1928–1929 birth cohorts), and the Oakland Growth Study (1920–1921 birth cohort; Eichorn et al., 1981).

Originally, these studies were meant to address intelligence and development (cognitive, physical, and social) among children, but all were re-funded for periodic follow-up until the 1980s or beyond, a remarkable feat for the time. Elder's primary interest in these data sources centered on the impact of significant historical events in the lives of men and women in different cohorts, from the Great Depression to World War II. Specific to this chapter is his interest in World War II and the timing of military mobilization in men's future life outcomes. Though attention to historical influence was inherently lacking in these studies, the Berkeley–Oakland data archives provided substantial empirical evidence on mobilization during World War II as a turning point in young men's lives (Elder, 1986, 1987b).

The Berkeley–Oakland sample included men who were mobilized for military duty at a young age, typically before age 23, before the men had established careers and families. Thus, mobilization gave them access to training, experience, and networks they otherwise might not have had. However, the Berkeley–Oakland data could not answer research questions about the disruptive effect of "late entry" into the military due to the timing of World War II in men's lives. By contrast, men in the Terman study at Stanford were relatively "old" for military duty at the time of Pearl Harbor: Nearly half were in their 30s and a preliminary analysis of the data revealed that 45% of the men in the Terman sample reported military service during World War II.

From the evidence at hand, the research team concluded that the Terman data provided the best fit with the late mobilization hypothesis and offered a rare opportunity to investigate more broadly the enduring life course effects of military service during World War II. This data archive is the result of a study by Professor Lewis Terman of Stanford University on gifted children in urban California, 1921–1922. His research team selected 857 boys and 671 girls, ages 3–19 years, with IQ levels above 135 (Minton, 1998a, 1988b; Terman & Oden, 1959b).

The original purpose of the study was to examine the stability of intellectual ability among gifted individuals after 10 years. However, follow-up surveys were carried out through 1992, covering up to 70 years of the study members' lives. The original 1922 and 1928 data collections focused on intelligence and achievement. The next waves of data collection (1936 and 1940) occurred at a time of educational attainment in the lives of study members and transition into adult roles (occupation, marriage). These topics were addressed in the subsequent follow-up (1945), along with questions on military service and involvement, including various service roles. Data on the postwar years (1950, 1955, and 1960) were collected during a time of family formation and development, career transitions, and mobility. The final waves (1972, 1977, 1982, and 1986) focused more on processes of aging, occupational career and retirement, family dynamics, and life evaluation toward the end of life, because the Terman sample had by then aged into older adulthood. The topics at each follow-up are listed in Table 5.1. Across all waves of data collection, very little information was collected on the historical contexts and social pathways of the study members. This became the research team's task.

The team soon discovered that the data were not originally set up to permit a life course study of the effects of wartime service into the later years. The Terman project had followed the same individuals

TABLE 5.1. Terman Longitudinal Sample and Data

Survey waves	Number of respondents	Primary topics
1922 1928	1,528: 857 men, 671 women	Home and school
1936 1940	1,256: 699 men, 557 women	Education, work, marriage
1945	1,334: 749 men, 585 women	Military experience
1950	1,271: 716 men, 555 women	
1955	1,286: 716 men, 570 women	Work, marriage, achievements
1960	1,127: 616 men, 511 women	
1972	927: 497 men, 430 women	
1977	821: 426 men, 386 women	Aging, work, and retirement
1982	813: 415 men, 398 women	Life review
1986 1991–1992	805: 404 men, 401 women	

over time, but the data were originally coded and stored in a manner consistent with repeated cross-sectional surveys. Linkages between individual data over time were not made; thus, longitudinal life histories were not available for study. Revisiting the archive was necessary to develop data for a life course study of military service in World War II. The research team led by Elder needed access to data files at Stanford University to create life records for each study member on achievement, marriage, parenthood, and health trajectories, in addition to wartime service.

Though wartime mobilization was directly addressed in the original data collections, cursory measures of service (timing of enlistment and exit, and branch) were gathered without details about the type of service undertaken, exposure to combat, or the heterogeneity of men's experiences during or in response to these experiences. These measures were not available in the original computerized data. However, over the years, study members voluntarily shared life experiences through open-ended questions, letters to the Terman study staff, newspaper clippings, and so forth. An inventory of these data archives indicated that the materials would provide a richer portrait of military experiences and address multiple aspects of service experience of interest to the project. Drawing from research on wartime activity, Elder and his research team at the Carolina Population Center created a codebook that served as an outline for inventorying the complete archive on men's wartime activities and experience. Six main areas were covered, along with well-defined measures:

1. *Lifetime military and military-related experiences*: veteran status and type; service before, during, and after World War II; entry and exit information, service career, branch, and unit; medals and education linked to the service (e.g., Reserve Officers' Training Corps [ROTC], GI Bill).
2. *Overseas experience before World War II or U.S. involvement*: duty for government, volunteer agency.
3. *Home front experience during World War II*: deferments, conscientious objector status, service with government.
4. *Wartime stress*: combat duration in weeks and months; experience of firing at the enemy and of being fired upon; exposure to wounded and dead (Allies and enemy); experiences of being wounded, held in a prisoner of war camp, and missing in action (also identified men killed in action, 3% of the total sample).
5. *Postwar experiences linked to the war*: civil administration duties during military occupation, medical care for Allied wounded, and medical evaluation for repatriation or emigration.
6. *Domestic exposure to care of American wounded and the dying*: experience of medical personnel in the sample, separation from those on the front line.

A summary sheet was created for each individual on these measures. Using all available information in the archive meant reviewing previously coded data, open-ended responses on the questionnaire forms, and supplemental materials from study members' files. Initially, 30 men in the Terman study reporting World War II involvement were chosen for preliminary testing of this coding scheme. A standardized form was necessary, because data were collected from multiple sources; some were reported directly by respondents themselves on surveys in closed- and open-ended questions, and others were evident through other volunteered materials (e.g., letters from spouses, newspaper clippings, etc.). The codesheets were then checked for inconsistencies or problems. After five trials and revisions, the finalized measures prepared for the codebook comprised the six areas of interest listed earlier.

Using these data the research team found that men who enter the service relatively late in life (after age 32) experienced a greater risk of divorce and negative physical health compared to men who entered at earlier ages (Elder, Shanahan, & Clipp, 1994). In addition, men reporting combat were likely to be younger, consistent with the literature on World War II recruitment and mobilization. Exposure to combat had a lasting negative effect on the health of men in later life, apart from time of entry, and this effect was especially strong among men with lower levels of both self-esteem and self-confidence before their war service (Elder, Shanahan, & Clipp, 1997).

The Stanford–Terman data bring up another valuable point in considering recasting and other strategies to breathe new life into archived data sources—the ability of existing and recasted data sets to produce new life course questions and hypotheses. For example, one of the original interests of the research team was the health of men in the Terman study, and especially health related to wartime experiences earlier in the life course. Upon examining the archive, the research team realized that a broad array of physical and mental health variables was available in the archive, but that these variables had not been coded in any systematic way for measures (see Elder, Pavalko, & Clipp, 1993). During this inventory of the data, they found that distinct patterns of health trajectories seemed to arise from both the quantitative and open-ended reports of the Terman study respondents. These multiple typologies of health trajectories are presented in Figure 5.1.

Thus, a new set of research questions was formulated in terms of health trajectories across the life course with reference to dominant patterns and their predictors (Elder et al., 1993). This shift to an interest in multiple trajectories of health was a novel approach at the time, because the only literature to chronicle such patterns at that time were case studies in medical research (Clipp, Pavalko, & Elder, 1992). In addition, the notion that certain health conditions would likely lead to specific patterns of functioning or overall health preceded by more than a decade a current and burgeoning interest in typologies of health trajectories in the public health literature (Lynn, 1997, 2001; Lunney, Lynn, Foley, Lipson, & Guralnick, 2003; Murray, Kendall, Boyd, & Sheikh, 2005; Taylor, 2005).

We found that among men in the Terman study, the largest pattern represented was that of constant good health (Trajectory 1: 36%), followed by decline at the end of life (Trajectory 5: 25%), decline and recovery (Trajectory 3: 22%), linear decline (Trajectory 4: 14%), and constant poor health (Trajectory 2: 3%). Younger cohorts were more likely not only to be in constant good health but also to experience decline and recovery, possibly reflecting the historical rise in medical intervention/technology before and during later life. Men with lower levels of education experienced trajectories characterized by decline (Trajectories 4 and 5). Although the health trajectories were spread somewhat equally by marital status among the men (married, divorced, widowed), never-married men were more likely to have trajectories of constant poor health (Clipp et al., 1992).

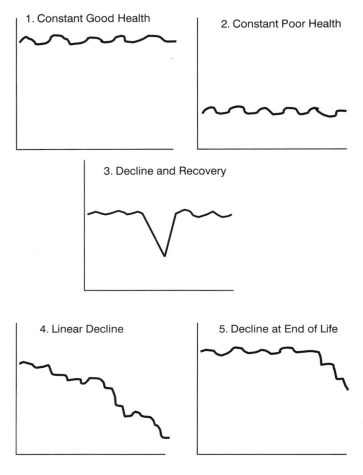

FIGURE 5.1. Physical health trajectories. From Elder, Pavalko, and Clipp (1993). Copyright 1993 by Sage. Reprinted by permission.

The measurement work of the research team in adapting the Terman sample to questions about World War II mobilization exemplifies recasting as a strategy that maximizes the fit between questions and available data. The Terman archive contained the information needed to address these questions during the historical period of interest, even though historical influences and military service were not topics that originally motivated the study. However, the limited data required a restructuring of the data set to address these questions and to use supplemental or volunteered materials from study members. In turn, the recasting process generated new research questions and hypotheses about health trajectories over the life course of men (the men's archives were originally chosen for recasting, owing to the study of service in World War II). In the section that follows we outline another strategy for maximizing the fit of question and data, the process of data supplementation. The decision to supplement arises from motivations similar to those leading to the recasting process. We discuss these motivations explicitly and move on to examples of supplementation of both completed data archives and those that are still active.

Linking Supplementary Information to Existing Longitudinal Data

The addition of supplemental data to existing archives can maximize the fit between a data archive and research questions, such as when extra information is needed or when outcomes of interest have occurred following the period of study using the original data. Alternate data sources (i.e., health, death, or criminal records) may be linked to the longitudinal archive to facilitate these new lines of inquiry. Like recasting, a discourse between question and data is needed, since the investigator is still working with what is available and may need to revise the question in a suitable manner.

Though potentially less arduous than recasting, the decision to supplement existing data comes with its own set of challenges, primarily because records of interest (e.g., death or health records) are often confidential and require a great deal of organization and clearance to obtain. Compounding this is the fact that informed consent may not be possible if study participants are deceased, have moved, or are otherwise not available. Nonetheless, if proper protocols are followed, it is possible to link supplemental information, even to large longitudinal data sets. Here we briefly discuss multiple motivations for undertaking this effort before moving on to examples from relevant life course studies in which the challenges and benefits are explained with specific examples.

One obvious motivation behind supplementation is that the information of interest is not available in the original data. As with recasting, the decision to supplement typically occurs when the data's original purpose diverges significantly from the research question at hand. In addition, supplementary data may provide an alternative source of information for comparison with self-reports in the study itself. For example, if we are interested in the perceived experiences of older adults while they were young adults, we may be able to compare self-reports of school performance with their retrospective reports. Finally, limitations in the data for certain research questions may be addressed with supplemental data. This would occur, for example, when the purpose of the study is in line with current research questions but aspects of survey design or unintended restrictions, such as limited coverage of a topic (e.g., military experience), make addressing certain research questions difficult.

In what follows, we discuss numerous examples of data supplementation that address one or more reasons given earlier for undertaking such a project. It is often the case that supplemental data are integrated with a data set, while data collection is still in progress to inform previous and upcoming waves. One example of this is the addition of transcript data from secondary schools and biomarkers to the National Longitudinal Survey of Adolescent Health. However, our focus is on examples in which investigators, independent of the survey design and collection, have gone back to existing longitudinal archives and merged supplemental records with them to address new lines of inquiry. We focus on this type of supplementation to highlight the use of existing longitudinal data archives.

The Terman Archive and Vital Statistics Records

Our first example of supplementary data linkage returns to the Stanford–Terman data archive described earlier in this chapter. Remember that the sample was the largest early longitudinal study at its first wave in 1922. It followed approximately 1,500 Californians from childhood for roughly 70 years. Also recall that the Terman data were originally intended to study the achievements of gifted children. Thus, detailed information on early achievement, personality and other psychological factors, and family structure were included. In the 1990s, Howard Friedman, a health psychologist at the University of California–Riverside, began to explore the long-term consequences of personality traits and childhood conditions for longevity. More specifically, he was interested in the types of pathways or processes that might explain the relationship of certain traits to differential longevity in middle and late life.

With a research team, Friedman collected information on reported deaths in the Terman sample and requested death certificates from state bureaus for those individuals. This meant trying to ascertain the state where the individual died, although most lived in California their whole lives (Peterson, Seligman, Yurko, Martin, & Friedman, 1998). The death certificates were then coded for cause of death by a physician-supervised, certified nosologist using the ninth revision of the *International Classification of Diseases* (ICD-9; U.S. Public Health Service, 1980). Of particular interest to Friedman and his team were deaths from particular chronic conditions (cardiovascular disease, cancer) and those due to injury (accident or violence; Friedman et al., 1995). Death certificates were not available for 20% of the deceased, so cause of death was imputed from next-of-kin reports when possible. This resulted in death records on roughly 1,200 respondents from the original sample of 1,528 (over 78% of the original sample had died).

With these supplemental data, Friedman discovered that known connections between personality traits (e.g., sociability, conscientiousness, and neuroticism) and health were not the product of direct linkages, but functioned as intermediary (causal) pathways in which certain traits were more likely to place individuals at risk of poor health behaviors and unstable marriage careers (Friedman et al., 1995). He also found a distinct and lasting link between parental divorce during childhood and the increased risk of mortality for all causes of death (Friedman et al., 1995). Although the original Terman sample contained much of the information that interested Friedman, the supplementation of death records enabled him to pursue a completely new line of inquiry that focused on effects of childhood and adult personality and health on longevity.

The Gluecks' Study and Crime/Vital Statistics Records

The second example of adding supplemental data to an existing longitudinal archive is provided by Sampson and Laub's examination of the Gluecks' *Unraveling Juvenile Delinquency* (1950) data set. With an interest in criminal careers over the life course, Laub and Sampson (2003) investigated how various childhood and adult factors (marriage, occupation) affect and are intertwined with trajectories of criminal offending throughout adulthood and into later life. This objective led them to supplement existing Gluecks' data with death and criminal records on the men through their middle and late adulthood. In a follow-up interview, they obtained life histories (ages 50–70) from a small percentage of the sample still alive in the early 1990s (see a later section for details of this life history follow-up).

The original *Unraveling Juvenile Delinquency* study was conducted by Sheldon and Eleanor Glueck, starting in 1940. Their research goals were to establish the sociocultural (family), somatic (health), and intellectual (intelligence) characteristics of delinquency, and how these factors related to patterns of delinquency into young adulthood (Glueck & Gleuck, 1950). The sample contained 500 persistently delinquent boys between ages 11 and 16 years, drawn from two correctional schools near Boston. The study also included a sample of 500 nondelinquent boys from Boston public schools that served as matched controls. Subjects were matched on age, ethnicity, IQ, and disadvantaged neighborhood. Two follow-up studies were conducted over the next 25 years, when the study members were ages 25 and 32, respectively. The Gluecks collected a vast amount of data over the 25-year period on individual characteristics (biological, psychological, and social); family structure and parental factors; achievement and activities in school; occupational mobility and details of work life; and other factors, such as leisure activities, networks and companions, and civic involvement (Laub & Sampson, 2002).

In 1993, using data from the original study, Laub and Sampson searched the Massachusetts Office of the Commissioner of Probation for 475 of the original 500 delinquent boys and their criminal record data up to that time (over 50 years after the baseline study). In this way, they were able to "update" the criminal records of the original study members and create trajectories of criminal careers across the life course. They then classified arrests into violent, property, substance-related, or other. Because the men could have had criminal records in states other than Massachusetts, "rap" sheets were requested and obtained from the Federal Bureau of Investigation, a process that took roughly 18 months. Simultaneously, a search of death records was undertaken from both the Massachusetts Vital Records and the National Death Index. At the last wave of the Gluecks' study, 25 of the men had died, but dates and other information were available for these subjects from the archived data (Sampson & Laub, 2005a).

With these supplements, Sampson and Laub (2005a) were able to construct criminal and health careers for men throughout their adulthood and in conjunction with the items collected in the Gluecks' original data. They found, for example, that childhood predictors of delinquency do not necessarily translate to adult patterns of offending, and that social bonds (most notably marriage) have strong protective effects (Laub, Nagin, & Sampson, 1998). They also found that there are distinct trajectories of individual offending over the life course rather than one average "crime" curve (see Doherty, Laub, & Sampson, Chapter 9, this volume). The data archive provided by the Gluecks was a theoretically relevant and remarkably comprehensive data source for investigating delinquency and the likelihood of its transition into adult criminal offending. But supplementation of these data enabled Laub and Sampson to extend the usefulness of the longitudinal data and address life course questions on the lifelong trajectories of men's offending and nonoffending behavior.

The National Long-Term Care Survey and Medicare and Vital Statistics Records

A third example of supplementation is provided by an ongoing project directed by Miles Taylor that merged two data archives, the National Long-Term Care Survey (NLTCS) and Medicare/Vital Statistics records.

Building on the work of Elder and colleagues (Clipp et al., 1992), Taylor's research interests covered trajectories of health and well-being over the life course and, specifically, into older adulthood. Using the NLTCS and other data, Taylor observed that disability trajectories among older adults follow multiple distinct patterns rather than an average linear increase, similar to the trajectories of health discussed earlier in this chapter (Figure 5.1). They vary significantly by demographic and social factors (Taylor, 2005). These findings led to her interest in whether certain chronic conditions predict patterns of disability in later life. However, Taylor soon recognized that supplementation of the existing longitudinal data was necessary to address the linkage of chronic conditions with both disabled and nondisabled trajectories.

The NLTCS was conducted in 1982, 1984, 1994, 1999, and 2004 to address the health and health care utilization of older adults. The rotating panel design of the survey included adults age 65 and older at each wave, making the study well suited for the comparison of true cohorts over time. Originally, the NLTCS was designed to report on prevalence and trends in disability, so an emphasis was placed on collecting detailed information from those reporting disability of some kind. The NLTCS represents a large data source (total $N > 42,000$), because it follows true cohorts of older adults for up to 20 years, but rich information on socioeconomic assets, chronic conditions, social support, kin networks, and so forth, was collected only for those who reported some disability until 1994, when these variables were also collected for a healthy supplement.

The NLTCS's original sampling frame drew from Medicare recipients, and Medicare and Vital Statistics files could be linked to every study member extending back to the early 1980s (see Table 5.2). The original data included self-reports of chronic conditions and utilization, but only for individuals reporting disability. With access to the Medicare and Vital Statistics files, ICD-9 chronic condition codes have been recoded into prevalent conditions, such as heart disease and diabetes, for both functional and disabled individuals.

This supplementation endeavor was difficult owing to changes in Medicare reimbursement over the last three decades and other potential sources of bias. Nonetheless, the Medicare and Vital Statistics supplement allow the quantitative, multivariate investigation of how chronic conditions lead to processes of disability and mortality for all individuals in the sample. Self-reports of conditions can also be compared to Medicare ICD-9 condition codes to determine whether older adults give reliable reports of their diseases, or whether objective reports are preferred. Although the supplementation effort entailed data cleaning, programming support, and decision rules on the part of the principal

TABLE 5.2. National Long-Term Care Survey Health and Mortality Variables

Measures	Year/survey available (see table note)
Sociodemographic predictors	
• Age, gender, race	1982S–1999S
• Education, marital status, living alone	1982CC–1999CC
• Income/assets	1982C, 1984C, 1989C, 1989I, 1994C, 1994I, 1999C, 1999I
Chronic conditions	1982C, 1984C, 1989C, 1994C, 1999C
Rheumatism/arthritis, cancer, diabetes, obesity, arteriosclerosis, heart attack, hypertension, stroke, broken hip, Alzheimer's disease, dementia	Medicare inpatient, outpatient, physician, hospice, home health, skilled nursing facility (ICDM-9-CM), Physician/Part B 1991–1999 yearly
Functional impairment	
• Activities of daily living	1982S–1999S, 1982C–1999C, 1984I–1999I
• Instrumental activities of daily living	1982S–1999S, 1982C–1999C
Mortality	
Date of death	Vital statistics records date of death

Note. S, screener; CC, control card; C, community; I, institutional.

investigator, the data effort has been invaluable in checking self-reports against more objective administrative reports, and for generally supplementing nondisabled individuals' reports of chronic conditions.

Following Up an Existing Study

Sometimes, desired measures of key concepts are not available unless they are actually obtained from respondents, a limitation that may warrant a follow-up of participants in an existing archive. Like the recasting process, this task should be undertaken only when other strategies to maximize the fit between the research question and data have been explored unsuccessfully. As with any of the strategies discussed previously, investigators should consider the gains and costs of primary data collection.

The major challenges in a follow-up study include significant financial and time costs, the skills required in designing a new or supplemental survey instrument, the availability or accessibility of the respondents, and various issues concerning response rates. Of the discussed strategies to make use of existing data, this strategy is by far the most challenging, and generally entails the heaviest costs in terms of finances and personnel time. In particular, an investigator with no experience in measure and instrument design or interviewing is faced with retooling existing instruments and perhaps consulting with experts before undertaking interviews of existing participants. Depending on the scope and depth of the follow-up, a pilot project may be necessary to obtain the necessary funding or manpower for a full-scale follow-up.

Two projects make a case for follow-ups that have the potential to address pertinent and timely research questions. Both are considered "catch-up" studies, in which members are reinterviewed many years after the original data collections took place (Kessler & Greenberg, 1981). Although these studies should be assessed for sources of bias (Henry, Moffitt, Caspi, Langley, & Silva, 1994; Janson, 1990), information obtained from them can uniquely address research questions on life course topics.

Life Histories of the Glueck Study Members

The Gluecks' *Unraveling Juvenile Delinquency* study (described earlier) was initiated in 1940, using a sample of 500 delinquent and 500 nondelinquent boys from the Boston area. Remember that the original study included two follow-up interviews of subjects at ages 25 and 32. In the early 1990s, Sampson and Laub supplemented these data with criminal records from both state and national sources, and death records that allowed them to capture offending behavior and health of the study members throughout adulthood and into later life. With data supplementation, Laub and Sampson (2003) could examine how life course trajectories of embeddedness and achievement (marriage, work) affected the criminal activity, health, and mortality of study members up to the age of 70.

This supplementation provided an already rich and influential data archive with extended capabilities to study trajectories of delinquency and offending throughout the entire life course. However, the investigators believed that quantitative data alone were not sufficient to answer questions regarding the lives of the study members. Thus, they set out to locate a subsample of the Gluecks' study men who were still living in the early 1990s to obtain their detailed life histories. The original goal was to select five individuals from each of the eight distinct trajectories of offending they observed at various life stages, resulting in 40 interviews. However, the final sample size of the life history interviews includes 12 additional men (Laub & Sampson, 2003).

Starting with a sampling frame of 500 individuals representing different experiences, Laub and Sampson (2003) sought to find the men, now about 70 years old, if alive. Roughly half of these men had died, and some of the original cases had data missing from the archive. Of the possible cases, the researchers were able to locate 79%. Of these, they selected 141 men who were most likely to be contacted and interviewed. Roughly one-third of these participated in the life history follow-up.

Laub and Sampson (2003) were interested in the timing and details of the men's various life stages, especially because certain offenders changed their behavior in early or later adulthood. Using a life history calendar as a study instrument, they asked study members about multiple domains of life, education, work, military service, marriage and family relationships, social activities, neighborhood characteristics, alcohol and drug use, and criminal behavior. They were specifically interested in the men's subjective views about the progression of their own lives and their evaluation of certain turning points (e.g., marriage) with respect to later criminal behavior. In this way, the project could study human agency in a way not possible with the available data. Although the men were asked to provide retrospective data stretching far into the past, the investigators believed that these life histories would provide important insight into histories of offending or desistence coupled with the quantitative data they had already obtained.

The life histories collected by Laub and Sampson replicated findings of heterogeneity displayed earlier in quantitative work and extended their knowledge of adult development and criminal offending over the life course (Laub et al., 1998). They found that more than half of the variation in the life history sample was explained by within- rather than between-individual differences. They also found that although childhood factors had a lasting role in predicting crime throughout the life course, adult experiences such as marriage, employment, or military service could serve as turning points for individuals predisposed to crime by childhood risk factors. Thus, the importance of certain transitions in adulthood was highlighted in changing the path of delinquent or criminal offenders across the life course (Laub & Sampson, 2003).

Also among their overall findings the researchers found an impact of historical, generational, and contextual factors (lives in time and place) that mirror Elder's findings from the Terman and Berkeley–Oakland studies. For example, living through the Great Depression stood out as a unique and notable factor in men's lives. In addition, service in World War II opened up "new horizons" for the men and served as a turning point in their lives (Laub & Sampson, 2003; Sampson & Laub, 1996).

Although the supplementation of criminal and death records undertaken by these authors led to significant findings on life course patterns and processes of criminal careers, the follow-up study allowed the authors to achieve a richness of information not available in the original study or the linked records. In this way, they were able to establish the importance of time and place for the men in the study, and to address important themes in theories of criminal offending.

Mothers and Daughters: The Cornell Women's Roles Study

Our second example uses a follow-up study of women's changing roles in the second half of the 20th century. In 1979, Donna Dempster-McClain and Phyllis Moen initiated the Women's Roles and Well-Being Project after a discussion with one of the original coauthors, Robin M. Williams of Cornell University. On this topic, Williams shared with the two younger scholars a "feminine independence scale" that he and colleagues had created for an archived cross-sectional study on women's roles in 1956. After an inventory of the archive, Dempster-McClain (then a graduate student) and Moen (an assistant professor) discovered that they had a rich data source on their hands. This led to a follow-up study to answer new questions on how women's roles had changed since 1956, and how the roles of women's daughters compared to their own.

Williams, along with original coinvestigator John Dean, designed and collected the original "Women's Roles" study with funds from the National Institute of Mental Health (Dean & Williams, 1956). The sample comprised 521 women who were wives and mothers in their 20s–50s in a midsized upstate New York community. The data included relevant measures of work, family, role involvement, autonomy, and attitudes about women's gender roles in general. Important control variables were included as well to make these data even more valuable, including work and status information, and health of the women. Unfortunately, the data were never fully utilized and lay dormant in the form of punch cards and original data analysis tables until Dempster-McClain and Moen (1977) undertook the challenge of following up a select portion of the sample in 1979. In this case, the original sampling frame was intact, which means that the original names, addresses, and telephone numbers of all the women participating in the survey were still available.

The largest challenge, of course, was to determine whether any of the original survey respondents could even be tracked in a follow-up, because the data were over 30 years old when tracking efforts began in 1980. The research team first used four "passive" tracking techniques to find respondents: searching the telephone directory, historical society obituary records, city directories, and checking on the nature of the neighborhoods originally sampled. These techniques, requiring little staff time and training, resulted in the location of more than half of the original respondents (280 women living in the community, 24 deceased).

With this encouragement, the investigators launched a more extensive tracking initiative and underwent training themselves to follow respondents systematically. They were also successful in obtaining research funds for a follow-up survey (Moen, Dempster-McClain, & Williams, 1989, 1992). In the research proposal to fund the study, the investigators limited the follow-up to only those women in the 1956 survey who had had children ($N = 427$). The process of tracking the original women spanned a time frame of 6 years and involved creative strategies, including returning to the field to recruit informants (neighbors, friends) and visiting churches and clubs in the sampled neighborhoods to gain information on the respondents.

Through these techniques and perseverance, the investigators ultimately found over 95% of the original sample of interest. Of these 408 women, 326 were located and 82 were identified as deceased. Of the located women, only 3% refused to participate in the follow-up. The nature of the follow-up study was such that relevant measures in the original project (i.e., role involvement) could be used to measure changes in the lives of women over the 30-year period. In addition, retrospective questions were included in the 1986 survey to form life histories of work and family careers. With these data, the researchers found that they could address topics of role involvement and women's well-being across the life course. For example, they found that occupying multiple roles in 1956 had a positive effect on women's subsequent health 30 years later, after they controlled for health status in 1956 (Moen et al., 1992).

Because the objective of the follow-up partially involved intergenerational differences between mothers and daughters, the analysis focused on comparing the sex roles of mothers from the original survey with those of their adult daughters (Moen, Erickson, & Dempster-McClain, 1997). They found that an intergenerational transfer of gender role ideology occurred between mothers and daughters, but that women's changing roles during the historical period 1956–1988 led to greater congruence in mothers' and daughters' reports of role ideology (Moen et al., 1997).

Like Laub and Sampson's follow-up of men in the the Gluecks' study, the follow-up of the Women's Roles study enabled Moen and Dempster-McClain to examine life course change in experiences and roles for the original sample of women. However, intergenerational relationships were also central to the Elmira follow-up and facilitated measurement of intergenerational transfer of women's roles between mothers and their adult daughters. This type of richness and methodological design could not have been established with a strategy that did not involve contacting the original members of the study. Although more tedious, difficult, and time consuming than the other strategies discussed, the follow-up studies in these examples have provided a rich payoff in terms of understanding life course processes.

Conclusion

Over the past five decades, longitudinal data have become the standard for examining psychological, social, and biological processes in the life course. The full significance of this trend is noted by Butz and Torrey (2006) in their description of longitudinal surveys as the "Hubble telescope" of the social sciences, a frontier development. Both enable scientific observers to "look back in time and record the antecedents of current events and transitions" (p. 1898). The growth of these surveys is truly stunning. Little more than half a century ago, there were less than a dozen studies of this kind in the United States, and they were small in size and local rather than nationwide. Today these studies number in the thousands and include major national samples. A similar trend has appeared in Northern Europe and Canada.

Many of these longitudinal studies have outlived the research questions that motivated them, as noted in this chapter. The greater the longevity of the study and sample, the greater the distance between currently relevant questions and such data. To extend their usefulness, we have discussed three strategies (recasting, supplementation, and a follow-up survey) that maximize the fit between research question and longitudinal data archives.

Through recasting, we can transform a data source to address a new topic by reshaping the existing data. Though the Terman Study data were originally created to study intelligence and life outcomes of gifted children, these data were recast in a way that allowed a thorough examination of wartime mobilization in World War II and its subsequent life outcomes. Although a substantial amount of effort and planning went into the recasting effort, the payoff was significant, especially given the fact that no new data had to be collected. In addition, this effort led to even more research topics once the potential of the recasted data was realized.

Supplementation is another way to revitalize a data source to answer current research questions. The Gluecks' data provide another example of an existing data source that has far outlived its original purpose. The original data were meant to study the antecedents and dynamics of delinquency as adolescent boys aged into young adulthood.

The efforts of Sampson and Laub to supplement the data with crime and Vital Statistics records led to the ability to track criminal behavior over a large portion of the life course. As with the men in the Terman study, the payoff of these strategies was substantial, because the resulting supplemented data enabled researchers to follow delinquent and criminal activity across the life span.

Finally, although a follow-up design does require some data collection, the result of these efforts can produce truly unique and telling information. Dempster-McClain and Moen's creative techniques led them to contact a significant portion of the original Cornell Women's Roles Study, even after more than 30 years had elapsed. The result is an examination of the identity and roles of women during a historical time of transition in this country and the transmission of the women's beliefs to their own daughters.

The strategies we have discussed often entail substantial financial resources, a large amount of hard work, and a steep learning curve about one or more existing data archives. Especially for young researchers, it may be useful to collaborate with others who have differential experience and skills. Overall, this is an extraordinary time to embark on longitudinal studies, and we trust that the strategies we have outlined will make this a more efficient path to longitudinal research.

Acknowledgments

Miles G. Taylor was supported by the National Institute on Aging (Grant Nos. F32AG026926 and K99AG030471).

PART II

MEASURING LIFE COURSE DYNAMICS

Eleven years ago at the time of our first book on *Methods of Life Course Research* (Giele & Elder, 1998b), some of the most prominent analytic techniques were event–history analysis and linear structure equation modeling to measure recursive effects of relationships between the individual's actions at time 1 and at time 2. Now the focus is not so much on specific events or transitions as on the way these elements are linked together into larger trajectories. With this change has come a new focus on how to classify and analyze trajectories, and a new family of methods for the classification of trajectories. These methods are variously termed growth curve analysis, latent class analysis, or latent growth curve analysis.

In his review of life course research since 2000, Mayer (2009) contrasts the earlier "analytic" strategies that measure the effects of discrete events and transitions with later "holistic" approaches that compare differences among entire trajectories. He sees the emerging interest in growth curve models as a way of bridging the analytic and holistic approaches. Growth curves are models of various types of trajectory. They also incorporate the causal factors that lead to one kind of trajectory or another. Mayer's observation is fascinating in light of the chapters on measurement in Part II of this book.

Chapter 6, "Cumulative Processes in the Life Course," by Angela M. O'Rand, provides a conceptual overview of the underlying logic that is common to a number of dynamic processes. She begins with an explication of the classic form of cumulative processes, which has been called the "Matthew effect," in reference to Jesus's saying that to those who have much, more will be given, and from those who have little, even that will be taken away. Efforts to measure cumulative advantage and disadvantage first gained prominence in the study of social inequality. The famous Blau–Duncan model of status attainment showed that unequal access to resources at an earlier stage in life led to better or poorer health, income, and education later on. O'Rand points out that the cumulative processes that stratify individuals into those who are better off or worse off are similar to the accumulation of daily hassles and tension in the stress process, which leads to better or worse physical and mental health. Important variables that determine the slope and level of accumulation are the time and sequence of exposure to favorable and unfavorable conditions, short or long duration, and continuity or discontinuity in the exposure.

Education turns out to be a pivotal factor in helping people to escape from early disadvantage. But for many, early disadvantage is a barrier to getting an education that will help them become upwardly mobile. O'Rand concludes with a consideration of some of the unanswered questions in the study of cumulative process, such as the challenges in identifying relevant causal variables, and the problem of unobserved differences among subjects. A particularly knotty and interesting question concerns identifying conditions that can lead to reversibility of a cumulative process compared with those that lead to path dependence (i.e., continuation in the same direction).

Chapter 7, "Life Transitions and Daily Stress Processes," by David M. Almeida and Jen D. Wong, illustrates very precisely how to measure accumulation of ordinary stress and its effects on individual happiness and well-being. The authors summarize research findings around a central thesis that life transitions require adaptations that inevitably produce positive or negative stress. They then develop a typology using the Elder–Giele four-factor schema to classify transitions related to time and place, social networks, sense of control (agency), and timing. They suggest that the interesting observation—that stress decreases over the life course—may be due to learning effective coping strategies. Another possibility is that losses connected with aging are expected and prepared for, whereas stress in young and middle-aged adults may be associated as much or more with positive events as with loss. Almeida and Wong use a daily diary method to record changes in stress over time. They then analyze the precursors and patterns of stress, using hierarchical linear modeling to chart the ways in which stress varies over time and between individuals, and where and when it is most likely to occur. These several methods for measuring stress and its impact can also be adapted for charting ups and downs in physical and mental health.

Chapter 8, "Conceptualizing and Measuring Trajectories," by Linda K. George, tackles the key methodological issues in analysis of dynamic processes over the life course. George calls trajectories the "premier tools for assessing the dynamics of change," and emphasizes that they refer to *intraindividual change.* A key purpose of trajectory analysis is to identify between-person characteristics that predict within-person patterns of stability and change. The mapping of trajectories can either be transition-based, by comparing sequences of transitions, or it can measure the increases or decreases in a given variable such as income or self-esteem. Especially helpful is George's discussion of the uses of latent growth curve analysis (LGCA) and hierarchical linear modeling (HLM), which is used by Almeida and Wong in Chapter 7 on stress accumulation, and latent class analysis (LCA), which is used by Doherty, Laub, and Sampson in Chapter 9 to generate trajectory solutions that account for the major patterns in criminal cases. George concludes with an instructive review of four different techniques of trajectory analysis in the life course field: qualitatively derived descriptions; investigator- and computer-generated trajectories; LCGA to identify single, dual, and triple trajectories; and LCA to find a classification that best fits the data.

Chapter 9, by Elaine Eggleston Doherty, John H. Laub, and Robert J. Sampson demonstrates the application of latent class analysis to construct "Group-Based Trajectories in Life Course Criminology." Using the growth mixture models that Nagin (2005) developed, they look for the patterns of experience within individuals that explain different patterns of offending over the life course. With the group-based trajectory method, Laub and Sampson (2003) had earlier demonstrated that not all cases fit into the two basic patterns of lifelong hardened criminal or adolescent delinquent. In this chapter the authors report connections between patterns of incarceration during adolescence and later trajectories of offending while "free." They have found five distinct trajectories—the Institutionally Raised, Hard Cons, Soft Cons, Latecomers, and Average Joes—that range from the earliest and most incarcerated offenders to those with the mildest pattern of offending and incarceration. These patterns of incarceration were linked to total offending while free. The Soft Con group had the best chance of avoiding further offending, and the Latecomers had the least chance. A steady but low level of incarceration during adolescence—the Soft Con trajectory—appears to produce the most positive outcomes, whereas later but high-level offending and incarceration is the most detrimental for future rehabilitation. The chapter concludes with a list of intriguing examples of trajectory analysis in other fields, ranging from the investigation of posttraumatic stress in Gulf War veterans to a comparison of women's employment patterns after childbirth, and pathways associated with low back pain and childhood obesity.

CHAPTER 6

Cumulative Processes in the Life Course

Angela M. O'Rand

Several research traditions in sociology have converged over the past 40 years to define what we currently consider to be the "life course framework"—an approach to studying lives over time that (in its broadest sense) adopts C. Wright Mills's conception of the intersection of biography and history, producing social heterogeneity and inequality. Social stratification and demography are among traditions that have influenced both the formation and development of the life course perspective, and have in turn been influenced by this progressive framework. More recently, medical sociology has adopted life course concepts and methods to understand the association between health disparities and mortality, and patterns of social inequality and social stress. These various traditions share an interest in cumulative processes over the life course that lead to inequalities in the well-being of populations over time.

The convergence in the topics of interest to scholars of inequality and the life course is understandable for several reasons. First, heterogeneity and inequality pervade the life course from birth until death and across the major interdependent life domains of family, education, work, and health. Unequal access to resources across individual life spans produces population-level inequalities in relative well-being that persist or accumulate over time. The idea of cumulative advantage (or disadvantage) powerfully expresses this central process that stratifies individual lives. The analytical appeal of this idea stems from its simplicity, falsifiability, and generativity. Its simplicity—like other provocative concepts, such as life cycle and heredity—stems from its parsimonious representation of complex phenomena. Its falsifiability—permitting the test of hypotheses regarding persistence or change in inequalities over time—is readily apparent. And, its capacity to generate competing hypotheses and new approaches to old questions spawns inquiries across a number of specialties and disciplines.

Second, the expansion and growing availability of panel data collected over extended periods of the life courses of several cohorts of the 20th century make the study of temporal processes of inequality more accessible to researchers. The growing availability of panel data, coupled with the improved (but not perfect) precision and standardization of the measurement of life course variables—including indicators of socioeconomic status, health status, and health behaviors—is permitting more rigorous comparisons of the results of different studies focused on similar questions. In addition, improved analytical methods for longitudinal data that adjust for data limitations, such as attrition, measurement error, missing values, selective mortality, and unobserved heterogeneity, are improving the processes of mapping and specifying cumulative processes.

This chapter reviews different conceptualizations and methods for studying these processes and considers the research challenges in this area. It begins with a brief review of several research traditions and their convergence, beginning in the early 1970s and continuing to the present. I take up the specific cross-fertilization of cumulative advantage and stress process theories for studying cumulative processes. The second major section of this chapter identifies major aspects of cumulative processes that can be examined with longitudinal data over phases of the life course, including the major mechanisms of selection, cumulative (or duration of) exposure, and persistence (or change), that appear to operate from childhood to old age. This survey reveals a diversity of concepts, methods, and results that, taken as a whole, have the paradoxical effect of both keeping this area of research in a formative stage and generating competing hypotheses and the application of new methodologies that signify a research frontier. The concluding section addresses the challenges faced in studying these processes, especially with respect to the construction of variables, attention to unobserved heterogeneity, and issues of causality.

One caveat regarding this review: Only a small sample of the enormous literature on these processes can possibly receive attention in this limited space. The literature since the early 1990s has exploded across specialties, and particularly in health-related research areas. The studies cited here are selected primarily because they illustrate different aspects of cumulative processes in the life course and apply different methods for their analysis.

Convergence of the Life Course Perspective, Status Attainment, and Social Gerontology

The core conceptual framework of the life course perspective was formed between the 1960s and early 1970s with the convergence of several research traditions, each with independent perspectives on the organization of social roles and statuses at different phases across the life span. Norman Ryder's (1965) classic study proposed a demographic basis of social change through the succession of cohorts who came of age under different historical conditions, leading to new kinds of lives and new institutional arrangements. Glen Elder's studies (e.g., 1974, 1975; Elder & Rockwell, 1979a) of adolescents and young adults coming of age under the specific conditions of the Great Depression and World War II identified the importance of life stage in the experience of history and of history in the formation of attitudes and temperaments, and in the patterns of later achievement of adult social roles. During the same period, Peter Blau and Otis D. Duncan's (1967) pathbreaking study of the importance of social origins and educational attainment for occupational status achievement among young men set the agenda for status attainment research that followed (e.g., Featherman & Hauser, 1978; Hauser & Featherman, 1977).

Social gerontology, another tradition that historically has focused on a much later phase of the life span, was energized by a new approach that sought to examine aging across the life span as a key process for understanding both individual lives within cohorts and social change across cohorts. The age stratification perspective championed by Matilda White Riley (1973) also set the groundwork for studying lives in time by calling for a framework that deemphasized age group–specific theories and promoted studies of lives across ages and life stages. Following her lead, researchers by the mid-1970s were applying status attainment models used earlier on younger samples only to mature samples to link earlier statuses to older statuses (e.g., Campbell & Henretta, 1980; Henretta & Campbell, 1976). By the 1990s, research in medical sociology, epidemiology, and delinquency both adopted and contributed to the developing life course perspective that links later life status to social origins and other earlier life exposures.

Theoretical Foundations for Studying Cumulative Processes

The convergence of these new approaches has matured as the life course framework. The "life course" is a lifelong manifold phenomenon of intertwining cumulative processes, in which earlier events and experiences are consequential for later events and experiences, and their management by individuals (Elder, Johnson, & Crosnoe, 2003). The key consequence of this complexity is the emergence, persistence, and widening or narrowing of inequality in different aspects of well-being— social, economic, physical, and psychological. The central puzzle for researchers is to identify the mechanisms that drive these processes from childhood (if not from the time of fertilization and *in utero*) to adulthood and old age to produce considerable heterogeneity in aging populations. No single mechanism has been identified. Rather, multiple, culmulative components appear to operate in different ways for different aspects of well-being. The major components are summarized below. However, the association of some of these concepts with alternative guiding theoretical frameworks for studying cumulative processes is discussed first.

Two middle-range theories are guiding the bulk of research on cumulative processes. The first is *cumulative advantage* (or *disadvantage*) *theory*, which provides the most frequently used vocabulary, if not the primary methodology, for researchers in this area. It is an extension of the status attainment model, traceable to Blau and Duncan (1967), that is now widely used across specialties to examine causal mechanisms of life course inequality over time (DiPrete & Eirich, 2006). And the second is the *stress process model*, developed by Leonard I. Pearlin and colleagues over nearly three decades (Pearlin, 1999; Pearlin, Menaghan, Lieberman, & Mullan, 1981; Pearlin, Schieman, Fazio, & Meersman, 2005).

Cumulative Advantage Theory

Cumulative advantage theory originated in Robert K. Merton's (1968) essay on the highly skewed distribution of publications and recognition among scientists. His argument, supported by early empirical investigations of inequalities in science (summarized in O'Rand, 2002), was that the reward system of science reflected a cumulative and widening inequality based on pervasive and inexorable social selection processes. Early small inequalities in productivity and recognition of achievement in science led to the growing concentration of resources among the few over time. The relevance of this theory for studying aging populations was proposed two decades later, when research started revealing patterns of increased heterogeneity and inequality, and growing health disparities within cohorts over time based on major social status attributes, such as race, gender, and class (Dannefer, 1987; Dannefer & Sell, 1988; O'Rand, 1996). To this point, it was commonly assumed that a leveling or narrowing of disparities occurred at older ages. However, as in the case of Merton's scientists, life course research revealed a "fanning out" of populations as they move through institutions across time, from family to education to labor market to nursing home, thereby suggesting a cumulative social process with sequential exposures to risks and rewards correlated with social origins (e.g., race and class) and systemically reproduced across social institutions (Dannefer, 2003).

However, as the discussion in the next section reveals, the patterns of cumulation observed by recent research provide a more complicated picture than the simple "rich get richer, poor get poorer" metaphor often ascribed to them. Some studies are identifying compensatory or pivotal mechanisms that slow or diminish negative cumulation processes (e.g., Ferraro & Kelley-Moore, 2003; Pampel & Rogers, 2004). Other studies find significant interactions of different cumulative trajectories, with different explanatory variables that generate diverse pathways of inequality. For example, factors other than its progression may influence the onset of a disease (e.g., Herd, Goesling, & House, 2007; Zimmer & House, 2003); educational attainment may be more important for the onset of disease, whereas income and/or health insurance coverage may be more important for the progression of disease. Finally, and no less importantly, "unmeasured heterogeneity" (or variables omitted from the analysis) may influence the results observed in potentially significant but unknown ways. Sample attrition through institutionalization or mortality or unmeasured indicators of illness in early life, hostile workplaces, hazardous neighborhood environments, poor schools, or the quality of diverse social relationships may contribute to observed cumulative patterns of well-being but typically are unmeasured (or cannot be measured) in surveys.

The modeling of cumulative advantage processes has depended on the application of diverse multiple regression–based methods (e.g., structural equation models; hierarchical linear models, including latent growth curve models; and latent class models and other mixture models) used widely in the social sciences but identified most strongly in their development with demography, social stratification and, now, the life course. These methods permit the specification of models that can deal with variable interactions, asymmetry of effects, and unmeasured heterogeneity, among other challenges.

A recent review of cumulative advantage research (DiPrete & Eirich, 2006) makes the case that the status attainment model (going back as early as Blau and Duncan, 1967) provides the basic tools for studying these cumulative processes of selection and exposure. The phenomenon of interest is inequality in the level and growth of an outcome variable (e.g., wages or health) that can be accommodated with the traditional status attainment model. This model measures and estimates the relationships among sequential statuses across the life course.

DiPrete and Eirich (2006) argue that two categories of cumulative advantage exist in the literature. The "*strict forms*" include exponential or contagious growth models that examine the impact of current (initial) differences (selection) in an outcome (e.g., wages) on differences in rates of growth or change in that outcome over time. Strict forms have right-skewed distributions in outcomes and, distinctively, reveal growing inequality in the outcome over time as a positive function of earlier levels of the outcome variable itself. A second strict form adds other explanatory variables besides the focal outcome (e.g., wages over time), such as race, education, employment, and so forth, to specify the effects of the accumulation of past events or patterns of "path dependence," which denotes a sequentially selective process whereby advantage or disadvantage in earlier life domains (e.g., childhood circumstances) condition later advantage–disadvantages in and across a range of sequential life course domains, such as education, work, family and health statuses across the life course. The path-dependent model implies that the impact of prior events increases across the life course.

"*Status attainment forms*" of cumulation are more widely applied in the literature of interest here and fall in two categories: The status-dependent form measures the effects of a fixed status (e.g., race, childhood poverty) in an additive framework, including other sequential explanatory variables to predict levels of an outcome (e.g., wages) or changes in levels of an outcome. According to DiPrete and Eirich (2006), one status attainment form, labeled the "status-dependent form," tracks the effects of cumulative exposure across the life course, as in the case of the cumulative disadvantage of being black over time within and across social domains. Dependence on status also reflects other aspects of social selection, captured by the enduring effects of childhood conditions well into adulthood, closely associated with path dependence in the previously discussed strict form category.

In the second status attainment form, labeled the "status resource form," a fixed status (e.g., race or childhood poverty) interacts with other explanatory variables (e.g., such as educational attainment) to estimate the extent to which explanatory variables behave differently across status groups. Hence, the interaction between race and education can specify the process whereby, all else being equal, blacks receive lower returns, from economic, personal, and health resources to years of cumulative education across their lives. Such information adds specificity (e.g., by race) and complexity (e.g., between races) to the social mechanisms of cumulation processes. These models, so described, permit the observation of selection, cumulative (duration of) exposure, and persistence or change as cumulative processes.

The Stress Process

Whereas the cumulative advantage framework is founded in social strat-ification research, the stress process framework is evolved from research on physical and mental health (Pearlin, 1999). It comprises several com-ponents: "stressors" (traumas, challenges, threats, hardships, debilita-tive conditions) that influence individuals' capacities to maintain nor-mal functioning; "stress proliferation" (the exposure to some [primary] stressors, such as economic hardship, that lead to other [secondary] stressors, such as illness); physical and psychological "health outcomes"; and "mediators" (economic, social or personal resources that can atten-uate or accentuate the effects of stressors) or "moderators" (statuses or resources that regulate the pattern of effects of stressors).

The cumulation of stress over time can be initiated by trauma or severe hardship or crisis at any time in the life course, or by repeated exposure to the same stressor (e.g., poverty) over an extended dura-tion or to a proliferation or cascade of stressors (poverty, poor health, trauma), especially in the absence of attenuating influences (Pearlin et al., 2005). Stressors can exhibit trajectories of persistence, of incline, or of decline that affect the onset and progression of outcomes such as depression or disability. As such, the stressor trajectories can influence the trajectories of outcomes. Like the cumulative disadvantage process, the stress process entails selection, extended duration of exposure, and growth or proliferation over time.

These two models of cumulative processes developed somewhat independently, but they now employ similar methodologies to reveal explanations for inequalities in all aspects of well-being in aging pop-ulations. The analytical tools are the same and, increasingly, the con-ceptual frameworks are effectively equivalent, linking early events and conditions to later events and conditions as multiple trajectories of the life course.

Cumulative Processes: Sequential Selection, Duration of Exposure, and Continuity

Cumulative processes can therefore be studied by the extent to which they are sequentially selective, involve cumulative or varying durations of exposure to favorable or unfavorable conditions, and are relatively per-sistent trajectories of advantage or disadvantage in salient life outcomes that are anchored in social origins. As such, social selection, cumulative exposure, and trajectories of continuity (persistence or change) are the major components of cumulative processes, and they are highly correlated over time. For predicting the effects of life course variables on cumulative trajectories for advantaged and disadvantaged groups, these processes require multiple observations over time and methods for identifying trajectories rather than point-in-time estimates.

Childhood Conditions

Selection processes contribute to cumulation by anchoring life course trajectories in initial conditions, with differential access to resources that in turn condition access to resources in subsequent social contexts, such as education, the workplace, marriage, and the health care system. This is the path-dependent status attainment process that has been revealed and continuously elaborated over five decades. Childhood conditions directly influence educational opportunities, and the timing and level of educational attainment. Economic adversity and family instability in childhood positively influence patterns of school leaving and negatively influence baccalaureate completion, which has persistent long-term influences on work stability and wage attainments (Bernhardt, Morris, Handcock, & Scott, 2001).

But the process of educational attainment, which is usually defined by a single variable measuring years of schooling, is complex and reveals in its complexity the dynamics of cumulation. Recent studies of school reentry patterns by adults reveal that although childhood origins tend to select students systematically into academic versus nonacademic tracks that are relatively impermeable and lead to interrupted educational careers among the most disadvantaged (Elman & O'Rand, 2007), adults are nevertheless reorganizing their lives to return to educational institutions well into the fifth decade of life. Analysis of longitudinal data from two waves of the National Survey of Families and Households reveals that those who return to complete baccalaureate degrees experience wage increases, but, following a pattern of cumulative advantage, those who complete these degrees earlier (i.e., who follow uninterrupted school schedules before entering the labor market) have significantly steeper wage trajectories (Elman & O'Rand, 2004). Selection processes operate to influence the timing of educational attainment, but the transition is not inexorable within cohorts, and educational reentry patterns reveal compensatory or discontinuous trajectories based on individual agency.

The longer-term outcomes of educational inequality in level and timing of attainment are apparent in levels of income inequality in middle-aged and retired populations. Race/ethnicity, educational attainment, and occupational history strongly determine components of income before and after retirement. However, Crystal and Waehrer (1996) found that both short-term and long-term factors influence retirement wealth and income. Five cohorts of older men were followed over a 15-year period in the National Survey of Older Men. Adverse life events in the short term served to derail earlier cumulative patterns for some men and illuminated volatile patterns of status maintenance and decline in aging populations. Health events, work dislocations, and family losses are stressors that mediate long-term cumulative processes, with effects as significant as those imposed by the long-term effects of childhood conditions and educational attainment.

Early life conditions affect long-term health outcomes as well (Hayward & Gorman, 2004), but highly disruptive, unexpected crises anytime in the life course also have consequences for health (Pearlin et al., 2005). Persistent exposure to poverty, beginning in childhood, constitutes what has been referred to as "a fundamental cause" of negative adult outcomes, including disease (Link & Phelan, 1995; Phelan, Link, Diez-Roux, Kawachi, & Lavin, 2004). Childhood conditions appear to have particularly formative and cumulative effects on long-term economic, social, psychological, and physical well-being (Luo & Waite, 2005; McLeod & Almazan, 2003). Childhood illness (Palloni 2006), childhood economic adversity (Hamil-Luker & O'Rand, 2007), and instability in family of origin (Elman & O'Rand, 2004) have resulted in lower educational attainment, disrupted work and family careers, lower socioeconomic achievement, early onset of illness, and early mortality in a path-dependent pattern strongly associated with these disadvantaged origins, whereas relative advantage in childhood with respect to health, economic security, and family stability has produced less disadvantaged, though more diffuse, outcomes.

A recent study of the persistent effects of childhood health and socioeconomic conditions is a good illustration of the operation of selection, cumulative exposure, and persistence (Haas, 2008). With longitudinal data from the Health and Retirement Study, the Haas study uses latent growth curve models to examine the baseline level and progression of functional limitations in a population in or near retirement. Latent growth curve models constitute a form of multilevel or mixture model analysis, which nests repeated measures of events or levels of economic status or health conditions (Level 1) within individuals (Level 2) over time. This method produces average trajectories of events and permits covariate estimates of these trajectories. This procedure corrects for biases in estimates due to clustering, thus providing correct standard errors, confidence intervals, and significance tests. Although these models have typically been used with interval- or ratio-level variables, they are readily applicable to binary data, such as those associated with health events and transitions (Guo & Zhao, 2000).

The study found that poor childhood health and adverse childhood conditions were related to baseline levels of functional limitations and higher rate of growth in functional limitations. Both childhood and adult factors influenced baseline levels, but only poor childhood health and socioeconomic conditions were associated with cumulative rates of change over time. As such, selection and cumulative exposure increase the initial levels of disease and their rates of increase after onset.

Other recent studies using multiple waves of the Health and Retirement Study, but applying latent trajectory models instead of growth curve models, found persistent effects of childhood adversity on trajectories of heart attack risk, particularly among women (Hamil-Luker & O'Rand, 2007; O'Rand & Hamil-Luker, 2005). Latent class models provide a disaggregated approach to trajectories, which assumes that heterogeneous patterns of repeated measures reflect a finite number of qualitatively distinct trajectories that represent latent classes in a population; that is, whereas growth curve models estimate the average trajectory of an outcome (e.g., wage growth or health decline) in a sample, latent class models reveal multiple latent trajectories within samples. Hence, patterned differences in age at onset and duration of diseases such as cancer (especially the more prevalent colon, breast, and prostate cancers), heart disease, and diabetes can be identified and the effects of different covariates estimated.

This method was applied in O'Rand and Hamil-Luker (2005) to uncover the latent classes of childhood health and socioeconomic status (SES) conditions that predicted trajectories of heart attack risk across six waves of the Health and Retirement Study. They identified three trajectories of heart attack risk within the sample: early high risk, increasing risk, and low risk. They found a persistent effect of childhood adversity on higher risks for heart attack even after adjusting for education, adult working and living conditions, social relationships, access to health care, and health behaviors. With respect to education, they found that introduction of the educational attainment variable actually amplified the effects of early childhood on heart attack risk. Using a related method (a nonparametric hierarchical model that incorporates latent trajectories as dependent variables), they also identified gender differences in trajectories of heart attack risk, which showed that women fall into only the increasing and low-risk trajectories, whereas men fall into the three trajectories defined earlier (Hamil-Luker & O'Rand, 2007). Women's increasing risks for heart attack were influenced directly by early childhood adversity, but men's high and increasing risks for heart attack were not. Workplace, social relationships, and health behavior variables were more important for men than for women in their placement into high and increasing heart attack trajectories. The analyses reveal strong selection and cumulative exposure effects for early child-hood adversity among women.

Caveat Regarding Biological Factors

The foregoing studies did not address potential biological factors that may emerge at birth or in early life and affect childhood and later adult health. The introduction of biological factors in the study of cumulation processes constitutes a promising frontier in life course research (McLeod & Almazan, 2003). Research projects are integrating social survey data with data on biological markers of health and DNA samples that should assist us in the long run in characterizing the dynamics among genes, environments, and behaviors across the life course (Shanahan, Hofer, & Shanahan, 2003). Progress in this area will probably assist in determining which biological differences matter for human development, vitality, and longevity. At this moment, these factors are potential sources of unmeasured heterogeneity, with possibly latent effects on behavior and development.

At least three key aspects of cumulative processes will benefit from these new data. One most certainly will include the sources of childhood illnesses and developmental trajectories (including cognitive resources and development that may have implications for later cognitive decline) that expose children to early stressors that may have long-term implications for adult achievement and health. The second area is stress research. The stress process is ultimately predicated on the assumption that the neuroendocrine system directly interacts with individuals' responses to and management of stressors. The third area focuses on sex differences in trajectories of physical and mental health, and in the interdependent physiological and social processes that account for them. Sex differences pervade cumulation processes and span the life course from childhood health to old-age frailty.

Race

These cumulative processes have been observed in a similar fashion in studies of black–white differences in health and mortality outcomes because of the high negative correlation between race and class; the life-long disadvantage and discrimination experienced by blacks in the educational, workplace, and health care sectors; and the higher levels and trajectories of morbidity and mortality among blacks (Shuey & Willson, 2008; Williams, Lavizzo-Mourey, & Warren, 1994). Some inconsistent findings have challenged the cumulative argument by observing a leveling or even a reversal ("crossover") in the black–white health gap, specifically among selected health conditions, such as disability. But corrections for selective mortality and sample attrition, and other sources of selectivity and unmeasured heterogeneity, have provided stronger support for the cumulative disadvantage argument for blacks (e.g., Kelley-Moore & Ferraro, 2004; Shuey & Willson, 2008).

An early hypothesis about the mechanism producing this racial gap was that blacks, especially those living in low-income neighborhoods, experience worsening health between childhood and young adulthood, with long-term implications for their own health and that of their children. The "weathering hypothesis" (Geronimus, 1996) suggests that the prevalence of early illness compromises the effective response of afflicted individuals to later exposures to illness, disability, or other stressors, and makes these populations vulnerable to early onset and increased progression of disease.

A recent study tests this hypothesis with a growth curve in a random-onset model to assess the black–white disability gap (Taylor, 2008). The dependent variable (disability level measured as a summary variable of activities of daily living and instrumental activities of daily living) was split into two outcome variables: first, a dichotomous indicator of disability onset at each wave, and second, a continuous variable measuring level of disability. In two bivariate models predicting the effects of age and race on disability trajectories, the traditional growth curve model revealed a divergence by race over time, with blacks demonstrating a more accelerated decline, but the growth curve with a random onset model revealed that the black–white difference was actually determined by the timing of the onset of disability and not by the intercept or the slope of the disability level trajectory. Hence, timing (early onset) was conditioned by selection and cumulative exposure.

Education

The positive correlations among educational attainment, SES, and health and mortality in adulthood have been even more widely reported over a longer period than those between childhood conditions and adult economic and health outcomes (e.g., Elo & Preston, 1996; Mirowsky & Ross, 2003). The predominant explanation for these observations is that human capital accumulation through schooling mediates the effects of social origins. The fundamental argument is that level of education is an achieved status that serves as a proxy for unmeasured factors, such as substantive learning, socialization, and more positive personal outlooks and attitudes toward the management of life course challenges and risks. And the argument is supported by some observations that marginal returns from each additional year of schooling are higher among the most disadvantaged populations (Mirowsky & Ross, 2003). Accordingly, such asymmetrical returns over time should reduce the disparities in economic, social, and personal resources observed in early life and compensate for adverse social origins.

With respect to health outcomes, education is positively related to better health and mortality at later rather than earlier ages, though House, Lantz, and Herd (2005) argue that education's effects are strongest in predicting the onset of disease, whereas other SES factors, such as income or health insurance, influence the course of disease. These and other mixed findings across studies suggest that educational attainment may reproduce (and perhaps amplify) the effects of childhood inequalities under some conditions (or for some status groups based on gender and/or race; see earlier discussion of O'Rand & Hamil-Luker, 2005) and mediate their effects for others.

Education, then, is a pivotal and multidirectional factor in cumulation processes; it both reproduces childhood inequalities and provides a means for escaping previous disadvantage. The mechanisms of its effects may include the unmeasured factors proposed by Mirowsky and Ross (2003). But other unmeasured selective factors, such as school quality, curriculum track, competing role demands, and other unknown factors that can perhaps better explain the ameliorative, compensatory or exacerbating effects of schooling, may be operating as well to affect health trajectories.

Adult Income and Poverty Status

The research reviewed earlier suggests that educational attainment and adult household income affect different components of trajectories of health and illness in later life. The central argument is that an adult income trajectories and its proximate correlates may influence the trajectories of subsequent inequalities in health rather than their onset. Other studies that focus on analyses of income and poverty trajectories in adulthood provide mixed support for these arguments that trajectories of illness in mid- to late life are sustained mainly by persistent (duration-dependent) patterns of low income (Willson, Shuey, & Elder, 2007) and poverty in adulthood (McDonough & Berglund, 2003) rather than initial inequalities.

Willson et al. (2007) addressed this inconsistency using the Panel Study of Income Dynamics (PSID) to examine these relationships, and they found conditional support for both path-dependent (educational effects) and duration-dependent (cumulative income effects) processes of inequality in trajectories of self-reported health. They found that the average overtime change in income is associated with a slow process of cumulative advantage–disadvantage that leads to sizable disparities in health. These disparities appear between advantaged and disadvantaged trajectories: Income trajectories of advantage across adulthood yield gradual rates of health decline, whereas long-term income trajectories of disadvantage yield steeper rates of health decline. These findings support the original Mertonian hypothesis that within a cohort, small, early inequalities cumulate into large inequalities at a later time in life. This study also confirms the earlier finding by Lynch (2003) that the overtime attrition of individuals of lower SES from longitudinal studies, such as the PSID, whether due to mortality or other reasons, can lead to underestimates of the effects of earlier disadvantage on health in studies that do not account for selective mortality or survey attrition.

An earlier study using the same data set (the PSID) examined poverty histories instead of average income trajectories. McDonough and Berglund (2003) observed also that health deteriorates over time, and that earlier and sustained experiences of poverty increase both the onset and persistence of health decline. Increasing incomes in adulthood improve self-rated health, but they do not attenuate the effects of earlier poverty on health.

Empirical Generalizations: Are Cumulative Processes Path-Dependent or Reversible?

One major generalization emerges from the literature sampled here: Cumulative processes work in a variety of ways to produce path-dependent patterns of inequality. Path dependence emerges as a result of the (1) timing of relative advantage or disadvantage, (2) sequential contingency of statuses with age, and (3) duration of exposure over the life span to advantaged or disadvantaged conditions. First, the *timing* of advantage or adversity is important. The repeatedly observed selective or anchoring effects of childhood health and SES provide evidence for path dependence. Similarly, the achievement of higher educational (postsecondary) status early in young adulthood also has long-term effects on later well-being. Across studies, the enduring net effects of these variables (after researchers control for other intervening factors) point to childhood and adolescent exposures and experiences as formative and as having persistent effects. The enduring effects of early timing may reflect both manifest (e.g., early poverty) and latent (e.g., biological factors or the proximate influences of early poverty on other, unmeasured early life conditions such as nutrition and health) aspects of social origins. As such, social origins are filtered through other social institutions that reinforce or even amplify, rather than attenuate, their effects.

Second, path dependence is evident in *sequentially contingent* relationships between statuses over the life course. Sequential contingency identifies chains of effects over the life course, which (after controlling for social origins) reveal trajectories linking different life course statuses across adulthood. Earlier statuses in a particular domain, such as education, are influential on statuses in subsequent life domains, such as work, which in turn influence old-age disparities in income and health.

Third, *duration of exposure* to advantageous or disadvantageous opportunity structures is also a principal mechanism of path dependence. The persistent exposure to a disadvantageous condition or status exerts a kind of social gravity that produces path dependence. The persistent effect of race on all aspects of population inequality in the United States is an example of the impact of duration of exposure. Other examples include duration of exposure to poverty, underemployment, poor health, and hazardous environmental conditions.

Potential for Reversibility of Cumulative Processes

I have demonstrated that path dependence denotes patterns of continuity or persistence. However, cumulative processes are reversible under selected conditions, as revealed by some of the studies cited earlier. McLeod and Almazan (2003) suggest that at least two other life course models accompany the (linear) path-dependent one, in which early life conditions have selective direct effects on later statuses or persistent indirect effects unmediated by intervening events and statuses. One model views the connection among childhood conditions, education, and later adult statuses as stochastic. Chains of experiences over the life course can have multidirectional, as well as path-dependent, potentials. In this process, positive or negative circumstances, and major and unexpected shifts in life conditions or personal aspirations, can potentiate discontinuities, whereas disadvantaged origins can be overcome, or the protective effects of advantaged origins can be eclipsed.

Following this logic, at least three kinds of experience can precipitate a downturn or an upturn of fortunes. Life course *events*, such as divorce or marriage, job loss, and occupational mobility, can bring either significant adversity or opportunity. Experience in *pivotal institutions,* such as schools or the military, can reproduce or diminish inequalities. And, more generally, *changing life conditions* may enable individual choices that introduce discontinuities that affect long-term trajectories by compensating for disadvantage (e.g., returning to school) or exacerbating disadvantage (e.g., the onset of a severe illness), or derailing advantaged trajectories (e.g., through divorce, unexpected job loss in an economic downturn).

In the second model identified by McLeod and Almazan (2003), which is more aptly defined as "personalogical," individuals are active in selecting and constructing their environments to support their needs and predispositions. These alternative models allow for consideration of the impact of chance and agency in the life course, following Glen Elder's model of life course dynamics (Elder et al., 2003). One body of research that has grown in recent years is well-suited to considerations of agency. It examines the life course conditions and effects of health behaviors on mortality and health disparities in later life. Health behaviors, such as smoking, drinking, and obesity—to the extent that they are not largely or exclusively determined by biological factors—are more likely than social origins or other structural opportunities to be matters of choice at different points in the life course. Information about the hazards of these behaviors is widely available to all SES groups, yet the association of these behaviors (and of changes in these behaviors) with social inequality provides a strategic site for examining path-dependent versus reversible cumulation processes. Recent studies in this area have proposed hypotheses that challenge strict path-dependent models of cumulation. Whereas long-term socioeconomic conditions may better represent fundamental underlying causes of life course inequalities, unhealthy lifestyle choices may serve as independent and potentially deflecting influences on health and mortality (Pampel & Rogers, 2004).

For example, the case of obesity or significant weight gain as a cumulative phenomenon is receiving increased attention in this regard. Well-documented trends reveal that levels of obesity in the U.S. adult population are reaching approximately 20–25% on average. Some subgroups of the population, especially those with disadvantaged and minority statuses, appear to have higher rates of overweight and obesity. A recent Alameda County study that tracked body weight trajectories over 34 years, beginning in 1965, found that all study subjects gained weight, but that the largest gains were among African American women who also displayed disadvantaged trajectories of SES, including cumulative measures of disadvantage in childhood, education, occupation, and income socioeconomic position over the period (Baltrus, Lynch, Everson-Rose, Raghunathan, & Kaplan, 2005). The study acknowledged that potential problems associated with selective survival and attrition, as well as unmeasured biological vulnerability to obesity, were limitations. However, the trends in early onset and persistent obesity are spreading across socioeconomic groups, and in spite of the cumulative disadvantage of African American women, the changes in diet and exercise behaviors within the population as a whole raise questions regarding selective perceptions and lifestyle choices.

Using a cumulative advantage framework, Ferraro and Kelley-Moore (2003) focused on the processes whereby trajectories of obesity can be modified by eliminating the health risk factor (through weight loss) or by compensating for it with countervailing practices (e.g., regular exercise) to diminish long-term disability outcomes. Interventions such as regular exercise raise the prospect that some cumulation processes are reversible, modifiable, or discontinuous. Ferraro and Kelley-Moore followed a national sample of adults over 20 years to estimate the effects of patterns of obesity on disability. They found that not only does obesity in early life increase levels of disability in later life, but also that regular exercise attenuates these effects. They argue that because obesity is a mediating variable between SES and later health outcomes, it provides some information about the cumulative disadvantage process—possibly following a stress proliferation model of cumulation in which persistent disadvantage leads to secondary stressors, such as overeating and not regularly exercising.

Studies of associations among SES, health, and other behaviors raise similar questions about the inevitability and extent of persistent cumulation processes. Smoking and excessive drinking are two of these behaviors that also are concentrated in disadvantaged populations. Pampel and Rogers (2004) tested competing theories of cumulative advantage in the effect of lifestyle choices on morbidity (a scale including activity limitations, disability days, and chronic conditions), self-rated health, and mortality in the 1990 U.S. National Health Interview Survey. They questioned whether unhealthy behaviors, such as smoking, drinking, and excessive weight gain, and lower SES influence health and mortality following an additive or multiplicative framework; that is, they asked whether lower SES and risky health behaviors contribute independently to poor health and death, or whether lower-status groups are more vulnerable in these outcomes to the harm inflicted by these behaviors. They divided socioeconomic factors into ascribed (age, gender, race/ethnicity) and achieved (education, occupational status, family income) statuses and observed different cumulative processes. Ascribed statuses (gender and race/ethnicity) and smoking have additive effects on mortality, whereas achieved status (occupational status and family income) and smoking have multiplicative effects on self-rated health and morbidity: Higher achieved status reduces the harmful effects of smoking on health. This suggests that resources and lifestyles do not always interact to affect health outcomes (in this study, mortality), but that "one disadvantage increases the harm of another disadvantage" (Pampel & Rogers, 2004, p. 316) for other health outcomes. The observation of different patterns for ascribed and achieved statuses, respectively, was not discussed in detail by the researchers. But, as in the previous study, it may also be interpretable by a stress proliferation model, in which cumulative exposure to lower relative positions in education, occupation, and income exposes individuals to a trajectory of stressors that generates or sustains risky behaviors that compound the effects of disadvantage on poor health.

Random Factors in Cumulative Processes

To some degree, the factors that precipitate loss or gain of advantage occur at random, and touch some individuals and not others as a result of chance. Who is affected can vary depending on the specific process, such as recessions leading to job loss or health crises in the family that precipitate income loss. These factors can have asymmetrical effects on the direction of cumulation (divorce can increase a woman's risk of poverty but motivate her commitment to the labor market; threat of job loss can increase not only stress but also investment in human capital through continued education).

Hence, turning points in lives can occur across the life course as a result of random structural opportunities, chance events, and human agency (Elder & Conger, 2000). Bad economic times can change lives, but in different directions—toward fractured families and wealth dissolution, or toward new resolve for solidarity and well-being. Similarly, higher educational attainment is strongly influenced by social origins. But increasing proportions of adults return to educational institutions not only to compensate for earlier disadvantages but also to adapt to proximate economic downturns that threaten or eventuate in actual job loss (Elman & O'Rand, 1998, 2002). Finally, increased exposure to information regarding the importance of smoking and diet to longevity and health or the unexpected onset of disease can motivate some people to adopt differential health behaviors that become turning points toward better health (Pampel & Rogers, 2004). The incidence and accumulation of such structural conditions for individuals motivate diverse individual actions for change in life conditions that often deviate from prescribed or predicted trajectories.

Advances and Challenges to Studying Cumulative Processes

The study of cumulative processes has been facilitated by the introduction of longitudinal designs for data collection and analysis that permit the tracking of lives over time using panels or pooled cross sections. The 1960s initiated multiple efforts in this regard. By the turn of the millennium, numerous data sets have made it possible to examine trajectories of inequality within and across cohorts over multiple decades. These data-collection strategies have been accompanied by the continuous development of analytical methods that are increasingly sensitive to the time-varying elements of social lives, and to the pervasive selective and cumulative exposure processes that sort subgroups of the study populations into relatively persistent economic and health trajectories over subjects' lives.

However, Lieberson (1985) and Winship and Morgan (1999) warn that social processes are intrinsically selective and generate differentiation within, as well as between, subgroups. Hence, more sources of heterogeneity probably exist than are predicted by theory or group differences, or are measured with existing methods. This argument alerts us to consider alternative hypotheses and counterfactual tests of our favorite models to determine whether, and under which conditions, cumulative processes are path dependent or reversible.

Counterfactual arguments are applied far less often in life course research and have not been used in studies of cumulation processes, which are prone to identify and explain between-group differences. These arguments lead us to ask whether presumed explanatory variables actually account for the outcomes that interest us. An exemplary counterfactual argument would ask the following questions: If childhood poverty had not occurred, would dropping out of high school not have occurred? Or if childhood poverty had not occurred, would increased heart attack risk at midlife not have occurred? Strong indications from previous research suggest that patterns of cumulative disadvantage are more readily apparent as path-dependent processes; earlier disadvantages breed later disadvantages in relatively consistent ways.

A counterfactual argument would also question whether the causal sequence comprises distinct, nonoverlapping events with unique effects on the outcome or, instead, overlapping and related events that stem from another, unaccounted for cause. Similarly, patterns of cumulative advantage, which appear less path dependent and more stochastic, often demonstrate weaker associations between causal variables and outcomes. Earlier advantages may permit more choices (greater agency) and other unmeasured behaviors that produce heterogeneity in well-being. In this regard, Lieberson (1985) compares the relative opportunities of wealthier and poorer children to attend private schools, and argues that within-group differences in private school attendance are likely to be ignored and, hence, important sources of selectivity left unmeasured within groups. As such, cumulative processes, as conceptualized, may be prone to differentiate populations prematurely, to overstate causal relationships, and to overlook or fail to consider important sources of variation in the outcome of interest.

The selected set of studies reviewed in an earlier section of this chapter reveals a common interest in studying the origins and consequences of cumulative processes over the life course. However, diverse strategies, competing hypotheses, and inconsistent findings contribute to a diversity of concepts and strategies. They are representative of the exploding literature on cumulative processes that extends to studies of deviance and delinquency; to many different aspects of physical and mental health, and cause-specific mortality; and to different national contexts that variably moderate the levels of social inequality and health disparities via social policies.

The future of life course research in general and research on cumulative processes in particular depends on the continued cross-fertilization of theories and methods, and the rigorous search for competing hypotheses and counterfactual comparisons to challenge the premises underlying the generalizations enumerated earlier. Theories of cumulative advantage and disadvantages have a provocative appeal. They are simple and have generated many questions that occupy researchers in our disciplines. They are falsifiable, but not without considered and considerable efforts to test their fit with reality. We are dependent primarily on quasi-experimental design using large data sets with many variables; this does not protect us. But studies reviewed here, and many others in the recent literature, are making substantial efforts to characterize these processes and to identify their contingencies and causes.

CHAPTER 7

Life Transitions and Daily Stress Processes

David M. Almeida
Jen D. Wong

Life transitions and daily stress have been studied extensively, though much research has neglected their mutual relevance. We know from past studies that major life transitions often have been used as markers of social development for the young, and as influences that shape adult health and well-being (Baltes & Baltes, 1990; Chiriboga, 1989, 1997; Elder, George, & Shanahan, 1996). In the life course, transitions denote "changes in status that are discrete and bounded in duration" (George, 1993, p. 358). Transitions not only entail changes in status but, in accordance with life course theory, also lead to changes in individuals' internal states that can be abrupt and disruptive or empowering, thereby resulting in some degree of stress, either positive or negative. From a stress perspective, these transitions also may require individual adaptation that depletes psychological and physical resources or even genetic resources. It has long been known that transitions such as job loss, marital disruption, and death of a loved one adversely affect psychological and physical health (Brown & Harris, 1989; Dohrenwend & Dohrenwend, 1974; Holmes & Rahe, 1967; Hultsch & Plemons, 1979). However, the transition into a marriage or new job may increase well-being through acquisition of new social and human capital (Sampson & Laub, 2003). Because transitions are embedded in life course trajectories that influence the transition experience, these contextual environments must be considered in assessing how transitions affect stress and subsequent well-being. We contend that stress increases during periods of uncertainty and that transitions, by their very nature, challenge past routines and invite new adaptation. Furthermore, experience over the life course results in people learning how to handle transitions and developing successful adaptations that they can call on again.

In this chapter we present a perspective on life transitions and daily stress processes by describing a model that applies key life course principles to the study of life transitions and daily stress processes (Giele & Elder, 1998a). This perspective highlights variations and differences within and between individuals as they develop in multidimensional social–historical contexts (Elder, 2000; Elder, Johnson, & Crosnoe, 2003). We use principles of life course theory to understand group and individual differences in the effects of life transitions on daily stress across adulthood, within the context of changing and stable personal and environmental factors (e.g., social–demographic factors, personality, chronic stressors, health status). We believe that applying the key life course principles to the analysis of life transitions and daily stress processes will enhance our understanding of the ways people manage the changing circumstances of everyday life to maintain their well-being, both physical and emotional.

Life Events versus Daily Stressors

There are two prominent ways to think about the stress of life transitions. One approach focuses on the molar impact of the life changes—this is the life event tradition (e.g., Holmes & Rahe, 1967). The other approach takes a microscopic dynamic approach to stressors, with a focus on the accumulation of daily stress (Bolger, Davis, & Rafaeli, 2003; Pearlin, 1999). The two approaches are complementary. For example, the transition from marriage into divorce may represent a long-term disruption, as well as an immediate change not only in one's social and economic situations but also in health behaviors (Morrison & Ritualo, 2000; Peterson, 1996). Lorenz, Wickrama, Conger, and Elder (2006) found that divorced women report significantly higher levels of psychological distress than do married women in the years immediately after their divorce. Psychological distress, however, corresponded closely to the event of getting a divorce, rising quickly and then declining as the event receded into the past. Depending on the context, the transition from marriage to divorce may substantially increase the stress level as a whole, but a daily history of this change is likely to show periodic peaks and valleys as individuals adapt to this transition. Wheaton (1990) has highlighted the importance of context, showing that distress decreases when individuals terminate an unsuccessful, conflict-ridden marriage. For those who exit satisfying marriages, distress increases. What is missing in these analyses is how divorce and subsequent social and economic transformations lead to disruptions, challenges, and perhaps opportunities in daily stress processes that may in turn play an important role in psychological distress.

An emerging literature has shown that day-to-day stressors, such as spousal conflict and work deadlines, play an important part in health and emotional adjustment (Zautra, 2003). Daily stressors represent tangible, albeit minor, interruptions that tend to have a more proximal effect on well-being than major life transitions. In terms of their physiological and psychological effects, reports of life transitions may be associated with prolonged arousal, whereas reports of daily stressors may be associated with spikes in arousal or psychological distress during a particular day (Almeida, 2005). In addition, minor daily stressors exert their influence not only by having separate and immediate direct effects on emotional and physical functioning but also by piling up over a series of days to create persistent irritations, frustrations, and overloads that increase the risk of serious stress reactions such as anxiety and depression (Lazarus, 1999; Pearlin, Menaghan, Lieberman, & Mullan, 1981; Zautra, 2003).

Daily Stressors and Diary Designs

The understanding of daily stressors has benefited from the development of diary methods that obtain repeated measurements from individuals during their daily lives. Using short questionnaires or telephone interviews, individuals report on the stressors they experienced on that day, as well as their behaviors, physical symptoms, and emotional states during that same time frame. The number of days and the number of respondents vary greatly across studies. For example, the Vienna Diary Study followed 40 couples every night over the course of an entire year (Kirchler, Rodler, Holzl, & Meier, 2001), whereas the National Study of Daily Experiences assessed the daily lives of 1,483 adults across United States on eight consecutive evenings (Almeida, Wethington, & Kessler, 2002). Diary methods have a number of virtues (Bolger et al., 2003). By obtaining information about individuals' actual daily stressors over short-term intervals, they circumvent concerns about ecological validity that constrain findings from laboratory research. Furthermore, diary methods alleviate retrospective memory distortions that can occur in more traditional questionnaire and interview methods that require respondents to recall experiences over longer time frames.

Perhaps the most valuable feature of diary methods is the ability to assess within-person stressor reactivity. "Reactivity" is the likelihood that an individual will show emotional or physical reactions to daily stressors (Almeida, 2005). In this sense, "stressor reactivity" is not defined as the converse of well-being (i.e., negative affect or physical symptoms) but is operationalized as the within-person relationship between stressors and well-being. This represents a shift from assessing mean levels of stressor and well-being between individuals to charting the day-to-day fluctuations in stress and well-being within an individual. Stress is a process that occurs within the individual, and research designs need to reflect this process. For example, instead of asking whether individuals with high levels of work stress experience more distress than individuals with less stressful jobs, a researcher can ask whether a worker experiences more distress on days when he or she has too many deadlines (or is reprimanded) compared to days when their work has been free of stress. This within-person approach allows the researcher to rule out temporally stable personality and environmental variables as third-variable explanations for the relationship between stressors and well-being. In addition, the intensive longitudinal aspect of this design permits a temporal examination of how stressors are associated with changes in well-being from one day to the next. By establishing within-person associations over time between daily stressors and well-being, researchers can more precisely establish the short-term effects of concrete daily experiences (Bolger et al., 2003).

Figure 7.1 illustrates how we statistically model daily stressor reactivity. The predictor variables are aspects of stressful events that occur on a given day (e.g., number and type of stressors, average severity of stressors). The outcome variables are measures of well-being the respondent experienced on a given day (e.g., negative mood, physical symptoms). Figure 7.1 is based on daily diary data, using the day of the week as the unit of analysis but repeated data for different intervals of time (e.g., hours or weeks) that can be fit to the model. This model is a prospective reactivity model in that it uses time lags to test whether stressors at one point in time predict well-being at a subsequent point in time. The data can be analyzed using hierarchical linear modeling (HLM; Bryk & Raudenbush, 1992), a method that allows simultaneous estimation of both (1) a separate within-person model of regression slope and intercept for each respondent; and (2) a between-person model in which the within-person slopes and intercepts are treated as dependent variables regressed on person-level predictor variables. The simple form of an HLM can be conceived of as two separate models, one a within-person model (Level 1) and the other a between-person model (Level 2). This model can be expressed as

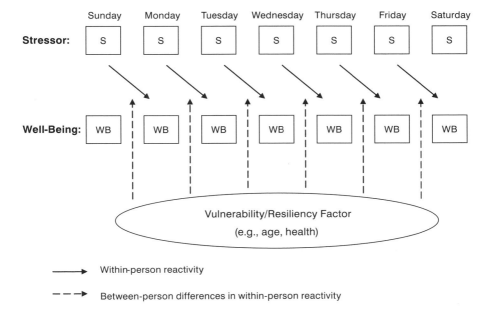

FIGURE 7.1. Prospective model of daily stressor reactivity.

Level 1: WELL-BEING$_{it}$ = a_{0i} + a_{1i}STRESSOR$_{it-1}$ + e_{it} (1)

where WELL-BEINGit is the reported well-being (i.e., psychological distress, physical symptoms) of person i on day t, STRESSOR$it - 1$ indicates whether a given daily stressor was experienced by person i on day $t - 1$ (coded 0, if no stressor occurred, and 1, if a stressor occurred), a_{0i} is the intercept indicating person i's level of well-being on days when STRESSOR = 0, a_{1i} is the reactivity slope indicating the emotional or physical reactivity of person i to the daily stressor, and e_{it} is the random component or error associated with well-being of person i on day t. To estimate average effects for the entire sample, the intercepts and slopes of the Level 1 within-person model become the outcomes for the Level 2 between-person equations as follows:

Level 2: a_{0i} = b_0 + d_i (2)

a_{1i} = b_1 + g_i (3)

Equation 2 shows that person i's average well-being score across the diary days (a_{0i}) is a function of the intercept for the entire sample—the grand mean of the sample (b_0)—and a random component or error (d_i). Likewise, Equation 3 shows that person i's reactivity slope (a_{1i}) is a function of the grand mean of the entire sample (b_1), and a random component or error (g_i). In this way, reactivity is operationalized as the slope determined by both the occurrence of daily stressors and well-being (a_{1i}).

Researchers can adapt this model to examine not only the occurrence of daily stressors but also other aspects of daily stressors, such as content of the stressor (e.g., overloads, interpersonal conflicts), dimension of threat (e.g., danger, loss), stressor severity, and primary appraisal of the stressors. Subsequent analyses can examine the extent to which reactivity to daily stressors differs as a function of social–demographic factors and personality. The following section describes a life course approach to studying predictors of daily stress processes.

Life Course Model of Life Transitions and Daily Stress

Advances in daily stress research have sought to identify sources of variation across stressors *within individuals*, as well as sources of variation in the stress process *between individuals*. In other words, certain stressors are unhealthier than other stressors, and certain individuals are more prone than other individuals to the effects of stress. Life transitions are likely to play important roles in both sources of variation. Recent improvements in the measurement of daily stressors and study design have allowed research to address (1) how different types of stressors, and personal meaning attached to these stressors, affect well-being; and (2) how life transitions account for group and individual differences in daily stressor processes.

Figure 7.2 applies a life course perspective to these two questions. The right side of Figure 7.2 represents daily stress processes that occur within the individual. Daily stress processes occur over relatively short time intervals, ranging from minutes to days and weeks. Our model of daily stress combines the environmental stress perspective that emphasizes objective characteristics of daily stressors and the psychological perspective that highlights individuals' subjective appraisal of stressors. Objective characteristics of the stressor include *frequency*, *content* classification (e.g., interpersonal tension, overload), a *focus* on who was involved in the stressor (e.g., family member, coworker), and the normative *severity* of the event (e.g., degree of unpleasantness, disruption for an average person). This model also takes into account individuals' perceptions and evaluations of the daily stressors. Individuals appraise stressors in terms of perceived severity of loss, threat, or challenge, as well as

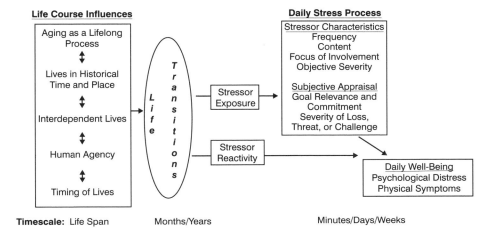

FIGURE 7.2. Life course perspective on life transitions, daily stress, and well-being.

disruption of daily goals and commitments. Both objective and subjective components of daily stressors are vital to daily well-being (Cohen, Kessler, & Gordon, 1997). The topic and severity of the stressor, as well as who is involved, may play an important role in how that stressor is appraised and, in turn, the distress it causes. Integrating these two components of the stress process allows researchers to ask whether certain types of stressors are associated differentially with varying components of well-being and the extent to which certain daily stressors elicit different appraisal processes and, hence, different well-being responses.

The middle of Figure 7.2 shows how life transitions influence daily stress processes. Life transitions occur over longer timescales than do daily stress processes, but they still play an important role in daily well-being. We contend that major life transitions affect daily well-being by increasing exposure and reactivity to daily stressors. "Exposure" is the likelihood that an individual will experience a daily stressor based on combinations of life course factors. Experiencing stressors is not simply a matter of chance or bad luck; rather, differences in stressor exposure more often emerge from individual social–demographic, psychosocial, and situational factors (Pearlin, 1999; Wheaton, 1999).

The stressor exposure path in Figure 7.2 illustrates that daily stress exposure processes may be precipitated by life transitions. It is during periods of uncertainty that stress tends to be higher, and transitions, by their very nature, challenge past routine and invite new adaptations. These transitions may entail older children leaving home (e.g., Lowenthal & Chiriboga, 1972), career transitions (e.g., Moen, 2003), and the renegotiation of family relationships (e.g., Blatter & Jacobsen, 1993). Life transitions often involve a transformation of multiple domains of responsibilities, such as when work responsibilities and caretaking are combined for aging parents and children. Normal and expectable life transitions do lead to changes in self-concepts and identities; however, they do not necessarily produce crises (Neugarten, 1979). Role changes that are unanticipated and unrehearsed are likely to expose individuals to unique daily stressors and require them to elect strategies for a successful adaptation. These stressors may mediate and specify the effects of life transitions on daily well-being. "Mediation" may occur when a life transition leads to increased day-to-day stressors that in turn add to the overall effect of life transitions on well-being. This process was illustrated by Rowlison and Felner (1988), who view major life events as transitional markers that often disrupt established daily activities, formerly shared responsibilities, and day-to-day social relations, thereby increasing the risk of psychological distress.

Life transitions also may play an important role in daily stressor reactivity, as depicted in Figure 7.2. Because resources of individuals and their environments (e.g., education, income, chronic stressors) limit or enhance the possibilities and choices for coping with daily experiences (Lazarus, 1999), reactivity to stressors is likely to differ across people, as well as across situations. The stressor reactivity path in Figure 7.2 illustrates that life transitions modify reactivity to daily stressors. The emotional and physical impact of minor day-to-day stressors may be magnified in the context of a major life transition either by representing the proverbial straw that broke the camel's back (e.g., an objectively small, but insurmountable, financial difficulty caused by a breakdown of the family's only car in the wake of the chief breadwinner's job loss) or by taking on new meaning in the context of a matching event that makes the minor event seem much more important than it would be to the average person (e.g., a minor disagreement with a coworker coinciding with a conflict-ridden marital breakup; Brown & Harris, 1978).

Finally, the left side of Figure 7.2 indicates that the effects of life transitions on daily stress processes are greatly shaped by life course influences. Life transitions may bring about disruptions of established roles and status that may be stressful and lead to distress in other areas of individuals' lives (Pearlin, Schieman, Fazio, & Meersman, 2005). However, the effects of life transitions on psychological and physical well-being depend on temporal and social characteristics of the individuals and their environment. Thus, each key principle of the life course perspective has important implications for the study of daily stress processes via exposure and reactivity to daily stressors, as depicted on the left side of Figure 7.2.

Life Course Influences on Daily Stress Processes

The following subsections describe how each of the key life course principles can be directly applied to the study of daily stress processes. We then provide an integrated example of a life course perspective on life transitions and daily stress processes by presenting recent studies on how the timing of retirement affects daily stress and well-being. Our examples come from the National Study of Daily Experiences (NSDE), a telephone diary study of a U.S. national sample of 1,483 adults ranging in age from 25 to 74 years. Interviews occurred over eight consecutive nights, resulting in 11,578 days of information.

The NSDE is well suited to examine daily stress from a life course perspective for a number of reasons. First, previous diary studies of daily stressors have relied on small and often unrepresentative samples, with restricted age ranges that limit the generalizability of findings. In contrast, the NSDE analyzes data from a national sample of adults who are a representative subsample of a general population survey, Midlife in the United States (MIDUS). Second, previous studies of group and individual differences in exposure and reactivity to daily stressors typically have examined only one source of variability, such as age, to the exclusion of others. The NSDE utilizes data collected in the larger MIDUS survey on a wide array of psychosocial and social–demographic characteristics of respondents to study the determinants of exposure and reactivity to daily stressors. Third, previous studies typically have relied on self-administered checklists of daily stressors that only assess the occurrence of a stressor. This study used a semistructured telephone interview instrument that measures several aspects of daily stressors, including objective stressor characteristics (e.g., type) and subjective stressor appraisals (e.g., perceived severity). Finally, the NSDE recently has obtained a second wave of information approximately 10 years after the original data collection. In the final section of this chapter, we use these longitudinal data to examine how the timing of a specific major life role transition, retirement, predicts daily stress processes.

Aging as a Lifelong Process

An overarching principle of the life course perspective is that human development is a lifelong process that must be examined across time (Elder et al., 2003). A primary focus of our research has been on adult development and daily stressors. It is well documented that younger adults report greater psychological distress than their older counterparts (Gurin, Veroff, & Feld, 1960; Mroczek & Kolarz, 1998). This age gradient in distress is most likely due in part to age differences in both exposure and reactivity to major life events and daily stressors. Compared to younger adults, older adults are more likely to experience certain life transitions that involve loss (e.g., retirement, widowhood) and less likely to experience others that involve new or expanded relationships (e.g., marriage, childbirth) (Hughes, Blazer, & George, 1988; Lowenthal, Thurnher, & Chiriboga, 1975). In terms of daily stressors, older adults tend to have fewer undesirable daily events (Zautra, Finch, Reich, & Guarnaccia, 1991). This decreased exposure may be due to a reduction in social roles and time commitments across the life course. Verbrugge, Gruber-Baldini, and Fozard (1996), for example, showed that with increasing age, time spent on personal and physical care, sleep, and personal activities increased, whereas time spent on work and sports participation decreased. Moreover, older individuals also may be less reactive to daily stressors, because they have fewer and less expansive expectations and life goals (Brim, 1992; Cross & Markus, 1991). Another possibility is that older individuals are less reactive to daily stressors because of the types of events they face. Brim and Ryff (1980) suggested that age-related life events, which have a strong likelihood of occurring (e.g., the "empty nest" or retirement), permit anticipatory coping that may mitigate their potentially stressful impact.

Using data from the NSDE, we examined *daily* stressor exposure by assessing age differences in objective and subjective characteristics of daily stressors (Almeida & Horn, 2004; Birdett, Fingerman, & Almeida, 2005; Neupert, Almeida, & Charles, 2007). These analyses revealed that young (25–39 years) and middle-aged individuals (40–59 years) reported a greater daily frequency of experiencing at least one stressor and multiple stressors than did older individuals (60–74 years), consistent with previous research documenting that older adults tend to experience fewer life events (Hughes et al., 1988; Lowenthal et al., 1975). Compared to older adults, young and midlife adults also experienced a greater proportion of interpersonal tensions (e.g., marital conflict or argument with a coworker) and "overload stressors"—stressors involving multiple demands and responsibilities. Older adults, on the other hand, reported a greater proportion of "network stressors"—events that happen to a close friend or relative and turn out to be stressful for the respondent (e.g., a spouse's illness). The age-related patterns of the content classification (overload and interpersonal tensions vs. network) of daily stressors can be interpreted through the social roles that these respondents were likely to inhabit. The results suggest that overloads and demands are a greater source of daily stressors for young and midlife adults compared to their older counterparts, although the source of the demands might differ by gender. Young men's daily stressors were more likely than stressors of respondents in the other groups to revolve around overloads and interactions with coworkers. Midlife women reported the same percentage of overloads as young women but had a greater proportion of stressors that involved other people (network stressors). Although overloads were not a common type of stressor for older adults, those respondents with overload had the greatest proportion of network and spouse-related events. Subsequent analyses used multilevel modeling to assess age differences in reactivity to daily stressors. Overall, younger adults were more emotionally reactive to interpersonal tensions, and older adults were more reactive to network stressors.

Historical Time and Place

A key principle of the life course perspective is that lives are nested in historical context and place (Elder et al., 2003). Historical and economic experiences can influence future life experiences and alter the trajectory of the timing and decisions made through the life course (Elder & Rockwell, 1979a; McAdam, 1989). In the study of daily stress process, it is important to consider that exposure and reactivity to stressors differ because of not only what people do in their lives but also the historical context and place in which they are embedded. For example, daily stress processes may be altered in the context of a national tragic event. Neupert, Almeida, Mroczek, and Spiro (2006) examined the effects of the Columbia shuttle disaster on the daily lives of older adults. When the Columbia shuttle exploded on February 1, 2003, the U.S. Department of Veterans Affairs (VA) Normative Aging Study (NAS) was carrying out a daily diary investigation of daily stressors and well-being among military veterans and their spouses. Findings from the study showed that respondents reported fewer daily stressors on the days following the shuttle tragedy. Given the enormity of the explosion and the unfortunate deaths of the astronauts on board, it is possible that the explosion led to a general recalibration of the definition of a "stressor," and people were less likely to report minor incidents. Perhaps, with the explosion as the reference point, being stuck in traffic or waiting in line at the grocery store paled in comparison. Respondents also reported a significant decline in positive affect, but there were no significant changes in negative affect after researchers controlled for the number of daily stressors experienced. The decrease in positive affect on days following the shuttle explosion could be attributed to the realization of the somberness of the event and its consequences. The participants in this study also were older (ages 59–89) and had served with the military or had seen their spouses serve. Their previous experiences with stressors and negative affect might have helped to minimize their negative response in this instance.

Specific historical events can impact individuals' lives directly; however, the broader historical context, such as membership in a specific birth cohort, also can shape daily lives. Take the work of Easterlin (1987), who connected cohort size among the low-birthrate generation of the 1930s and the high-birthrate generation of the 1950s to the fortunes and future of personal welfare. Upon reaching adulthood, those born in the 1930s experienced a labor market in which younger workers were in short supply. These members of the 1930s generation were able to find employment with good wages and to ascend the career ladder. These individuals also experienced little unemployment. In contrast, those born in the 1950s faced a labor market in adulthood in which younger workers were abundant and employment competition was high. Difficulties in finding a job, especially a job with good wages and benefits, undoubtedly affected marital, as well as childbearing, decisions. Thus, according to Clausen (1986, p. 8), "a cohort's placement in historical time tells us much about the opportunities and the constraints placed upon its members."

Our research has explored the daily stress processes among the birth cohorts of the baby boom generation. Significant historical changes (e.g., Vietnam War, education opportunities) and economic conditions (e.g., employment rate) associated with birth year have altered the life course of baby boomers in distinct ways. Using data from NSDE, Almeida, Serido, and McDonald (2006) assessed differences in exposure and reactivity to daily stressors among early and late baby boomers. Baby boomers were classified into two groups: early baby boomers—born between 1946 and 1954, and late baby boomers—born between 1955 and 1964. The average age of early baby boomers was 45 (age range, 41–49), whereas that of late baby boomers was 36 (age range, 31–40). Early boomers were more likely to have graduated from college and less likely to have children under the age of 18 in the household. Furthermore, more early baby boomer men had college degrees in comparison to late baby boomer men. These differences could be attributed to early baby boomers who graduated from high school having had the option of entering the armed forces, in addition to continuing their education or entering the workforce. Young adults who could afford an education may have decided to continue their education to avoid military service. In contrast to the early baby boomers, by the time the late baby boomers were making a similar life decision, the specter of military service no longer was present.

Next we examined whether these demographic differences translated into differences in daily stress processes. Although, both groups experienced a similar number of work, home, and health-related stressors, late baby boomers reported more other-focused stressors (i.e., stressors that happened to another person but impacted the respondent) than did early baby boomers. It may be that younger baby boomers are impacted more directly by stressors that involve others, such as younger children. Late baby boomers' stressors also presented more of a risk to finances than did those of early baby boomers. There are several possible explanations for this finding; perhaps older baby boomers have had a greater number of years than late baby boomers to establish their financial security. Another explanation might be that having children in the household may be a potential financial drain for late baby boomers. Late baby boomers also reported experiencing significantly higher levels of psychological distress than did early baby boomers. Finally, comparison of education level within each cohort revealed that respondents without a college degree report higher levels of distress on both stressor and nonstressor days. Among late baby boomers, that effect was exacerbated on stressor days, in that on days when late baby boomers experienced a stressor, those with a college degree reported lower levels of distress than did late baby boomers without a college degree. These findings highlight that examining cohort effects simply is not adequate without considering the social–demographic context of individuals such as education.

Interdependent Lives

Another key life course principle is that developing lives are lived interdependently. The principle of linked lives suggests that different levels of social actions interact and mutually influence each other (Giele & Elder, 1998a). Social networks shape and are shaped by major life transitions (Elder et al., 2003). Similar processes also are present at the daily level. People's daily lives are characterized by interactions with family members (e.g., spouses and children), acquaintances (e.g., neighbors and coworkers), and friends. Although these social exchanges often are positive, they also may be negative. Family relationships, especially those that are characterized by higher quality and reciprocity, may be sources of social support and function as buffers against stressors by providing emotional support, advice, and assistance (Rossi & Rossi, 1990). However, these social exchanges also may be conflicted, demanding, and sources of worry or concern (Kiecolt-Glaser & Newton, 2001; Pearlin & Skaff, 1996). Of all daily problems encountered, interpersonal problems are the most detrimental source of stress, taxing an individual's emotional, physical, and cognitive resources (Almeida, 2005; Bolger, DeLongis, Kessler, & Shilling, 1989; Clark & Watson, 1988). Indeed, interpersonal tensions are better predictors of psychological well-being than other types of everyday stressors, such as work overloads (Almeida

& Kessler, 1998; Bolger et al., 1989). The experience of interpersonal tensions, furthermore, varies from early adulthood to old age. The adulthood and aging literatures postulate that as people grow older, they have fewer problems in their relationships, experience less distress, and become less aggressive and more conciliatory, because they are exposed to different social contexts and perhaps are better able to regulate reactions to problems (Blanchard-Fields & Cooper, 2004; Carstensen, Isaacowitz, & Charles, 1999; Lazarus, 1996).

Our research using the NSDE has investigated whether younger and older adults differ in exposure and reactivity to interpersonal problems in day-to-day life (Birdett et al., 2005). We defined "exposure" as the number of interpersonal problems that individuals experienced and the type of social partners (e.g., spouse, child, and acquaintance) with whom they experienced problems. "Reactivity," on the other hand, involved how a person responds emotionally and behaviorally to that tension. To examine these issues, we used daily reports of tensions, which allowed us to assess the variety of social partners who irritate adults of different ages, and how they respond to those irritations. In addition, by examining daily reports, we were able to assess whether differences in exposure accounted for variations in reactivity. These analyses revealed that older adults, compared to younger adults, reported fewer interpersonal tensions, were more likely to report tensions with spouses, less likely to report tensions with children, experienced less stress, and were less likely to argue and more likely to do nothing in response to tensions. Age differences in emotional and behavioral reactions did not appear to be due to variations in exposure to tensions.

Another example of the role of linked lives on daily stress process comes from an analysis of adult caregivers (Savla, Almeida, Davey, & Zarit, 2008). Past research on routine assistance to older parents is based primarily on retrospective accounts of assistance provided over long time spans. Very little is known about the association between providing routine assistance amid everyday circumstances and the psychological consequences for the adult child over shorter time spans. From the NSDE, we used 3,668 daily diary interviews of 529 participants who provided assistance to their parent. A unique question accessible with this design was whether adult children were more distressed on days they provided assistance to a parent than on days they did not. Even after controlling for situational variables, such as time spent on daily chores at home and work, and network stressors, psychological distress was found to be higher on days when one provided assistance to a parent than on days when one did not. Social–demographic and psychosocial variables, such as being African American, unmarried, having a high school degree or less, and being highly neurotic, were found to be important vulnerability factors. Results highlight the importance of examining micro-level daily data to understand the enactment of the caregiving role.

Human Agency

Although historical and interpersonal contexts play important roles in daily experiences, it is imperative to consider the agency of human beings in constructing their daily lives. Individuals are not passive recipients of their environment. As active agents, individuals construct their lives within the constraints of their social and historical contexts (Elder et al., 2003). Such decisions and choices, undoubtedly, have important consequences for long-term future trajectories, as well as short-term daily experiences (Ong, Bergeman, & Bisconti, 2005). Our research has examined agency by assessing two types of control beliefs, mastery and constraint. "Mastery" often is described in terms of one's judgments about his or her ability to achieve a goal, whereas perceived "constraints" refer to the extent to which people believe that factors interfere with goal attainment (Lachman & Weaver, 1998). Pearlin and Schooler (1978) suggested that personal mastery is an important psychological resource that mitigates the effects of stress and strain. When faced with stressful situations, a strong sense of control also has been linked to low levels of self-reported perceived stress (Cameron, Armstrong-Stassen, Orr, & Loukas, 1991) and lower risk of depression (Yates, Tennstedt, & Chang, 1999). Higher levels of perceived control also buffered recently bereaved wives from anxiety when they were faced with daily stressors (Ong et al., 2005).

We were particularly interested in examining both mastery and constraint in the NSDE because they could be differentially important across the adult lifespan. For example, as younger adults are striving toward goals in their work lives, a sense of mastery may be particularly important. Because midlife represents a time when work status and expertise may be at its peak (Clark-Plaskie & Lachman, 1999) and differences in sense of control within the work domain exist between young and middle-aged adults as a function of progress along the career path at different stages in the life course (Heise, 1990), we examined whether control beliefs would be particularly important for middle-aged adults' well-being in response to work stressors. Based on prior research findings that younger adults who are invested in establishing interpersonal relationships more often employ active problem-solving strategies to their daily interpersonal problems than do older adults, we predicted that perceived control (both constraints and mastery) would have a stronger relationship with well-being (both emotional and physical) among younger adults than among older adults. Finally, we wanted to examine whether there were age and control belief differences in emotional and physical reactivity to home and network stressors. Findings from the NSDE showed that age and control beliefs both play an important role in reactivity to interpersonal, network, and work stressors (Neupert et al., 2007). Specifically, older age and lower perceived constraints were each related to lower emotional and physical reactivity to interpersonal stressors. High mastery buffered the physical effects of work stressors for younger and older adults, and high mastery was important for middle-aged adults' emotional reactivity to network stressors. Furthermore, when network stressors were examined, high constraint was found to be detrimental for younger and older adults' physical symptoms in comparison to those of middle-aged adults.

Life Transitions, Daily Stress, and Timing

According to George (1993), a study of "timing" has been largely ignored in stress research and is much needed. The principle of timing refers to the idea that "developmental antecedents and consequences of life transitions, events, and behavioral patterns vary according to their timing in a person's life" (Elder et al., 2003, p. 12). Depending on when it occurs in the life course, the meaning of a transition differs and affects an individual differently (Wheaton, 1990). A good example of the effect of transition timing and well-being is Quick and Moen's (1998) research on the transition to retirement. These researchers first conceptualized timing of retirement by defining retirement transitions as *early* (before age 60), *on time* (between ages 60 and 65), or *late* (after age 65). They then categorized retirement timing according to the difference between respondents' expected and actual retirement age, resulting in those who retired earlier than, later than, or at the time they expected. Women who retired on time were more likely than those who retired early or late to be very satisfied with retirement. Furthermore, those women who retired early (before age 60) were more likely to rate their retirement years as better than their preretirement years on the job than were women who retired on time or late. As for men, the expected timing of retirement mattered more than actual timing of retirement transition. In comparison to men who retired when they expected, men who retired earlier than expected were more likely to indicate that the years since retirement were better than the 5 years prior to it.

This study illustrates the importance of accounting for timing of transitions, whether through age expectations or social timetables, in understanding the social and personal meanings attached to life transitions. By investigating the context of life transitions, one can obtain a more complete understanding about the experiences of individuals undergoing them.

We have begun to examine how transitions in social roles affect daily experiences of respondents in the NSDE. It is important to mention that the NSDE examples presented thus far to illustrate the key components of the life course on daily stress processes have relied on cross-sectional data. The study of transitions, however, requires longitudinal data. Fortunately, the NSDE recently completed a second wave of data collection, approximately 10 years after the first. Respondents in the second wave ranged from 35 to 84 years of age and answered a protocol similar to the original: They completed daily telephone interviews about time use, psychological distress, physical symptoms, productivity, and daily stressors over 8 consecutive days. The newly collected longitudinal data enabled us to study life course transitions and coinciding changes in daily stress processes. The following are new findings on how the timing of the transition from employment to retirement predicts changes in daily psychological distress and the nature of daily stressors over the 10-year interval between the first and second waves.

We chose retirement because it is a very salient marker of adult development. Although not all workers will make the retirement transition, entitled programs, such as Social Security, have made retirement possible for more Americans. Conceptualized as the exit from one's *primary* career occupation, "retirement" also has been defined as the *final* exit from the labor force or *when* one receives a pension (or early retirement package) from a career employer and/or Social Security benefits. Retirement can also be a self-definition of *being retired*. Although the definition of retirement continues to be an unsettled issue, most researchers view retirement as a *process* that occurs in *context*. According to Moen (2003), retirement is an occupational career transition, as well as a family transition. For some, the exit from one's primary career occupation represents a transformation in one's social and physical worlds (e.g., changes in social role). The transition from employment to nonemployment may lead to increased opportunities for participation in unpaid volunteer work and leisure activities, thereby resulting in changes in one's daily life.

Data were from 79 respondents (average age 66.5, $SD = 6.7$; 34 men) who reported being employed at Wave 1, then classified themselves as being retired at Wave 2. As noted earlier, timing of retirement was classified into three categories utilized by Quick and Moen (1998). In addition to timing of transition, we also examined the effects of gender and education (less than a high school degree, high school or some college, and a college degree or more). A series of hierarchical multiple regressions, including transition timing, gender, and education (Step 1), and interaction between transition timing and gender, and transition timing and education (Step 2) were estimated for each psychological distress and daily stressor variable. Change scores in psychological distress and daily stressor variables were computed by subtracting scores at Wave 1 from Wave 2, in which a positive value denotes higher value at Wave 2.

Gender played an important role in how timing of retirement affected daily experience (see Figure 7.3). Men who transitioned into retirement early (before age 60) experienced the greatest increase in negative mood in comparison to their male and female counterparts who retired on time (between ages 60 to 65) or late (after age 65). For these men, moving into retirement too early may have represented a violation of societal norms and expectations about work, as well as the masculine role. Although not explored in the current analysis, future analyses also should examine the push-and-pull factors (e.g., health, job satisfaction) associated with employment. In contrast to the pattern observed for men, women who transitioned into retirement late (after age 65) reported the greatest increase in negative mood when compared to women who transitioned into retirement early or on time.

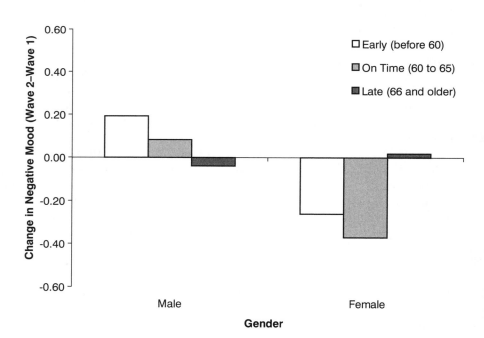

FIGURE 7.3. Retirement timing and gender interaction on change in negative mood.

We also were interested in respondents' appraisals of their daily stressors; however, gender and timing of transition did not predict appraisals of daily stressors. Nor did gender and timing of transition predict changes in stressor severity. Education level also was explored, but there was no significant interaction between education and transition timing, and psychological distress or daily stressors. Although the transition to retirement may represent an opportunity to depart from psychological, physical, and social stressors associated with one's employment (e.g., a difficult employer, irritable coworkers, or a physically demanding job), these findings suggest that researchers must go well beyond whether a transition was experienced, however disruptive, to examine the *timing* of the transition and its impact on individual well-being.

Future Directions: Earlier Stages of the Life Course

Throughout the chapter, we used examples of daily stress processes during middle and later adulthood, but this perspective may also be useful for other periods of the life course. Young adulthood, for example, is a time with multiple life transitions, including moving out of the parents' home, starting careers, and becoming parents. Each of these transitions brings a unique set of daily stressors. For example, parenthood, with associated and ongoing changes in roles, relationships, routines, responsibilities, identities, and task demands (Fish, Stifter, & Belsky, 1993), represents a paradigmatic life change with potentially serious consequences. A host of new and intensified challenges emerge during the transition to parenthood: physical changes, symptoms, and pregnancy/delivery complications; sleeplessness; concerns about financial stability; managing infants' crying or nearly continuous need for physical care and monitoring; and time-related pressures, including work–family balance.

It is important to acknowledge that the interfaces between parental transitions are greatly shaped by life course principles we describe earlier. Many of these principles are featured in Linda Burton's (1996) important work documenting family role transitions among African American women. The principle of linked lives is illustrated in the way that the transition to parenthood transforms the caregiving responsibility of not only mothers but also grandmothers and even great-grandmothers. The timing of childbearing had a profound effect on the whole extended family, because "family timetables for childbearing, marriage, and grandparenthood provided clear directives for these women as they moved from one family role to the next" (p. 201). Members in families with "on-time lineage" timetables expected these role transitions, were prepared for them, and willingly assumed their role responsibilities. However, in "early lineages," in which accelerated child-bearing resulted in early transitions to grandmotherhood and great-grandmotherhood, these lineages were "thrown off track," in that these women "did not expect, nor were they prepared for, the roles into which they had been propelled" (p. 205).

Life transition and daily stress research can also be applied to even younger ages. Research on adolescent development, for example, has highlighted the transition to middle or junior high school as a time of special significance for youth well-being. This transition has been linked to increases in psychological distress (Blyth, Simmons, & Carlton-Ford, 1983; Simmons, Rosenberg, & Rosenberg, 1973), and risky and aggressive behavior (Nansel, Haynie, & Simons-Morton, 2003; Pellegrini, 2002). As such, the life course model of life transitions and daily stress would allow researchers to illuminate micro-stressors and well-being processes, and their development over a period of dramatic change.

Conclusion

In this chapter we have documented the ways in which five main life course principles can be integrated into the study of life transitions and daily stress processes. Life transitions are often major, life-changing events requiring adaptation and causing depletion of individual psychological and physical resources that may result in stress. Transitions also may increase well-being to the extent that they bring new opportunities and desired social roles. Daily stressors, on the other hand, reflect the minor irritations and frustrations of daily life that may have a more proximal effect on well-being than major life transitions. In terms of their physiological and psychological effects, reports of life transitions can be associated with prolonged arousal, whereas reports of daily stressors can be associated with spikes in arousal or psychological distress that day. Both life transitions and daily stressors are embedded in multiple layers of temporal and social contexts that shape individual well-being. In this chapter we have presented a perspective on life transitions and daily stress processes by describing a model that links key principles of the life course to the study of life transitions and daily stress processes. By utilizing life course principles, we can better understand the opportunities, as well as vulnerabilities, that individuals experience as they undergo life transitions that are both important markers of development and important predictors of daily stress and well-being.

This approach relies on daily diary methodology to capture daily stress. Repeated measurements of *daily* stressful events, as well as health behaviors, symptoms, and psychological well-being, increase ecological validity, reduce memory bias, and permit the dynamic assessment of stressor reactivity (i.e., within-person correlation of stressors and well-being). Thanks to new statistical approaches, such as multilevel modeling, it is possible to assess within-person stressor reactivity and between-person differences in stress reactivity. This statistical method can be used to examine how life transitions and the key principles of the life course perspective predict exposure and reactivity to daily stressors.

Using data from the NSDE, we have provided several examples linking life course principles to daily stress processes, showing how age, historic events, and birth cohort membership shape exposure and reactivity to daily stressors. In addition, we have demonstrated how the social context in terms of interpersonal tensions and caregiving status, as well as how perceptions of personal control, play important roles in shaping daily stress processes. The final set of analyses showed how the timing of the transition into retirement translated into different levels of daily well-being for men and women. These findings, we hope, will serve as a template for more analyses that combine life transitions and daily stress processes using a life course perspective.

The life course perspective reminds us of the importance of studying human development in context. This reminder is more important than ever as we move further into the 21st century, where we see the life course changing in several ways, with implications for the study of life transitions and daily stress processes. First, not only have parts of the life course been redefined (e.g., emerging adulthood, midlife), but time spent in major stages of the life course also have increased due in part to longer life expectancy and social changes (Moen, 2003). The major life transitions of adulthood, such as age at first marriage and first childbirth, have been rising since the 1960s (Knaub, Eversoll, & Voss, 1983) and have become dispersed over a broader age range. In comparison to the early 20th century, people are getting married and having their first child in their late 20s, which once was the period of career establishment (Knaub et al., 1983). Nor is the immediate transition from a single career to complete withdrawal from the labor force the norm any longer for most Americans. Workers are moving from one or several short-duration or part-time jobs (bridge jobs) between their full-time career employment and complete labor force withdrawal. These social changes present new challenges for researchers, as well as policymakers, in understanding how the timing of life transitions is changing and what the new norms determine what is deemed "early" or "late." We believe that linking the timing and transitions of the life course to the real-life, day-to-day experiences of individuals will help to illuminate their meanings and consequences for the well-being of individuals.

Acknowledgments

The research reported in this chapter was supported by National Institutes of Health Grant Nos. P01 AG0210166-02 and R01 AG19239, and by the Research Network on Successful Midlife Development of the John D. and Catherine T. MacArthur Foundation.

CHAPTER 8

Conceptualizing and Measuring Trajectories

Linda K. George

The language of trajectories, pathways, and similar dynamic descriptors have become standard fare in life course research over the past quarter-century. The notion of studying life course patterns of change and stability over time has great appeal. And the increasing availability of longitudinal data covering large portions of the life course, as well as methods for acquiring reliable, albeit retrospective, life histories creates the data infrastructure required for life course research. Many sociological theories imply process; thus, trajectories can be important for theory development and hypothesis testing. Indeed, trajectories are arguably the premier tools for assessing the dynamics of change. Despite the obvious appeal of studying trajectories, one need not delve very deeply into the topic—as either an investigator or a consumer of research—to see that the intuitive lure of trajectory-based research is neither simple nor straightforward in practice.

The purpose of this chapter is to examine conceptualization and measurement of trajectories and the substantive implications—including the costs and benefits—of measurement choices. It is organized in five sections. The first section addresses the definition of trajectories and the importance of trajectories for two broad theoretical frameworks. The second section describes various ways of measuring trajectories. The third section provides empirical illustrations of how the multiple ways of constructing trajectories have been applied in life course research. The last two sections address emerging issues in trajectory analysis, including illustrations of the wide range of research questions for which trajectories have been useful.

Trajectories and the Life Course

It is important to define the term "trajectory" as it is used in this chapter. In research to date, the term "trajectory" is used in multiple ways, ranging from a heuristic, global way of talking about all longitudinal analyses, to time trends based on aggregates (e.g., patterns of unemployment over historical time), to individual patterns of stability and change. A major inconsistency in trajectory-based research is lack of clarity about whether trajectories are *intraindividual* phenomena, *interindividual* phenomena, or both.

Clearly, stability and change can be observed both within and across individuals, but this does not mean that the term "trajectory" should be used indiscriminately. For my purposes here, trajectory refers *only to intraindividual change*. There are research questions for which it is appropriate to trace patterns of interindividual stability and change (e.g., average income levels or rates of disability across the life course) but clarity is maximized if the definition of trajectory is quite specific. There is general agreement that the life course perspective involves examining temporality in social and historical context. Therefore, although trajectories are based on intraindividual temporal patterns, the *meaning* of intraindividual change can only be understood by examining its relationship to social and historical context. For example, a trajectory of prolonged unemployment may have a very different meaning during economic prosperity than during major economic recessions. Thus, a key feature of life course theory is identifying the interindividual (i.e., between-person) characteristics and experiences that predict intraindividual (i.e., within-person) patterns of stability and change.

Two additional distinctions must be addressed at the outset. First, trajectories can be either transition-based or level-based. In early life course research, most trajectories were transition-based and frequently defined as sequences of transitions that form a trajectory that gives meaning to the sequence (Elder, 1985b). And transition-based trajectories remain the appropriate choice for many research questions. Level-based trajectories index patterns of increase, decrease, or stability for a variable of interest (e.g., declining health, increasing self-esteem). Ideally, the choice of a transition-based or level-based trajectory relies on the research question. But the metric of the variable of interest can restrict this choice. Categorical variables only permit transition-based trajectories. Continuous variables are typically used to construct level-based trajectories, although it is also possible to recode continuous variables to construct transition-based trajectories.

Second, trajectories can be constructed along two possible temporal templates. In some studies, trajectories are time-dependent—that is, the temporal axis is determined by date of measurement. For example, in a longitudinal survey with five times of measurement, trajectories would be based on patterns of stability and change from the first to the last survey. It also is possible, however, to construct age-dependent trajectories in which the temporal axis is age. For example, an age-based axis might include the ages 50, 60, 70, and 80. The related trajectory would represent patterns of stability and change observed between the ages of 50 and 80. If all the participants in a study were exactly the same age at baseline, there would be no difference between a time-based and an age-based trajectory. Obviously, however, this is an unlikely scenario. Recasting time-dependent to age-dependent observations is often very labor-intensive. Nonetheless, choice of an age-based or time-based trajectory should be dictated by the research question. Empirical examples presented later in the chapter illustrate transition-based and level-based trajectories, as well as age- and time-based trajectories.

Two broad theoretical perspectives underlie research on trajectories. First, life course theory highlights a variety of temporal issues that can be examined using trajectories. Measurement and analysis of trajectories require investigators to specify the temporal characteristics relevant to their research questions. Second, most life course research involves cross-fertilization of life course principles with other theories (e.g., theories of crime, stress process theory). Cross-fertilization is often challenging precisely because most social science theories have been framed in terms of between-person differences rather than within-person changes. For example, the hypothesis that socioeconomic status (SES) is negatively associated with health has been a core research topic since the origins of sociology. This hypothesis is usually tested by comparing a health outcome across individuals who vary in social status. Trajectory analysis would determine whether intraindividual trajectories of SES predict intraindividual trajectories of health. Conventional conceptualizations of the relationship between SES and health assume a between-person design and fail to consider issues such as the amount of change in SES required to change health, and the length of time between a change in SES and a change in health—issues inherently confronted when examining intraindividual dynamics of SES and health. Thus, in trajectory-based research, investigators often must reframe their theories before selecting a strategy for measuring trajectories. Both of these perspectives are detailed below.

Temporality

Life course theory focuses on time—biographical time and historical time. These temporal patterns have multiple characteristics. The importance of such characteristics varies depending on the research question being addressed. In this section, I briefly discuss four temporal characteristics that answer different questions about stability and change across the life course.

Timing and Critical Periods

The crucial issue in some life course studies is timing. The assumption in such studies is that events, experiences, or contexts may affect individuals differently depending on their timing in the life course. For example, Elder, Shanahan, and Clipp (1994) hypothesized that serving in the military during World War II would have different effects on subsequent socioeconomic achievements depending on the age at which one entered the military. Similarly, Turnbull, George, Landerman, Swartz, and Blazer (1990) predicted that the life course consequences of mental illness would differ depending on the age of onset of psychiatric disorder, with onset at younger ages generating greater difficulties in socioeconomic achievement and family formation/stability.

The notion of "critical periods" also rests on issues of timing. Most research on critical periods rests on the developmental postulate that if specific developmental tasks are not completed during a specific segment of the life course, subsequent development will be delayed or precluded. For example, Erikson's (1963) stage theory of adult development is based on the sequencing of developmental tasks across the life course. The theory also posits that failure to achieve a developmental task precludes the fulfillment of subsequent developmental tasks.

To test hypotheses about timing or critical periods adequately, trajectories must be constructed to meet two criteria. First, age-dependent trajectories must be constructed. Second, the trajectories must be constructed to highlight the outcomes of interest before and after the time/age hypothesized to be important. Issues of timing can be examined without relying on trajectory analysis (e.g., by comparing outcomes between/among groups that differ on timing). But trajectories are required to address many questions about timing (e.g., whether stable vs. unstable occupational or marital histories have different health consequences).

Duration

Duration is an inherent, though often unmeasured, component of trajectories. Two types of research questions focus on issues of duration.

First, many studies test hypotheses about the effects of *length of exposure* to specific conditions or contexts on outcomes of interest. For example, it is well established that individuals who regularly attend religious services are healthier and live longer than those who never attend religious services (George, Larson, Koenig, & McCullough, 2000; Musick, House, & Williams, 2004). Despite the use of longitudinal data in which religious attendance is known to precede the health outcome, nothing is known about how long one must attend religious services before health benefits can be observed. Trajectories of religious attendance over long periods of time would be the ideal way to link length of exposure to the timing and magnitude of health benefits.

Second, for some research questions the key issue is "duration dependence," a pattern in which the likelihood of change varies depending on length of time in a specific status or environment. The likelihood of marrying exhibits clear patterns of duration dependence in the United States. Between the ages of approximately 18 and 40, every year that one is unmarried increases the likelihood that one will marry the following year. But duration dependence also can change direction—and does so for marriage. After the age of 40 or so, every year that one is unmarried decreases the odds of marrying the following year. Many research questions can be framed in terms of duration dependence. For example, is divorce duration-dependent, such that every year one is married decreases the likelihood of subsequent divorce? Similarly, is job change duration dependent, with every year in a given job decreasing the odds of changing jobs?

Note that duration can be studied using time-dependent or age-dependent trajectories. In the previous examples, trajectories of religious service attendance would probably be time based, and trajectories of the probability of marrying would be age dependent. Depending on the research question, either level- or transition-based trajectories would be appropriate. Trajectories of exposure to religious services would be level based; trajectories of getting married would be transition based. In addition, measurements must be sufficiently frequent to permit accurate conclusions about differing lengths of exposure or changes in duration dependence.

Sequencing

Sequencing is used to determine whether the order in which discrete events occur affects an outcome of interest. Barrett's (2000) examination of the effects of marital history on mental health is a prime example of sequence trajectories. Barrett's study begins with the well-documented finding that married individuals are, on average, healthier than unmarried persons. She notes, however, that current marital status masks considerable heterogeneity in marital history. Currently married individuals, for example, include persons in first marriages and those in higher-order marriages. Among the remarried, some previous marriages ended in divorce and others by widowhood. Using detailed marital histories, Barrett identified the full range of marital trajectories in an adult community sample. There were two stable trajectories: persons who never married, and persons who married once and remained married. Other trajectories comprised sequences of marital transitions; approximately 40 unique sequences were identified.

Barrett's (2000) analyses were based on eight trajectories that (1) captured the vast majority of study participants and (2) highlighted trajectory characteristics that were expected to be most closely related to mental health (i.e., number of transitions and type of dissolution). The eight trajectories were used as dummy variables in regression equations predicting mental health outcomes. Specific contrasts were used to highlight the effects of number of transitions and type of dissolution (divorce or widowhood). Analyses were performed separately for men and women, and included a wide range of covariates, including a measure of mental health status prior to marriage that provided a partial adjustment for selection effects. Although there were minor differences for various mental health outcomes, the results generally suggest that number of transitions has significant consequences for mental health, such that remarried persons report more psychiatric symptoms than the once-married. Type of dissolution, however, had little effect: Both divorce and widowhood were associated with higher levels of psychiatric symptoms. Barrett also included duration of current marital status as a predictor, showing that (1) the disadvantage associated with remarriage lessens as years in that marriage increase, and (2) for women, but not men, increased years spent divorced or widowed are associated with reductions in psychiatric symptoms.

In their basic form, sequence trajectories are easily constructed: The investigator simply arranges events of interest in the order they occurred. At least two issues can complicate sequence trajectories, however. First, the number of sequences observed in a sample is typically so large that all sequences cannot be included in analysis. In this situation, the investigator is well-advised to select a subset of sequences especially relevant to the research question. Second, in their basic form, sequences ignore duration. Barrett's (2000) study of marital history illustrates ways to avoid both of these complications. As noted earlier, Barrett identified more than 40 marital history sequences in her sample but selected eight for hypothesis testing. She also incorporated differences in the length of time spent in current and former marital statuses in her analyses.

Turning Points

Some research questions focus on "turning points"—on specific events or milestones that substantially alter the direction and/or slope of a trajectory. In personal biography, turning points are often described as "defining moments" or "watershed experiences." There is a general expectation that turning points affect specific outcomes. For example, psychiatrists view the traumas that result in posttraumatic stress disorder (PTSD) as turning points in mental health. Sampson and Laub's research on criminal careers (1993) illustrates the potential importance of identifying turning points in the life course. Using life history data from the Gluecks' longitudinal study of 1,000 men, who were first interviewed as children and followed until age 70 or death, Sampson and Laub identified two turning points that led to desistance in criminal behavior: military service and marriage. Military service in early adulthood enhanced socioeconomic achievement and reduced criminal behavior (Sampson & Laub, 1996). Importantly, the benefits of military service were greater for men who served earlier rather than later in life, and for those who had officially been labeled delinquents. Marriage during early adulthood also was associated with decreases in criminal behavior. In some cases, marriage led to rather dramatic discontinuities in desistance (Laub & Sampson, 1993); in others, reductions in criminal behavior were more gradual and cumulative (Laub, Nagin, & Sampson, 1998).

Several factors associated with the identification of turning points need to be considered. First, and most important, turning points can only be identified retrospectively; that is, it is not possible to know whether an event or experience will be a turning point until there are long-term data afterward that permit the investigator to link a change in the form of the trajectory of the dependent variable to an earlier event or experience. A corollary of this is that a turning point cannot be identified unless the researcher has data prior to, and for a considerable period of time after, the event that comprises the turning point. Second, turning points can be observed in either age- or time-dependent trajectories. In general, developmental turning points are more easily identified in age-dependent trajectories, and turning points triggered by external events are more visible in time-dependent trajectories. Third, because nondevelopmental turning points are relatively rare (i.e., they are not experienced by a large portion of the population or at a specific age), between-person analyses are unlikely to reveal them, which is additional evidence of the utility of trajectories that measure intraindividual patterns of stability and change.

Cross-Fertilizing Life Course and Other Social Science Theories

Outside the life course framework, most social science theories implicitly assume that tests of their veracity will be conducted using between-person analyses. As a result, cross-fertilizing life course principles with other theories can be difficult, because life course theory focuses on within-person change and stability. Life course theory recognizes the importance of between-person differences, but a core assumption of life course theory is that the most profitable analyses of temporal issues examine between-person predictors or correlates of within-person trajectories.

Life course principles can be incorporated into between-person research designs in a variety of ways. Specific temporal characteristics, such as the age at which a transition occurs or the duration of a specific status, can be treated as between-person variables. These kinds of strategies for incorporating temporal variables are rather easily implemented given adequate data and do not challenge the variable-centered approach to understanding human behavior. I would argue, however, that these designs fall short of the ideal for understanding temporality. As several authors have observed (e.g., Singer & Ryff, 2001; von Eye & Bogat, 2006), the focus on intraindividual stability and change transforms research to a person-centered focus.

A specific example helps to clarify between- and within-person differences in methods of framing a research problem. The theory I discuss is part of social stress theory, specifically, the differential exposure versus differential vulnerability hypotheses. By now, probably thousands of studies support the general hypothesis that social stress is a robust predictor of negative physical and mental health outcomes. Stress theory includes attention to the antecedents of stress, the role of stress in explaining status differences (e.g., gender and socioeconomic status differences) in health, and the factors that mediate and moderate the effects of stress on illness.

The differential exposure versus differential vulnerability hypotheses address the question of health inequalities (i.e., why some groups are less healthy than others). Both hypotheses are simple and straightforward. The differential exposure hypothesis posits that some groups are less healthy than others because they are exposed to higher levels of stress. The differential vulnerability hypotheses contends that some groups are less healthy than others because they are more vulnerable to stress; that is, at equal levels of stress, the vulnerable groups will experience more negative health effects than the less vulnerable ones. These are not mutually exclusive hypotheses, but they are frequently pitted against each other in empirical tests.

A very large literature base addresses the effects of differential exposure and differential vulnerability. Nearly all previous research, however, is based on between-person designs in which persons experiencing varying levels of stress are compared to determine whether high exposure to stress is associated with subsequent increases in physical or mental health problems. Studies based on a within-person design would frame the question differently: Are increases in stress followed by decreases in health? Instead of comparing people who vary in levels of stress, the within-person design would determine whether increases in stress over time lead to health decrements.

In two previous papers, Scott Lynch and I (Lynch & George, 2002; George & Lynch, 2003) reframed the stress exposure versus stress vulnerability question as a within-person issue and analyzed three waves of longitudinal data using latent growth curve analysis (LGCA). The dependent variable was individual trajectories of depressive symptoms. Trajectories of stressful life events also were constructed; both trajectories exhibited substantial heterogeneity. We then determined whether trajectories characterized by "growth" in stress over time predicted trajectories in which depressive symptoms also "grew" over time—and they did. In a between-person component of the analysis, demographic factors were related to both the "intercepts" (or starting points) and the "slopes" (or rates of change) of the trajectories of depressive symptoms.

The key issue is that between-person and within-person designs answer different questions. In the previous example, a between-person design asks whether individuals who experience more stressors are more likely to become ill than persons who experience fewer stressors. A within-person design asks whether individuals who experience an increase in stress results subsequently experience a decrease in health. Life course theory combines the two, permitting investigators to determine whether between-person social characteristics are associated with varying intraindividual patterns of stability and change.

Measuring Trajectories

The factors involved in measuring trajectories can be usefully conceptualized as involving three major bifurcations based on (1) the metric of the trajectory variable, (2) choice of an aggregate trajectory or disaggregated trajectories, and (3) whether the trajectories are constructed by the investigator or empirically derived.

The Metric of the Trajectory Variable

This issue is closely linked to the distinction between transition-based and level-based trajectories, so the discussion here is brief. As noted earlier, transition-based trajectories are based on categorical measures; level-based trajectories are based on continuous measures. Ideally, the choice of transition- or level-based trajectories will be determined by the research question under investigation. In many cases investigators have the option of selecting the type of trajectory, because the variable to be analyzed can be coded either categorically or continuously. Take, for example, depression. Some research questions focus on trajectories based on the onset of, recovery from, and recurrence of episodes of clinically diagnosed depressive disorder, thus requiring transition-based trajectories. Other research questions focus on increases and decreases in levels of depressive symptoms. Addressing these questions requires level-based trajectories.

It is always possible to break a continuous variable into relevant categories (though the possible cut points may not be ideal or, too frequently, are arbitrary). It is not possible to transform categorical data into continuous form. Moreover, these two types of trajectories answer fundamentally different research questions. Consider the example of two survey questions that ask respondents about their participation in voluntary organizations. One question asks whether respondents belong to one or more voluntary organizations and is coded dichotomously (i.e., yes or no). The other question asks respondents how frequently they attend meetings of voluntary organizations in an average month. Trajectories based on the original metrics of these two questions would describe quite different phenomena.

Aggregate versus Disaggregated Trajectories

Another primary issue in measuring trajectories is whether to examine the aggregate trajectory that best describes the sample as a whole or multiple trajectories that represent discrete patterns of change and stability within the sample. Again, selection of an aggregate trajectory or of disaggregated trajectories is best determined by the research question. Consider, for example, the hypothesis that average age-earnings profiles are flatter for recent cohorts than in the past. Testing this hypothesis requires longitudinal data covering a substantial period of time from at least two cohorts (i.e., an earlier cohort and a recent cohort). The best strategy for testing this hypothesis would be to construct an aggregate age-dependent income trajectory for each cohort. The investigator is interested not in variability within cohorts, but in differences across cohorts. Nonetheless, the analysis would be based on intraindividual differences in income across time–age in each cohort.

Disaggregated trajectories should be used when the investigator expects (1) substantial variability within the sample, (2) a finite number of distinctive patterns of stability and change, and (3) that these distinctive patterns will be meaningful (e.g., will have different predictors or correlates). Consider, for example, the dynamics of disability over time. In the older population, the dominant pattern is clearly one of increasing disability over time. But other trajectories also are observed (Gill, Allore, Hardy, & Guo, 2006; Jagger et al., 2007). Some sample members "recover" from disability over time (e.g., after joint replacement). Because a "recovery" trajectory would characterize only a small proportion of the population, it would not be observed in an aggregate trajectory of disability over time. Different rates of change also could generate distinctive patterns, even when the direction of the change is the same. For example, disaggregated trajectories may allow the investigator to observe multiple patterns of disability increase. Some sample members may exhibit a gradual increase in disability over a period of years; others may exhibit precipitous increases in disability over short periods of time.

Aggregate trajectories are probably used more frequently than is desirable. Two major issues underlie this conclusion. First, one cannot know a priori the extent to which an aggregate trajectory is hiding distinctive patterns of stability and change; that is, only by using disaggregated trajectories can an investigator demonstrate that an aggregate trajectory does justice to the data. Second, precisely because social scientists are more accustomed to thinking in between-person terms, few of our theories, and relatively little previous research, have examined intraindividual change. Thus, in the absence of relevant previous research, we cannot dismiss the possibility of multiple patterns of stability and change.

Constructed vs. Empirically Derived Trajectories

Trajectories can be constructed in two ways: investigator constructed and empirically derived. One option is for investigators to construct trajectories. In some cases, investigators literally print the values of a variable for each sample member, visually inspect them, and sort them into trajectory categories. For example, Martijn and Sharpe (2006) interviewed 35 homeless youth, ages 14–25 years. In earlier cross-sectional studies, high rates of both mental illness and criminal behavior were observed among homeless youth. The investigators collected in-depth retrospective data to determine whether these problems were causes or consequences of homelessness. The investigators read the interview transcripts and sorted them into trajectories. Two raters independently sorted the data and resolved discrepancies. They observed several patterns in the data. First, almost all sample members described experiencing one or more severe traumas (e.g., physical or sexual abuse) prior to homelessness. A majority of sample members also reported mental illness, including substance abuse/dependence, prior to homelessness. Episodes of mental illness were reported to increase after homelessness, regardless of preexisting psychiatric problems. Only one respondent had a history of criminal behavior prior to homelessness, but most participants reported frequent criminal activity after homelessness.

In another form of constructed trajectories, investigators develop a set of decision rules that is used to create trajectories. The decision rules may be based on conceptual criteria or on a review of raw data. The decision rules are typically implemented with the use of computer software. Constructing trajectories by using decision rules has several advantages relative to the more informal procedure, in which the investigator sorts raw data into trajectories. First, for larger samples, computer-implemented decision rules are much more efficient. Second, and more important, computer-based construction is performed with perfect reliability. In contrast, when trajectories are created via visual inspection of raw data, some amount of subjectivity or "drift" in coding decisions is likely. Barrett's (2000) study of the effects of marital history on mental health, described earlier, illustrates the use of computer-implemented decision rules to create trajectories.

As new forms of analysis have become available (new for social scientists, at any rate), investigators increasingly use statistical techniques to derive trajectories based on empirical criteria. Two forms of analysis dominate empirically derived trajectories: latent growth curve analysis (LGCA) and latent class analysis (LCA). Both techniques require data from at least three times of measurement, and their statistical properties are even better when there are four or more times of measurement.

LGCA, also referred to as hierarchical linear modeling, generates an aggregate trajectory that best describes a sample, and analysis takes place in two stages. In the first stage, individual trajectories of the variable of interest are constructed for every sample member and the trajectory that best describes the sample as a whole (i.e., the average trajectory) is produced. The aggregate trajectory includes two important types of information: the "intercept," which is the starting point for the trajectory, and the "slope," which represents the direction and rate of change over time. In the second stage of analysis, factors that may explain variability around the aggregate trajectory are added to the model. As a simple example, age and gender may be used to predict an aggregate disability trajectory. Each independent variable may be significantly related to the intercept, the slope, both, or neither. Significant predictors of the trajectory intercept indicate that those variables predict different starting points. Thus, in the example used here, if age were a significant and positive predictor of the intercept, this would mean that older sample members had significantly higher levels of disability at baseline than younger participants. Significant predictors of the trajectory slope indicate differential rates of change. Thus, if age were a significant positive predictor of the trajectory slope, this would mean that older sample members experienced significantly more rapid increases in disability than younger ones.

The other statistical technique commonly used to derive trajectories is LCA, also called growth mixture models. In contrast to LGCA, LCA identifies the *set* of trajectories that best fits a longitudinal distribution. Specifically, LCA generates multiple discrete or disaggregate trajectories (a one-trajectory solution, a two-trajectory solution, etc.). Goodness-of-fit statistics allow the investigator to select the solution that best fits the data, although interpretation or conceptual clarity of the trajectories also can be taken into account. A one-trajectory solution would yield the same trajectory as LGCA. But unlike LGCA, LCA evaluates whether multiple trajectories better fit the data than one trajectory. Each sample member receives a score on each trajectory, indicating degree of resemblance to that trajectory. Some respondents score high on a single trajectory and low on all others; other respondents' scores are more similar across trajectories. In this sense, LCA is different from traditional cluster analysis, in which sample members are each assigned to only one cluster.

Unlike LGCA, LCA is not a two-stage process. Once the set of trajectories that best fit the data has been derived, the investigator chooses how to use it in subsequent analyses designed to identify the antecedents and/or outcomes associated with each trajectory. When the dependent variable is a set of trajectories, multinomial logistic regression, which can accommodate multiple dependent variables, is typically the analytic technique of choice. But many other analytic techniques are used as well.

Advantages and Disadvantages of Constructed and Empirically Derived Trajectories

Nagin and Tremblay (2005a) present an extensive critique of constructed trajectories, which they term "ad hoc classification." They identify four limitations of constructed trajectories relative to those empirically derived using LCA. First, when trajectories are defined by the investigator, their existence is not statistically verified. Second, there is substantial likelihood that ad hoc classification will fail to identify rare but "real" trajectories. The authors note that although rare trajectories characterize a small proportion of sample members, they may document the most severe and/or policy-relevant pattern in the data. Third, LCA provides investigators with estimates of the probabilities of group membership for each sample member on each trajectory. With constructed trajectories, each sample member either fits or does not fit each trajectory. Fourth, age-dependence and duration are likely to be neglected in ad hoc classifications. When constructing trajectories, investigators are likely to focus on sequences of transitions or global patterns of change (e.g., increasing disability) and to ignore other, temporal elements of change, such as varying lengths of time between events in a sequence or slow versus fast increases in the variable of interest.

In light of these criticisms, it is tempting to assume that empirically derived trajectories are superior to constructed trajectories. This is probably an accurate general conclusion, but empirically derived trajectories also have limitations, of which two are primary. First, empirically derived trajectories are atheoretical. Thus, if an investigator desires to test hypotheses about specific patterns of stability and change, empirically derived trajectories may or may not be ideal—or even appropriate. Second, when an independent variable is related at different levels of strength or in opposite directions with multiple trajectories, it is not clear *what property* of the trajectory is responsible. Any number of explanations is possible, including the following: One trajectory had a turning point and the others do not, rate of change differs across the trajectories, duration of exposure to the independent variable differs across trajectories, and so on. In contrast, investigators can construct trajectories in ways that permit comparison of trajectories that differ in a specific property that is expected to be differentially related to the independent variables.

Measuring Trajectories: Life Course Applications

In this section, empirical illustrations of four approaches to measuring trajectories are provided: qualitative studies, studies using computer-assisted trajectory measurement, LGCA, and LCA, also known as mixture models. Note that the primary goal of these empirical examples is not to review the results of the selected studies, but to illustrate the links between research questions and methods of trajectory construction.

Qualitative Studies

Although few qualitative studies are longitudinal per se, investigators frequently obtain retrospective accounts that focus on process. Setting aside concerns about the accuracy of retrospective data, trajectories can be a useful tool for summarizing the dynamics of change and stability, as reported in qualitative studies. Investigator-constructed trajectories seem quite "natural" in this research milieu for two reasons. First, sample sizes are typically small, which makes it feasible for investigators to construct the trajectories reliably. In addition, small samples usually preclude empirically derived trajectories, such as those generated by LGCA or LCA. Second, generating theory is frequently a goal of qualitative research, and the intense scrutiny of the data involved in constructing trajectories can further that goal.

Blair-Loy (1999) studied the careers of 56 women in high-status, finance-related jobs. Her analysis focused on three research questions:

1. Did women who "made it to the top" have orderly or disorderly careers?
2. Are there cohort differences in the career trajectories of female executives in the finance industry?
3. Did the social and legal changes in labor practices experienced during the 1970s affect women's pathways to executive finance jobs?

Women in the sample, reported their place of employment and occupation for each year from the age of 22 to the time of the interview. Blair-Loy constructed trajectories using three pieces of information: size of the company (four values ranging from small to very large), job level (a range of nine, including out of the labor force), and duration (number of years spent in each job/organization combination). She also calculated "slopes" based on the length of time required to move from one job level to a higher one. To gain precision, Blair-Loy used an optimal matching technique (Abbott & Hrycak, 1990) to identify common patterns in the sequences of jobs reported by sample members. This technique generated five trajectories: Two represented relatively orderly careers in large corporations; one included less orderly careers in medium and small companies; one represented disorderly careers; and the smallest trajectory identified women who left corporate employment to become self-employed entrepreneurs.

Blair-Loy (1999) reports that women's career trajectories were sharply different depending on cohort, with cohort membership based on distance from the social and legal pressures exerted by the women's movement in the early to mid-1970s. Members of the oldest cohort entered the labor market in the 1960s, had the most disorderly careers, and, did not profit from the women's movement until the later years of their careers. Members of the second cohort entered the labor market in the 1970s, had more orderly careers than the previous cohort, and gains generated by the women's movement allowed them to enter the finance industry early in their careers. Members of the third cohort entered the labor market in the 1980s, had the most orderly careers, and although they frequently changed companies, had a general pattern of sustained and steady advancement. The qualitative data also indicated that the youngest cohort of women had little understanding of the more difficult career paths of their predecessors. This study incorporates statistical analysis, via the optimal matching technique, to a greater degree than most qualitative studies. Nonetheless, the trajectories were constructed by the investigator, who chose the specific factors on which the trajectories would be based.

Investigator-Designed versus Computer-Designed Trajectories

The other primary form of "constructed" trajectory involves the investigator developing a set of decision rules and applying it to the data by using computer software. This form of trajectory is similar to the investigator-designed typologies developed in qualitative studies, but the categorization is performed by software application of the decision rules. In studies using this approach, there is a close match between the research question and the trajectories themselves (which may not be the case when trajectories are empirically derived).

Hallqvist, Lynch, Bartley, Lang, and Blane (2004) used data from a large Swedish case–control study to disentangle the effects of life course accumulation, critical periods, and social mobility on the incidence of myocardial infarction (MI). The investigators began with the observation that life course accumulation (i.e., cumulative disadvantage), critical periods, and social mobility imply different trajectories that can be compared to assess their relative importance for a given outcome. Hallqvist et al. coded respondents' occupations into manual versus nonmanual labor at three points in time based on retrospective occupational histories: (1) childhood, using the father's occupation; (2) young adulthood, using the respondent's first occupation between the ages of 25 and 29; and (3) late middle age, using the respondent's last occupation between the ages of 51 and 55. Combinations of manual versus nonmanual jobs at three points in time yielded eight trajectories that were used to predict the incidence of an MI. Analysis was restricted to men.

The findings supported all three temporal patterns. First, the longer the exposure to a manual, as opposed to nonmanual occupation, the higher the odds of MI, which supports the life course accumulation hypothesis. Respondents' manual occupations in young adulthood were stronger predictors of MI than were the manual occupations of their fathers in childhood or in late middle age, suggesting that young adulthood is a critical period of risk. In a comparison of respondents' occupations to those of their fathers, upwardly mobile respondents had reduced odds of MI; those who were downwardly mobile had increased risk.

This study illustrates both the potential and limitations of constructed trajectories. On the positive side, the investigators nicely demonstrate the links between various theories (e.g., cumulative disadvantage, critical periods) and specific trajectories. On the negative side, coding occupations as either manual or nonmanual is a crude summary of a heterogeneous mix of occupations. In addition, using this coding scheme required researchers to omit self-employed respondents and farmers from analysis. Missing data about occupation at one or more of the three time periods also resulted in substantial respondent loss. The specific effects of respondent loss and the unmeasured heterogeneity in occupations cannot be assessed but are surely nontrivial. Finally—and this is inherent in investigator-designed trajectories—there is no independent verification that the trajectories are statistically defensible.

Identifying Trajectories in LGCA

LGCA analyses are now very common in the social and behavioral sciences. One way that studies using LGCA differ is in the number of growth curves included in analysis. Organizing illustrative studies according to the number of estimated growth curves highlights the range of research questions for which LGCA is a useful analytic technique.

Single-Trajectory Analysis

In one form of this LGCA design, the dependent variable is modeled as an aggregate trajectory, and the effects of independent variables on both the intercept and slope of that trajectory are estimated. Note that this form of analysis is most appropriate when the predictors of interest are not time-varying.

Strohschein (2005) examined the impact of parental divorce on children's mental health trajectories over a 4-year period. At baseline, all the parents were married. There were significant differences in the intercepts and slopes of children whose parents divorced during the 4 years of observation compared to those whose parents did not divorce. At baseline, children whose parents later divorced reported significantly higher levels of depression, anxiety, and antisocial behavior than did children whose parents remained married. The "growth" in symptoms of depression and anxiety (but not antisocial behavior) also was significantly larger for children whose parents divorced.

In the other form of single-trajectory analysis, trajectories of an independent variable are used to predict a dependent variable. Barrett's (2000) previously described study of the effects of marital history illustrates this research design. Note that in this form of analysis, the dependent variable can be measured only at the final time of measurement (e.g., if mortality is the outcome), or baseline levels of the dependent variable can be included as an independent variable (as in Barrett's study). The latter case is residualized change analysis, and the independent variables predict direction and amount of change over time.

Dual-Trajectory Analysis

In most LGCA studies, trajectories of an independent variable are used to predict trajectories of the dependent variable. As in single-trajectory LGCA analysis, the independent variable can be a significant predictor of the intercept and/or slope of the dependent variable. In addition, the effects of fixed characteristics (e.g., gender, race/ethnicity) on the intercepts and slopes of both the independent and dependent variable are estimated.

Silverstein and Long (1998) used dual-trajectory analysis to examine the associations between trajectories of grandparents' perceived affection toward their adult grandchildren and trajectories of contact/proximity to grandchildren. Trajectories were based on five times of measurement spanning 23 years. The aggregate trajectory of affection toward grandchildren exhibited a linear decline for 14 years, followed by a modest rebound. The trajectory of contact/proximity declined at an accelerating rate over time. The investigators also compared older and younger cohorts of grandparents and found more rapid declines in contact/proximity in younger cohorts of grandparents. Because "independent" and "dependent" variables cover the same periods of time in LGCA, causal inference can be problematic. This study illustrates this point. Does grandparents' affection for their grandchildren decline as a result of declines in contact with and proximity to them? Or does declining affection for their grandchildren lead to declining contact with and proximity to them? Silverstein and Long carefully and appropriately avoided the language of causal inference in their interpretation of findings, and used the language of "association" rather than causality.

Triple-Trajectory Analysis and Beyond

In theory, LGCA can incorporate any number of trajectories. Taylor and Lynch's (2004) study of disability, depression, perceived social support, and received social support illustrates the use of more than two trajectories. Between-person longitudinal analyses indicate that disability is frequently an antecedent of depression in later life. Taylor and Lynch began their analysis by demonstrating that this finding also applies to trajectories of intraindividual change (i.e., trajectories of disability are strong predictors of trajectories of depressive symptoms over four times of measurement spanning 10 years). They then added trajectories of two forms of social support—perceived and received—to the analysis. Results revealed that trajectories of perceived support mediated the relationship between trajectories of disability and depression, but trajectories of received support did not. Thus, for persons who perceived increases over time in the amount and quality of social support available to them, growth in disability was not associated with growth in depression. In the absence of this perception, growth in support actually received did not prevent increasing disability from leading to increasing depression.

The studies reviewed here illustrate the potential of growth curve models to further our understanding of intraindividual patterns of stability and change over time. In particular, they provide evidence of the importance of identifying both differences in baseline levels of the variables of interest (i.e., their intercepts) and rates of growth over time (i.e., their slopes). LGCA is indeed a powerful method of identifying trajectories and their correlates, and for incorporating trajectories for multiple variables into a single analysis. Recall, however, that LGCA estimates a single aggregate trajectory for each variable and does not permit identification of distinct trajectories within a sample.

Identifying Trajectories in LCA

LCA, also known as mixture models or growth mixture models, is arguably the most flexible method for identifying empirically derived trajectories and modeling their antecedents and consequences. LCA analyses remain relatively rare in the social and behavioral sciences, but they are steadily increasing in volume.

Nagin and Tremblay (1999) used LCA to support a major challenge to conventional theories of physical aggression in early life. Previous studies of physical aggression typically focused on (1) children
of school age and older, and (2) levels of antisocial behavior during
the interval between school entry and late adolescence. Results of these
studies supported the view that physical aggression is a learned behavior—a perspective endorsed by two "blue ribbon panels": the National
Research Council (Reiss & Roth, 1994) and the Human Capital Initiative Coordinating Committee on Reducing Violence (1995). Nagin and
Tremblay (1999) suspected that research results supporting the conclusion that physical aggression is learned behavior were largely an artifact
of the ages of the samples investigated. In one of the rare studies of
physical aggression before age 6, Tremblay et al. (1999) demonstrated
that physical aggression peaks at approximately age 2 and declines
until age 6.

Nagin and Tremblay (1999) contributed further to the debate about
age-related patterns of physical aggression in a study that used LCA to
generate multiple trajectories of aggressive behavior among boys for
whom teachers reported physical aggression at ages 6, then annually
from ages 10 to 15. Previous between-person studies and LGCA analyses suggested an aggregate decline in physical aggression over time. It
was possible, however, that a small subset of boys increased in physical
aggression over time—a pattern that would not be observed using LGCA
but might emerge as a distinct trajectory using LCA. A four-trajectory
model fit the data best. The first trajectory comprised low levels of physical aggression at all ages. The second trajectory represented moderate
levels of aggression at age 6, with a decline to very low levels of aggression by age 10 and stability thereafter. The third trajectory represented
high levels of aggression at age 6, followed by steep linear declines in
aggression until age 15. The final trajectory, which described only about
5% of the sample, comprised chronic high levels of aggression from
ages 6 to 15. There was no evidence of a trajectory of escalating aggression over time, which would be expected if aggression is learned behavior. On the basis of their accumulated evidence, Nagin and Tremblay
posited that aggression is not a learned behavior, but an innate one, and
that children are socialized to suppress aggression as they age.

These studies illustrate two important features of trajectory analysis in general and LCA in particular. First, LCA can determine whether
a hypothesized trajectory that is not observed using LGCA is exhibited
by a small proportion of a sample. Second, this research reminds us
that the number and shape of trajectories differ depending on the number of times of measurement and the specific ages observed. The most

convincing evidence that physical aggression is innate and not learned is that aggressive behavior peaks during very early life and typically declines steadily thereafter.

Emerging Issues in Trajectory Analysis

As innovative statistical techniques are introduced to the scientific community, an evolutionary process typically occurs. In initial expositions, investigators devote considerable effort to describing the novel technique and illustrating its application. Over time, applications of the technique proliferate, and both description of the method and interpretation of results become relatively straightforward. It is during this period that investigators come to recognize the advantages and disadvantages of these techniques as well as subtleties that often are missed during initial—and often highly enthusiastic—explorations. In this section, I briefly review several aspects of LGCA and LCA that have emerged as their applications in the social sciences have increased.

The Importance of Time-Varying Dependent and Independent Variables

Several authors discuss the problem of using static characteristics to explain the trajectories generated by LGCA and LCA (e.g., Collins, 2006; Osgood, 2005). In some cases, investigators are interested in the effects of fixed statuses, such as race and gender. Too frequently, however, investigators predict trajectories on the basis of time-varying predictors that are measured at a single point in time. Both LGCA and LCA can model time-varying predictors and it generally makes sense to take full advantage of longitudinal data by modeling the dynamics of both predictors and outcomes. An efficient way to incorporate time-varying independent and dependent variables is to use trajectories of an independent variable to predict trajectories of the dependent variable.

Some scholars argue that even when fixed or early life characteristics are significant predictors of trajectories, they seldom *explain* patterns of change; rather, they anchor intervening but unmeasured explanatory processes. Sampson and Laub (2005a), for example, reported that the impetus for their application of life course theory to criminal behavior was their conviction that long-term patterns of criminal behavior could not rest solely on conditions in the distal past, as hypothesized by developmental theorists.

Turning Points and Path Dependencies

Adequate modeling of discontinuities over time can be challenging, even with sophisticated statistical techniques. In part this is because both LGCA and LCA generally model a polynomial function that is constrained to be smooth and to limit the number of directions in a given trajectory (Osgood, 2005). The likelihood of identifying trajectories with turning points or other discontinuities is greater in LCA than in conventional LGCA, because LCA generates multiple trajectories. Also, although I have seen few applications of it, Cudeck and Klebe (2002) describe a variant of LGCA called "piecemeal growth curve analysis," which can be used to identify discontinuities in continuous change models. In brief, it is specifically designed to capture nonlinear change adequately.

Path dependencies are similar to, but more specific than, turning points. A path dependency exists when patterns of change and stability differ for sample members who have and have not reached a specific state (Nagin & Tremblay, 2005a). For example, trajectories of sexual behavior may differ before and after puberty. Similarly, income trajectories may differ before and after divorce. Nagin and Tremblay argue that LGCA cannot identify path dependencies, but LCA can. Because investigators may not hypothesize path dependencies in advance, LCA provides a flexible strategy for observing them. This is especially important when the factor that creates the path dependency is age-related, yet not perfectly measured by age (e.g., puberty).

Recognizing the "Sensitivities" of LGCA and LCA

Investigators need to be aware that specific features of the temporal design of a study can have large effects on the results of LGCA and LCA. Eggleston, Laub, and Sampson (2004) demonstrated the substantial effects that three factors can have on the results of LCA. The first factor is length of follow-up and/or times of measurement. They convincingly demonstrated that even one additional time of measurement can substantially change the number and shape of trajectories generated by LCA. The second factor is inclusion of length of exposure or duration for the independent variables. Modeling duration of the independent variables, in terms of either specific levels of a continuous variable or time in a given state, can substantially change associations between predictors and trajectories. The third factor, including death as an outcome, can alter the number and shape of the observed trajectories.

Investigators often use secondary data to examine patterns of change and stability over time. In such cases, the investigator has no input into the temporal design of the data. Nonetheless, investigators should be aware that because their results may be specific to the temporal design of the study, they should empirically explore the implications of the temporal design to the extent possible.

Limits on the Temporal Specificity of LGCA and LCA

Finally, interpretation of the results of LGCA and LCA must always be tempered by the knowledge that neither technique captures all the change that occurs in a sample over time. As sophisticated as these statistical techniques are, they capture only a portion of the change that actually occurs. There are two primary reasons for this. First, as noted earlier, these techniques test various polynomial distributions and smooth results to describe the best-fitting trajectory (in LGCA) or trajectories (in LCA). Although LCA often reveals patterns of change not observed using LGCA, the measurement of true change remains incomplete. Second, because phenomena are not measured continuously in "real time," longitudinal data always miss some change and only estimate the timing of change. Obviously, this problem is greater for long intervals between measurements than for shorter intervals, but it is always present to some degree.

Osgood (2005) cautions against reification when interpreting the results of LGCA and LCA. One form of reification is to confuse the predicted, smoothed trajectories with the complex dynamics that the trajectories imperfectly measure. A second form of reification occurs when investigators take trajectories as actual entities rather than probabilistic patterns—especially when applied labels suggest that the trajectories represent homogeneous groups of people (e.g., early vs. late offenders). Thus, the cautionary lesson for investigators is to be wary about attributing a finite reality to complex patterns that do not exist.

Final Thoughts

Framing research questions about the life course in terms of intraindividual change is a relatively new era in social and behavioral research. By examining the effects of between-person characteristics on trajectories of intraindividual change, we employ a powerful analytic method for understanding how social factors shape personal biography. Trajectories also are a potent way to better understand heterogeneity—heterogeneity in life course patterns and the effects of heterogeneous social contexts. These sources of heterogeneity are unmeasured in more traditional between-person research designs.

Trajectories can generate significant theoretical and empirical contributions, but great care is needed in measuring and analyzing them. There are frequently tensions between how investigators desire to measure and analyze trajectories on the one hand, and data constraints on the other. Mastering the sophisticated statistical methods available for studying change over time is but a part of the investigator's responsibility. Theories may need to be reframed. Research questions must be well-crafted and carefully matched to relevant data sets and methods for answering those questions. Perhaps the most exciting aspect of trajectory-based research on the life course is that we have only begun to scratch the surface of its potential and promise.

CHAPTER 9

Group-Based Trajectories in Life Course Criminology

Elaine Eggleston Doherty
John H. Laub
Robert J. Sampson

A person's life course comprises multiple behavioral and social pathways, such as a marital trajectory, a work trajectory, and a criminal trajectory, to name a few. Trajectories depict long-term patterns of behavior and are marked by a sequence of transitions—events and roles—that evolve over shorter time spans. What has intrigued life course researchers is the variability among individual trajectories with respect to the timing, sequencing, and duration of these transitions and accompanying behaviors over time. (For a more detailed discussion on the concept and measurement of trajectories, see George, Chapter 8, this volume.)

Statistical methods that can model the variability in these developmental pathways have become more prevalent in life course research over the past several decades. Hierarchical modeling and latent growth curve analysis within a structural equation modeling framework are two such methods that traditionally have been used to identify and estimate within-individual change in a longitudinal perspective (for a review of these and other trajectory methods, see Raudenbush, 2001). One relatively recent addition to the list of methods that estimate developmental pathways over time is the group-based trajectory method, which is the focus of this chapter. In contrast to the previously mentioned traditional methods, the group-based trajectory method captures the heterogeneity of trajectories in a population by identifying distinct latent classes of meaningful subgroups of individuals who experience similar developmental patterns.

The technical components of group-based trajectory models, such as latent-class semiparametric mixture models (Nagin, 1999, 2005) and general growth mixture models (see Muthén, 2001, 2004; Muthén & Muthén, 2000), have been presented in several books, articles, and chapters over the past decade. In this chapter we focus on one group-based method—the semiparametric group-based method developed by Nagin and Land (1993; Nagin, 1999, 2005)—to examine the use of the group-based approach in life course criminology, with emphasis on the explanation of stability and change in offending, especially within-individual offending over time. In doing so, we draw on applications of this method in a long-term project examining crime over the life course (for background and details, see Laub & Sampson, 2003; Sampson & Laub, 1993).

The chapter plan is as follows: First, we describe the group-based trajectory method and trace the emergence of this technique in criminology. Second, we describe longitudinal data from the Gluecks' *Unraveling Juvenile Delinquency* study (1950, 1968) and subsequent follow-ups by John Laub and Robert Sampson. Next, we draw on these data to illustrate two different applications of group-based trajectory models. In the first application, we highlight how this method can be used to test group-based or taxonomic theories of crime, and specifically seek to uncover theoretically distinctive trajectories of offending (e.g., life course persistent offenders vs. adolescent-limited offenders). Then we illustrate how this method is used in assessing within-individual change, in which the growth patterns are hypothesized to be group based or to follow a multinomial distribution based on qualitative data. The chapter concludes with an overview of some extensions of group-based trajectories in disciplines outside of criminology that highlight the potential of this method for life course research.

The Group-Based Trajectory Method

A group-based trajectory method assumes that there are different groups of individuals whose patterns of behavior over time are homogeneous and enable a disaggregation of these trajectories to reveal the variability among groups in a population (e.g., Muthén, 2001, 2004; Muthén & Muthén, 2000; Nagin, 1999, 2005); that is, trajectory groups are meant to represent clusters of individuals who exhibit similar patterns of behavior throughout the life course. The method estimates the trajectory parameters (e.g., level, slope) for a fixed number of groups and determines the optimal number of groups based on goodness of fit with the data. Individuals are then assigned to the group to which they are most likely to belong based on their actual behavior patterns. The final result is a number of different temporal groups, each comprised of individuals who demonstrate similar patterns of behavior over time.

Although there are variations in group-based trajectory methods using different statistical packages, this chapter focuses primarily on Nagin's semiparametric group-based method using the Statistical Analysis System (SAS) PROC TRAJ macro (Jones, Nagin, & Roeder, 2001). This particular method has become quite popular, if not somewhat controversial, in the field of developmental and life course criminology.[1] However, the general discussion in this chapter applies to all group-based trajectory modeling techniques.[2]

The Emergence of Group-Based Trajectories in Criminology

Age is a key determinant in many human behaviors that develop over the life course, and crime is no exception. In the field of criminology, the age–crime curve is commonly recognized as a unimodal distribution of offending characterized by an increase in criminal activity in late childhood, followed by a peak in the teenage years and a decline in the early adult years that continues declining throughout adulthood (Hirschi & Gottfredson, 1983). This long-standing relationship provides the starting point for studying the longitudinal sequencing of an individual's criminal behavior over time (see Blumstein, Cohen, Roth, & Visher, 1986).

In the late 1980s, the question of whether this curve comprised a large number of offenders committing a few crimes or a few offenders committing a large number of crimes became a topic of great debate in criminological research (see Blumstein et al., 1988a; 1988b; Gottfredson & Hirschi, 1986, 1988; and, more recently, Osgood, 2005). One important contention in the debate was whether the criminal careers of individual offenders need to be elucidated. According to criminal career researchers, the age–crime curve should be disaggregated to reflect both participation in offending and frequency of offending at the individual level to understand criminal behavior better. In other words, the traditional approach of studying offending versus nonoffending in the aggregate should be abandoned in favor of examining the unique dimensions of each individual's offending career—onset, frequency of offending, career length, and termination (see Blumstein et al., 1986).

Drawing on the life course perspective (Elder, 1985b), Sampson and Laub (1993) developed what is now known as life course criminology. In general, life course theories of crime seek to explain stability and change in offending over time. Theoretical interest in understanding the longitudinal patterning of individual offending spawned a variety of methodologies to analyze these longitudinal data. As Land, McCall, and Nagin (1996, p. 409) stated, "It is now generally agreed that models of delinquent/criminal careers should be formulated, estimated, and tested at the individual level in order to take advantage of all the information available in longitudinal data sets of panels of individuals." To examine the developmental trajectories of offending and the factors that may affect these patterns of offending, analytic techniques to model criminal careers are needed to control for the individual variability in offending (i.e., take into account unobserved heterogeneity). The group-based trajectory approach is one such method used to assess stability and change in offending over time, while controlling for this unobserved heterogeneity. Before we turn to specific examples of criminological questions that the group-based trajectory approach is best suited to address, we describe the Gluecks' longitudinal data to illustrate the application of this method.

The Glueck Project

From 1930 to 1968, Sheldon and Eleanor Glueck, prominent researchers at Harvard Law School, spent much of their academic life conducting research on the causes of juvenile delinquency, adult crime, and the effectiveness of correctional systems (see Sampson & Laub, 1993). Their most famous project was the *Unraveling Juvenile Delinquency* study, which began in 1939 and sought to study the nature and development of delinquent and criminal behavior. In this study, the Gluecks identified 1,000 Boston males born between 1925 and 1932, and studied their criminal offending from childhood through age 32 (see Glueck & Glueck, 1950, 1968). They collected and analyzed family, school, attitudinal, behavioral, and life event data for the boys from childhood through young adulthood, drawing from several sources such as the boys themselves, their parents and teachers, employers and spouses, and others (e.g., social workers and psychiatrists), as well as a wide range of official data sources.

A matched sample of 500 males selected from two reform schools in Massachusetts, and 500 nondelinquent males selected from the Boston public school system was constructed. Each delinquent and nondelinquent pair was matched on age, ethnicity, IQ, and neighborhood socioeconomic status. All the boys were white, but their ethnicities ranged extensively, with the majority (69.2%) being English, Italian, or Irish

(Glueck & Glueck, 1950, p. 38). The average IQ score was approximately 93 (92.3 for the delinquents, and 94.2 for the nondelinquents). The majority of the sample came from neighborhoods with a delinquency rate of 10 per 1,000 to 24.9 per 1,000 (59.2% of the delinquents and 54.6% of the nondelinquents; Glueck & Glueck, 1950, pp. 36–38).

In 1987, John Laub and Robert Sampson began to reconstruct, augment, and reanalyze the Gluecks' *Unraveling Juvenile Delinquency* data. This effort resulted in the development of their age-graded theory of informal social control, as described in *Crime in the Making: Pathways and Turning Points through Life* (Sampson & Laub, 1993). The general organizing principle of this theory is that crime is more likely to occur when an individual's bond to society is attenuated or broken. Briefly, the theoretical framework was organized around three major themes: (1) Structural context is fundamentally mediated by informal family and school social controls, and it is weak informal social controls that explain delinquency in childhood and adolescence; (2) there is strong continuity in antisocial behavior from childhood through adulthood across a variety of life domains; and (3) informal social control in adulthood explains changes in adult crime, independent of prior individual differences in criminal propensity. Specifically, the stronger the adult ties to work and family, the less crime among both delinquents and nondelinquent controls (Sampson & Laub, 1993).

Crime in the Making addressed issues regarding the onset, continuation, and desistance from crime into early adulthood, but Sampson and Laub wanted to extend their investigation to crime in later life (i.e., middle and old age). Also, they sought to embark on a more person-based exploration of offending over the life course. Thus, in 1994, to add to the archived arrest and incarceration data from males ages 7 to 32, Sampson and Laub began a follow-up data-collection effort for the delinquent sample of the Glueck men, who then ranged from ages 62 to 70. In part, this follow-up included collecting annual criminal histories and death information for the delinquent sample to age 70. Laub and Sampson (2003) coded the newly collected criminal arrest data from ages 32 to 70 based on their in-depth search of Massachusetts and national criminal databases. The criminal history records include arrests for each age categorized as one of four offense types—violent (e.g., homicide), property (e.g., burglary), alcohol/drug offenses (e.g., drunkenness), and an "other" category (e.g., disorderly conduct) (Laub & Sampson, 2003, Chapter 4, Note 2). Mortality information from Massachusetts Vital Statistics and national death records were integrated into the longitudinal criminal histories to safeguard against presuming someone had stopped offending who had instead died—referred to as "false desisters" (Reiss 1989). Thus, the resulting long-term criminal history data include the annual number of arrests from ages 7 to 70 (including information up to age of death for those who died) and the annual days incarcerated from ages 7 to 32.

The follow-up effort also included interviewing 52 of the original delinquent men who were still alive at age 70. The purpose of these life history narratives was to "capture the heterogeneity of life-course experiences and uncover the dynamic process surrounding salient life-course events, turning points, and criminal offending" (Laub & Sampson, 2003, p. 66). This approach allowed Sampson and Laub to embrace a person-centered approach, to discover unanticipated hypotheses, and to integrate the quantitative criminal histories with narratives in an attempt to identify fully the mechanisms that connect salient life events with offending patterns across the life course (for more information on the full follow-up effort, see Laub & Sampson, 2003, Chapter 4). As seen below, these narratives help to illustrate how the group-based trajectory method can be used to empirically identify subgroups in a population when qualitative data reveal that distinct subgroups might exist.

Uses of the Group-Based Trajectory Method

In general, group-based trajectory methods are well-suited to research questions that seek to contrast discrete groups of individuals who are homogenous within their trajectory, yet distinct from those following other trajectories (see Nagin, 2005).[3] As with any method, there are advantages and disadvantages to using the group-based method, and the decision to use this particular application is based on the balance of these pros and cons (for a review, see Eggleston, Laub, & Sampson, 2004; Nagin, 2005; Piquero, 2008; Sampson, Laub, & Eggleston, 2004a). Instead of reiterating a list of these advantages and disadvantages in detail, we focus on research questions that, we believe, capitalize on the unique aspects of the group-based method.

The most basic distinction between traditional growth curve models and group-based growth models is that traditional methods assume that the developmental growth of a population is similar across all individuals. Thus, a population's trajectories can be best described by estimating the average trajectory and the deviations from that average. In contrast, the group-based approach assumes that individuals within a population do not change similarly, and the population is best described by estimating the trajectories of two or more subgroups within that population to capture the different developmental pathways. In other words, the group-based trajectory model does not assume a continuous distribution of growth but rather a multinomial distribution that can be approximated with a number of points of support (i.e., a number of groups; Nagin, 2005).[4] Thus, one advantage of the group-based approach is that it hypothesizes that there are several distinct groupings of individuals who display similar behavior over time. The group-based method, then, seems best suited to (1) test group-based or taxonomic developmental theories and (2) analyze questions of within-individual change, in which growth patterns are known or explicitly hypothesized as being distinct and different across a small number of groups (i.e., they do not follow a continuous distribution).

In the past few years, there has been concern about the seemingly widespread use of the group-based trajectory method in situations in which there is no a priori rationale to assume the existence of groups (see Raudenbush, 2005; Sampson & Laub, 2005a). Therefore, we seek to focus this chapter on research questions that call for the unique characteristics of group-based trajectories and in which the assumption of groups can be exploited to inform our understanding of criminal offending over the life course. To this end, we first draw on published work to illustrate how group-based trajectories are well suited to testing taxonomic theories. Second, we use the Gluecks' *Unraveling Juvenile Delinquency* study (1950, 1968) and subsequent follow-ups to age 70, conducted by Laub and Sampson (2003), to estimate group-based trajectories of incarceration and criminal offending. Our interest is in analyzing questions of within-individual change when qualitative data indicate that there are two or more groups of individuals with distinct patterns of offending.

Testing Group-Based Theories

A prime example in which group-based trajectories are particularly useful is the research question that seeks to test a group-based theory. In the 1990s, developmental psychologists and criminologists promoted the idea of typologies of offenders, positing that there are two groups of offenders in the population, with different ages of onset, different offending patterns over the life course, and different causes linked to their offending. For instance, Terrie Moffitt introduced her dual-taxonomy theory (1993), which explicitly theorizes about two distinct groups of offenders—a life course persister group and an adolescent-limited group. Although there are other group-based theories of delinquency, such as Patterson's theory of early- and late-onset offenders (Patterson & Yoerger, 1993), Moffitt's theory is the most well developed and empirically tested taxonomic theory. Thus, we discuss Moffitt's theory in detail here and review a select set of studies using the group-based approach that has focused on testing her theory (for a more extensive and comprehensive review of studies using the trajectory method, see Piquero, 2008).

According to Moffitt, a small percentage of the population begins exhibiting antisocial behavior in childhood and is involved in crime throughout the life course. This group of offenders is aptly labeled the life course persister group. Neurological deficits and negative environment–person interactions characterize this group of offenders, who display difficult behavior as early as age 3 in everyday interactions and manifest this difficult behavior as offending throughout adolescence and adulthood. The second group of offenders, who comprise the vast majority, are in the adolescent-limited group, whose offending careers are limited to adolescence as a result of peer influence and social mimicry. The motivation to offend stems from a gap between societal age and biological age in a struggle for mature status that is unattainable through prosocial means. In summary, the adolescent-limited offender mimics the delinquent behavior of his or her life course persistent peers to attain a sense of maturity and independence. However, as adult status is achieved naturally, the adolescent-limited offender desists from offending. Thus, the life course persister has an early age of onset and is characterized by behavioral continuity over the life course, whereas the adolescent-limited offender has a postpubertal onset and is characterized by behavioral change over the life course, with his or her offending restricted to the adolescent years (see Moffitt, 1993).

Several studies to date have used the group-based trajectory method to investigate the existence of these hypothesized groups and their corresponding etiologies. For instance, Nagin, Farrington, and Moffitt (1995) analyzed the Cambridge Study of Delinquent Development conviction data for men ages 10–32, using the group-based trajectory method to identify the two distinct groups of offenders statistically and to determine whether the groups have different etiological paths. Rather than two groups that best describe the sample's offending over time, the study found *three* groups of offenders with distinctive life course trajectories of offending—a high-level chronic group, a low-level chronic group, and an adolescent-limited group—along with a group of nonoffenders. These groups did manifest important cross-group differences, yet the results were not entirely in agreement with the theorized hypotheses. For instance, although the adolescent-limited group demonstrated an official decline in offending after adolescence, they also showed a continued self-reported pattern of employee theft, drug use, heavy drinking, and fighting, which is inconsistent with Moffitt's theory.

Similarly, Fergusson, Horwood, and Nagin (2000) used a group-based modeling approach for individuals followed from birth to age 18 to test the predicted hypotheses put forth by Moffitt and Patterson.

Again, rather than finding two groups, their analysis identified *four* groups including a group of nonoffenders and a group of moderate-level offenders, in addition to the hypothesized adolescent-limited and chronic offender groups. Moreover, they found mixed evidence in favor of the group-based theories with respect to the distinguishing etiological characteristics of each trajectory group.

This heterogeneity in offending and its relationship with group-based theories was also studied by Chung, Hill, Hawkins, Gilchrist, and Nagin (2002), who found *five* trajectories to best characterize offending from ages 13 to 21 in the Seattle Social Development Project sample. In addition to a group of chronic offenders and a desister group, this study also identified a group of nonoffenders, a group of late-onset offenders, and a group of escalating offenders. Although analysis of childhood predictors of these offending patterns revealed some evidence in favor of Moffitt and Patterson's group-based theories, the researchers conclude that, overall, different etiological theories do not seem necessary to distinguish between the various trajectories of offending.

Sampson and Laub (2003) used their data for 500 delinquent boys from age 7 to age 70 in the Gluecks' study and the group-based trajectory method to test the validity of the life-course-persistent component of Moffitt's theory (see also Laub & Sampson, 2003). Based on their analysis of the total offending trajectories for these men, Sampson and Laub reached three primary conclusions. First, they identified *six* offending trajectories, again rejecting Moffitt's notion of only two offending groups. Second, although there was a small group of high-rate chronic offenders, all six trajectory groups, including the high-rate "chronics," displayed a declining pattern of offending as they entered middle and late adulthood. Thus, there was no flat trajectory pattern of a true life course persister, as Moffitt's theory would predict. Third, after establishing the groups of offenders through the group-based trajectory method, Sampson and Laub tested whether the common childhood predictors among life-course persisters could distinguish between the trajectory groups. They included 13 individual risk factors that are characteristic of life course persistent offenders, as theorized by Moffitt, such as measures of IQ, aggression, and early onset of misbehavior. However, none of these numerous hypothesized risk factors could distinguish the chronic offender (or life course persister equivalent) from the other five groups of offenders. Sampson and Laub concluded that desistance processes are at work even among predicted life course persistent offenders, and that childhood prognoses account poorly for long-term trajectories of offending.

In a more recent work, Sampson and Laub (2005b) revisit the idea that developmentally distinct groups of offenders can be explained by unique causal processes. More specifically, they use a group-based trajectory model for "other" crimes (i.e., crimes that are minor from a legal perspective but capture important dimensions of deviant or antisocial activities). These other crimes include disorderly conduct, vagrancy, gambling, speeding, lewdness, desertion, and family nonsupport. Again, heterogeneity in offending trajectories is present, and the data firmly reject a simple typology of two offender groups. There are instead *five* groups of offending patterns by age that emerge for other offenses. Note that these results generally conform to the patterns for total offending, as well as crime-specific trajectories (see Laub & Sampson, 2003, pp. 104–106). Most important to our discussion is that the differences across groups seem to be age at desistance and rate of offending, but regardless of these differences, all groups eventually declined in offending with age. Moreover, there is little evidence of categorical groupings of men with distinct offender trajectories that can be accurately or meaningfully predicted in the prospective sense among high-risk adolescent delinquents. Although these analyses focused on Moffitt's theory, the most detailed and articulate theoretical statement of a taxonomic criminological theory to date, these results have implications for all group-based theories of crime (see Loeber & Hay, 1997; Patterson & Yoerger, 1993).

Taken together, these studies find that between *three* and *six* trajectory groups best fit the data, with some combination of not only a relatively small, high-rate chronic group and an adolescent-peaked desister group, as predicted by Moffitt, but also a variety of other trajectory groups that she did not predict.[5] Importantly, each of these empirical tests of group-based hypotheses was facilitated by the group-based trajectory model, founded on the notion of testing whether specific groups of offenders can be identified (see Nagin & Land, 1993).

Assuming the Existence of Distinct Groups

The second ideal situation for use of group-based trajectories occurs when extant data indicate that groups of individuals within a population exhibit behavioral trajectories that are similar to others in their group but distinct from those in other groups. To illustrate this situation, we draw on life history narratives regarding juvenile incarceration experiences among the men in the Gluecks' study and examine the impact of juvenile incarceration on future criminal offending. By design, all members of the delinquent sample in the Gluecks' study were confined in reform school at some point between ages 7 and 16. In the narrative data collected in old age, the impact of juvenile incarceration on future offending emerged as salient, yet the effect was not uniform. Whereas some men viewed reform school as a transformative experience that led in part to their desistance from crime, others reported that it was a negative experience that translated in part into later crime. The following excerpts from the men themselves illustrate these contrasting perspectives.

For men like Leon, reform school was perceived as a positive experience. At the time of his interview at age 70, Leon thought that the Lyman School for Boys was a "turning point in his life." He described the reform school as offering a "learning environment" (see also Laub & Sampson, 2003, pp. 122–123). Leon recounted:

> "I mean it might sound silly—I thought it was great. I mean they taught you a lot of things there. They taught you to respect yourself, and no matter what you did you were dressed up every day, you were clean, you went to school.... I might have been one out of a thousand that got anything out of it, but still, I go back to that whenever I think of a change in my life."[6]

For others, like David, it was the negative aspects of reform school that served as a turning point. In his interview at age 68, David stated that staying at Lyman was a "horrible experience" and could be viewed as having a deterrent effect (see also Laub & Sampson, 2003, pp. 130–131). David elaborated:

> "It was bad. Real bad. You see these pictures [today] about torturing the kids. Well, they did then, let me tell you. Well, we'd come in from a march out in the cold, and ... and you were walking beside him [another inmate] and I says 'How is everything going today?' and if the counselor heard you he'd take you back in the room and take your shoes off and you had to hold your feet up with no shoes on and he had a stick that big [about 2 feet long] and that thick [about 2 inches] and he'd give you 10 whacks. Now you can't walk. And if you dropped your foot down you'd get another 10. I mean the pain was right up through your leg. And then they'd take you in the corner and they'd pound the living shit out of you."

In a nutshell, both men reported that their desistance from crime was, at least in part, due to their juvenile incarceration experiences, even though Leon reported that it was the positive aspects of reform school and David expressed that reform school was a negative influence.

For other men, the juvenile incarceration experience was seen as criminogenic and a contributing factor in adult crime and imprisonment. Especially deleterious was the view that reform school fostered cynicism and defiance of the criminal justice system. For example,

Buddy thought that the reason he kept getting in trouble was that the Lyman School experience made him "so mad" that he "just hated society for the rest of his life" (see Laub & Sampson, 2003, p. 174). At age 69, he told the following story:

> "I was threw in with guys your size [6 feet, 2 inches, 200 pounds] and I'm only a kid 12 years old. They'd punch you right in the face, you know. Beat the hell out of you; like if you pissed in bed, which I used to do when I was a kid. I was very nervous or something. They'd scrub you with scrubbing brushes and stuff like that. They'd scrub you until you was raw; your skin was all raw. So I got so aggravated because of this experience that I hated any kind of rules or regulations, you know, when I got out. And I'd do things just because I wanted to aggravate people. You know what I'm saying? I wasn't mean. I wouldn't try to hurt people. But I'd take their money away from them. Like walk into a store and stick them up or something like that. But the only reason I did that—I don't think it was because I was so greedy. Because I didn't look for a whole bunch of money. It was just that I wanted something and that was where I was going to get it."[7]

In contrast to Leon and David, Buddy cites his juvenile experiences as being instrumental in his persistence in crime.

Taken together, these life history narratives indicate that the method necessary to investigate the impact of juvenile incarceration on future offending needs to allow for multiple trajectories of offending in adulthood that may be linked to the varying juvenile experiences. Using the juvenile incarceration data and young adult criminal offending data, we can begin to address two key questions:

1. Can we identify different patterns of juvenile incarceration among the full delinquent sample?
2. Can these patterns of incarceration be meaningfully linked to the divergent trajectories of persistence and desistance in offending over time, as reported by the men interviewed later in life?

Linking Incarceration and Offending with Group-Based Trajectories

Although all of the delinquent boys were incarcerated as juveniles, official records indicate considerable variability in their patterns of incarceration time during these years (see Sampson & Laub, 1993; Sampson, Laub, & Eggleston, 2004b). To test whether the differences in future offending patterns are associated with heterogeneity in the juvenile incarceration experiences of the men, we first modeled their trajectories of incarceration to capture simultaneously the timing and duration of the men's reform school experiences using the group-based trajectory method. This technique allowed us to identify distinct groups of boys who display similar trajectories of incarceration over time. We then estimate the trajectories for total adult offending for ages 17 to 32, taking into account time incarcerated.[8]

One method to address whether juvenile incarceration fosters recidivism or leads to termination in offending is to identify the relationship between the identified incarceration trajectories during adolescence and offending trajectories in adulthood. It is then possible to calculate the probability of being in a specific adult offending trajectory for those in each juvenile incarceration trajectory. A second method to test the relationship between the juvenile incarceration trajectory and future offending patterns is to analyze the trajectories of young adult offending separately for each juvenile incarceration trajectory group. These models allow us to control for any latent or unobserved heterogeneity in incarceration experiences, while studying whether there is heterogeneity in future offending. The key question here is: Within each group of individuals who display a similar juvenile incarceration experience, is there heterogeneity in future offending trajectories?[9]

Group-Based Trajectories of Incarceration

We begin the analysis by modeling the boys' incarceration experiences from ages 7 to 16, and estimating intercept and slope parameters for each trajectory group.[10] The trajectory method estimates these model parameters using maximum likelihood for a fixed number of groups. Although every individual in each group is constrained to the same slope and intercept of that trajectory, the level and shape of the trajectory are free to vary by group (Nagin, 2005, p. 33). To begin the estimation process, an incrementally larger number of groups is estimated, and the optimal number of groups is determined by the Bayesian Information Criterion (BIC), which can inform the selection of the best model for comparison of both nested and unnested models (for equation information, see Nagin, 2005, p. 64; see also D'Unger, Land, McCall, & Nagin, 1998). This procedure then assigns each individual a probability of membership in each group (for equation information, see Nagin, 2005, p. 79). Based on these probabilities, each individual is assigned to the group to which he is most likely to belong based on his incarceration pattern. These probabilities can also assess model fit using a number of model diagnostics, such as average posterior probabilities and odds of correct classification.[11] After evaluating all of these diagnostics as a group, we concluded that five groups were optimal to characterize the juvenile incarceration patterns of these men. These incarceration trajectories are described in detail in the next section.

Group-Based Trajectories of Offending

A similar procedure is used to estimate trajectories of offending in young adulthood.[12] Specifically, we estimate the offending trajectories, while accounting for incarceration time at each age. The simplest model of offending trajectories assumes that exposure time for everyone is equal (i.e., everyone is "free" to offend all 365 days of each year). However, prior research shows that the negligence of incarceration time in the rate of offending could result in an underestimation of the actual offending trajectory (Eggleston et al., 2004) and we know that several of the men in the Gluecks' study were incarcerated for extended periods of time between ages 17 and 32. Therefore, because exposure time is not equal, we included a parameter in the estimation that accounts for the time a person was in the community and "free" to offend each year. This added parameter incorporates the amount of time each person spent in the community each year. With this additional parameter, the predicted number of offenses for each person is weighted, such that it represents the number of offenses a person is predicted to commit had he been free 365 days of each year. For instance, if a person is incarcerated for half the year at age 26 and incurred two arrests in that year, he would be predicted to have committed four offenses had he been free that whole year. The BIC, along with other model diagnostics, again determines the optimal number of groups, which is six offending trajectories. The results of these trajectory groups are described in detail below.

Results

   Trajectories of Juvenile Incarceration. Figure 9.1 depicts the trajectory patterns for the five juvenile incarceration trajectories identified using the group-based trajectory method.[13] We have named the trajectory groups based on their incarceration patterns and placed the estimated proportion of the population belonging to each group in parentheses next to each group's label.[14]

   What is clear from Figure 9.1 is that although everyone in the sample was incarcerated at least once before age 17, their patterns over time are quite distinct with respect to timing and length of incarceration. The first, very small group comprises boys whom we considered to be "institutionally raised" youth. These boys began their incarceration

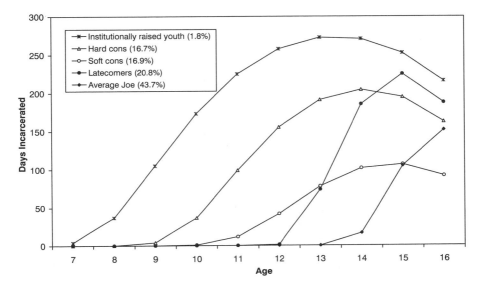

FIGURE 9.1. Incarceration trajectories: Ages 7–16.

experiences at a very young age and spent well over half of each year incarcerated, beginning around age 11. These boys were the first to be incarcerated and spent an average of over 5 years of incarceration out of the possible 10-year juvenile period. The second group, labeled the "hard cons" group, comprises 16.7% of the population. These boys also spent a considerable amount of time incarcerated beginning at a young age. However, their experiences were not as extreme as those of the "institutionally raised" youth. We labeled the third group "soft cons." This group also spent a number of years incarcerated. However, the boys spent many fewer days of each year in reform school than the other two chronically incarcerated groups, averaging approximately one-fourth of each year, beginning at age 13.

The fourth and fifth groups were incarcerated at a later age but spent a considerable amount of time incarcerated once they entered reform school. The "latecomers," who comprise 20.8% of the population, were incarcerated, beginning at age 12, and spent over half of each year on average in reform school, starting at age 14. This amount of time in confinement is comparable to that of the "hard cons" for these 3 years of adolescence (ages 14–16). Finally, the "average Joe" group, which is the largest group (43.7% of the population), included boys who were the oldest upon first incarceration yet were very close to reaching the level of the "hard cons" and "latecomers" groups in average number of days incarcerated per year by age 16 (150 days on average).

Overall, what is clear from this trajectory analysis is that although each juvenile delinquent was incarcerated, the actual amount of time, number of years incarcerated, and trajectory of incarceration vary considerably. Therefore, one hypothesis is that the differences in the offending patterns reported by the interviewed men are a result of these varying juvenile incarceration experiences. To test this hypothesis, we next analyzed the trajectories of young adult offending for the total sample, then separately for each juvenile incarceration trajectory group.

Trajectories of Young Adult Offending While Free. Figure 9.2 shows total offending trajectories while free, from ages 17 to 32—that is, the total predicted number of offenses for each individual weighted by the amount of time that person was "free" to offend in the community each year from ages 17 to 32.[15] Overall, as expected, there is considerable variability in the offending trajectories of these men who experienced different juvenile incarceration experiences. There are several general trends of offending, such as nonoffending (34.5% of the population), low-level offending (16.2% of the population), decliners I and II offending (19.6% and 13.7%, respectively), and high- and low-level chronic offending (8.8% and 7.1%, respectively).

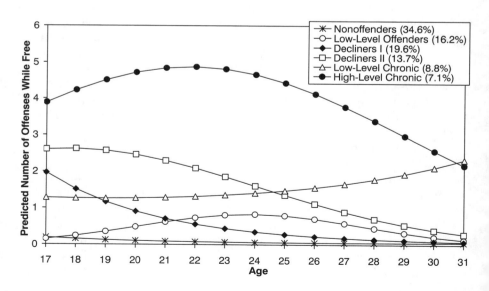

FIGURE 9.2. Young adult total offending while free: Ages 17–32.

One statistical advantage is that the group-based trajectory analysis assigns each person to the trajectory group to which he is most likely to belong, based on the posterior probabilities from the trajectory analyses. Thus, each man was placed into a juvenile incarceration group and a young adult offending group based on these probabilities (see Nagin, 2005, for more details). From these two sources of data, we then calculated the conditional probabilities of belonging to a certain adult offending trajectory group given membership in a certain juvenile incarceration group. This analysis provides information such as the following: What percentage of the juvenile "hard cons" were nonoffenders in adulthood? What percentage were high-rate offenders?

Linking Incarceration and Offending Trajectories. Table 9.1 displays these conditional probabilities. For ease of interpretation, we collapsed some of the groups. First, because the "institutionally raised youth" have such a low sample size and display a similar trajectory to that of the "hard cons" (although at a higher level), these men are combined with the "hard cons" for the following analyses. Second, we combined the two declining offender groups in the young adult offending model, because they also displayed similar patterns of offending, with differences only in level.

As Table 9.1 shows, there is a significant relationship between juvenile incarceration and young adult offending while free, based on a chi-square test ($p < .001$).[16] However, although the majority of the

TABLE 9.1. Conditional Probability of Young Adult Offending Group by Juvenile Incarceration Group

Juvenile incarceration trajectory group (ages 7–16)	Total offending while free trajectory group (ages 17–32)					
	Nonoffenders	Low-level offenders	Declining offenders	Low-level chronic	High-rate chronic	Total
Hard cons	29	9	41	4	6	89
	32.6%	10.1%	46.1%	4.5%	11.2%	100%
Soft cons	40	12	15	5	2	74
	54.1%	16.2%	20.3%	6.8%	9.5%	100%
Latecomers	23	10	44	9	15	101
	22.8%	9.9%	43.6%	8.9%	14.9%	100%
Average Joe	81	42	62	20	11	216
	37.5%	19.4%	28.7%	9.3%	5.1%	100%

Note. Chi-square = 44.397, $p < .001$.

"soft cons" and "average Joe" groups are nonoffenders, in general, the majority of the men in either the nonoffending or the declining groups regardless of their juvenile incarceration trajectory. In addition, the "soft cons" group has the highest chance of nonoffending (54.1%) and the lowest chance of high-level chronic offending (2.7%) in young adulthood compared to those in the other juvenile trajectory groups. In contrast, the "latecomers" have the lowest chance of nonoffending (22.8%) and the highest chance of chronic offending in young adulthood (14.9%) compared to those in the other juvenile trajectory groups. These findings imply that a steady but low-level incarceration over adolescence—the "soft con" trajectory—may produce the most positive criminal justice outcomes later, whereas later but high-level incarceration—the "latecomer" trajectory—is the most detrimental for future offending. Similar analyses on the crime-specific trajectories of young adult offending while free concur with these conclusions (Sampson et al., 2004b).

To investigate this issue further, we next analyze the trajectories of adult offending while free separately for each juvenile incarceration trajectory group. Figures 9.3a through 9.3d show the adult offending rates for the "hard cons," the "soft cons," the "latecomers," and the "average Joe" groups when analyzed individually.[17] As Figure 9.3a shows, for the group of "hard cons," five distinct developmental trajectories of adult offending while free emerged as the optimal number. Interestingly, these trajectories show that 30% committed no offenses while free (Group 1), 22% desisted by age 26 (Group 3), and another 30% followed a desisting pathway throughout adulthood (Group 4). The remaining 7% were chronic offenders to age 32. Thus, for those who were incarcerated at an early age and for much of their juvenile years, such experiences seemed to reduce recidivism for some but "backfire" for others and not dissuade them from future offending.

This result is evident for each of the juvenile incarceration trajectories. For instance, among the "soft cons" (Figure 9.3b), a sizable group of offenders continue to offend throughout adulthood (13.3%, Group 3) yet the majority are either adult nonoffenders (52.6%, Group 2) or adult desisters (19.9%, Group 4). Among the "latecomers" (Figure 9.3c), a wide variety of patterns is evident. First, there is a group that increases in its offending while free between ages 17 and 32 (Group 6) and a high-rate, although declining group (Group 3), in addition to the adult desister groups (Groups 4 and 5) and a nonoffending group (Group 1). Finally, the members of the "average Joe" group (Figure 9.3d), who were incarcerated later in adolescence but at a high rate, also show considerable variability in offending patterns, with two groups of stable offenders, one with 3.5 offenses per year free up to age 32 (Group 2) and

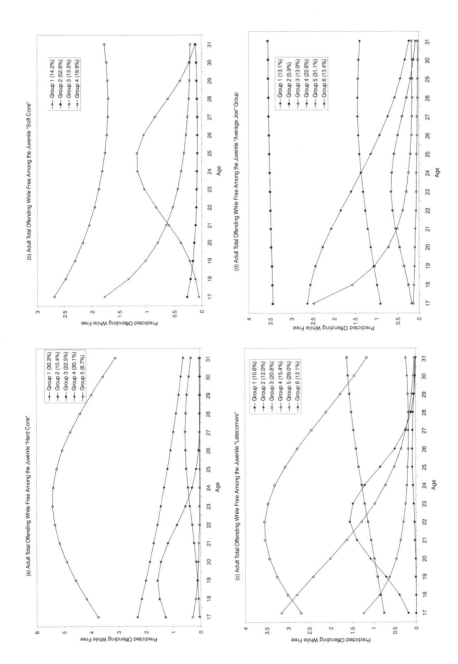

FIGURE 9.3. Young adult total offending while free, by juvenile incarceration group.

another that averages one offense per year free. Overall, one-fifth of this large group does not desist from offending in adulthood to age 32, whereas almost one-third remains nonoffenders.

Taken together, the analysis indicates a considerable amount of heterogeneity in offending, regardless of the juvenile incarceration pattern. Thus, the quantitative data may not be tapping into the complexity of juvenile incarceration revealed in the life history narrative accounts regarding reform school. Perhaps the persistence and desistance patterns among men with similar incarceration experiences (i.e., timing and duration of incarceration) depicted in Figure 9.3 depend on their individual characteristics and perceptions. These individual factors may interact with the reform school experiences in a way that would predict whether a person persists in offending or desists. Although a test of this and other, future hypotheses regarding the impact of juvenile incarceration on future offending patterns are beyond the scope of this chapter, what these analyses do convey is that the group-based trajectory method is a useful tool in understanding the complexity and heterogeneity of behavior.

We now step back from illustrations of how this method has been used within life course criminology and examine its application in other disciplines that investigate within-individual stability and change over time.

Group-Based Trajectories across Disciplines

Group-based trajectory methods are applicable to a wide range of populations within a variety of disciplines beyond criminology, such as those found in psychology, education, sociology, and medicine/public health, to name a few. In fact, group-based trajectories have already gained popularity in many of these disciplines, as evidenced by their regular appearance in the literature. Group-based trajectories have been used to examine a diverse array of outcomes among a variety of populations.

In the field of psychology, the group-based method has been applied to phenomena such as psychological well-being among retirees (Wang, 2007), posttraumatic stress disorder symptoms among Gulf War veterans (Orcutt, Erikson, & Wolfe, 2004), and depressive symptoms after the loss of a spouse or parent to Alzheimer's disease (Aneshensel, Botticello, & Yamamoto-Mitani, 2004). Prevention scientists have also used this method in an attempt to identify at-risk youth in need of targeted interventions, for instance, aggressive youth (Schaeffer et al., 2006). In education, the development of number skills among kindergartners has been modeled (Jordan, Kaplan, Olah, & Locuniak, 2006).

In sociology, researchers have investigated issues such as women's employment patterns after the birth of their children (Hynes & Clarkberg, 2005), patterns of welfare receipt among female high school dropouts (Hamil-Luker, 2005), family poverty trajectories among children (Wagmiller, Lennon, Kuang, Alberti, & Aber, 2006), and the educational outcomes of children and adolescents with varying developmental trajectories of internalizing and externalizing problems (McLeod & Fettes, 2007). The medical and public health fields have also begun to use group-based methods to examine the progression of medical conditions and treatments, such as chronic low back pain (Dunn, Jordan, & Croft, 2006), childhood obesity (Mustillo et al., 2003), and nighttime bedwetting in children (Croudace, Jarvelin, Wadsworth, & Jones, 2003). Therefore, although this chapter focuses on criminological patterns of offending and incarceration, the method is clearly not restricted to criminology or to behavioral sciences in general, because it can be applied to modeling patterns over time among many disciplines and types of phenomena.

Conclusion

Since the group-based trajectory approach was introduced to the field of criminology, there has been an ever growing number of substantive studies using the method, numerous articles and books on the statistical intricacies of the method, as well as heated debates about the advantages, disadvantages, and misconceptions of this technique. In this chapter, we have sought to outline some unique advantages of group-based trajectories and their value over other methods for understanding factors that affect individual variation in the life course. To this end, we have described one group-based trajectory method, Nagin's semiparametric approach, and have illustrated two key uses of this method in life course criminological research from a long-term project studying the stability and change in crime over the life course.

In light of the growing use of group-based trajectories across a wide variety of disciplines with diverse populations and phenomena, we offer one fundamental caution. Researchers may all too easily be lured into using a new method, such as the group-based trajectory method, for the sole reason that it is, indeed, a new and seemingly exciting way to analyze within-individual change in behavior over time. Thus, the general lesson of this chapter is that users of the group-based trajectory method need to think about how they can exploit the method's unique characteristics and advantages to benefit the body of knowledge within their disciplines. After all, statistical models are tools for theory and research, and are not ends in themselves. To embrace any method without theory leads to disciplinary bankruptcy through simple-minded research (see Curran & Willoughby, 2003; Laub, 2006). That said, we look forward to seeing how the group-based trajectory method and its extensions can advance our knowledge about criminological and non-criminological phenomena and ultimately enhance our understanding of the life course.

Notes

1. The reader is encouraged to read the exchange between Nagin and Tremblay (2005a) and Raudenbush (2005) in the special issue of the *Annals of the American Academy of Political and Social Science*, and the exchange between Nagin and Tremblay (2005b) and Sampson and Laub (2005a) in *Criminology* to gain a better understanding of the theoretical and methodological nuances affiliated with the group-based method.
2. The methodological differences between the variety of group-based models and accompanying software programs are not discussed. The reader is encouraged to read Nagin and Land (1993), Nagin (1999, 2005), Muthén and Muthén (2000), Muthén (2004), and Kreuter and Muthén (2008) to obtain a sense of the methodological differences in modeling change over time using these popular group-based approaches.
3. The group-based methods we discuss in this chapter were designed for quantitative data containing at least four data points over time. The emphasis is on creating empirically derived groups rather than groupings based on ad hoc subjective constructions.
4. There is considerable debate regarding the optimal number of groups, whether or not trajectory groups can be derived from a continuous but non-normal distribution, and whether trajectory groups actually exist (see Bauer & Curran, 2003; Raudenbush, 2005).
5. In a review of over 80 empirical studies, Piquero finds that "on average, between three and five groups tend to be identified by trajectory methodology" (2008, p. 49).
6. For additional life history narratives describing the positive influence of reform school, see Laub and Sampson (2003, pp. 125–131).
7. For some additional life history accounts describing the negative experiences (i.e., violence and abuse) and the "backfiring" effect of reform school and prison, see Laub and Sampson (2003, pp. 167–169, 188–189, 218–219).
8. To estimate the incarceration trajectories, we use the semiparametric censored normal model. This model is appropriate when a large portion of the sample is concentrated at the lowest end of the observed measure (i.e., 0 days incarcerated per year) and/or a smaller portion of the sample is concentrated at the maximum point of the observed measure (i.e., 365 days incarcerated per year). To estimate offending trajectories we employ the

semiparametric mixed Poisson model, which is appropriate for modeling count data such as number of arrests per year, taking into account incarceration time (i.e., arrests per year while free; Nagin, 1999, 2005).

9. The measures used in these analyses are described in detail in Sampson and Laub (1993) and Sampson et al. (2004b).

10. To model the incarceration trajectories, we use the censored normal distribution within the group-based trajectory framework. In this model, each developmental trajectory assumes a quadratic relationship that links age and incarceration days, truncated at 0 and 365. Incarceration days are assumed to be an indicator of a latent or unobserved variable of behavior (y_{it}^{*j}), which is illustrated by the equation $y_{it}^{*j} = \beta_0^j + \beta_1^j age_{it} + \beta_2^j age_{it}^2 + \varepsilon_{it}$ where y_{it}^{*j} is the latent variable as observed through incarceration time for person i in group j for time period t, age_{it} is the age of person i for time period t, age_{it}^2 is the squared age of person i for time period t, and the coefficients β_0^j, β_1^j, and β_2^j structure the shape of the trajectory for each group j. The error term ε_{it} is assumed to be normally distributed.

11. Nagin (2005) describes several diagnostics to better assure the user that the selected model is adequately capturing the heterogeneity in the sample and not identifying nonsensical groups. The first diagnostic is the average posterior probability of assignment for each group. This measure reflects the accuracy or certainty of group assignment. The closer the average posterior probability is to 1, the more certain a researcher can be about the group assignment. Also, a simple comparison between the group probabilities that are estimated for the population and the actual proportion of individuals assigned to the group can be informative. The closer these proportions are, the more adequate the model. A related diagnostic is the odds of correct classification (OCC), which measures the predictive capacity of the average probability of assignment beyond random chance (Nagin, 2005, p. 88). This diagnostic uses the average posterior probability and the estimated proportion of the population for each group to estimate the odds of correct classification. The larger the OCC, the better the assignment accuracy.

12. Specifically, the group-based model used for arrest data is the semiparametric mixed Poisson model, in which the predicted number of offenses at each age for each trajectory group is estimated; each developmental trajectory assumes a quadratic relationship that links age and offending. This estimation is illustrated by the equation $\log \lambda_{it}^j = \beta_0^j + \beta_1^j age_{it} + \beta_2^j age_{it}^2$, where λ_{it}^j is the predicted rate of offending for person i in group j for time period t, age_{it} is the age of person i for time period t, age_{it}^2 is the squared age of person i for time period t, and the coefficients β_0^j, β_1^j, and β_2^j structure the shape of the trajectory for each group j.

13. The mean group assignment probabilities for this incarceration analysis range from .90 to .99.

14. It should be noted that these labels are not meant to reflect groups that occur in reality. The technique is used as a heuristic device to cluster the data with respect to their developmental trajectories over time. Also, these labels are assigned relative to other groups in the sample. For instance, the

label "hard cons" is relative to others in this delinquent sample, who arguably all might be considered "hard cons."

15. The mean classification probabilities for the offending analyses range from
.82 to .92.

16. Although there is inherent classification error in the group assignments,
the errors of inference using conventional methods are small as long as the
classification is high (see Nagin, 1999, footnote 11).

17. Again, because there are only eight people in the "institutionally raised"
group, we collapsed the "hard cons" and the "institutionally raised" youth
and labeled them "hard cons." When the institutionally raised group was
analyzed separately, the latent class analysis identified only a single trajectory as the optimal number of groups. The offending trajectory for this
group shows steady offending between 0.4 and 0.5 offenses, which begins to
decline slowly at age 23. However, it should be noted that two of these eight
men spent the vast majority of their adulthood to age 32 incarcerated, and
one of the eight men died at the age of 23.

INVESTIGATING EXPLANATORY FACTORS

Whereas Part II of this volume is focused on conceptualizing and measuring life course outcomes as represented by differently shaped trajectories, Part III is concerned with the explanations or causal factors that produce one kind of trajectory rather than another. These chapters consider causal factors in a reverse hierarchical order from micro to macro. Although we, as editors, did not set out with a plan to get chapters that would parallel the four-factor paradigm of life course development, each in fact turns out to focus on one of the four dimensions. Chapter 10, on the interaction between an individual's genetic predispositions and environmental forces corresponds with the *timing* factor. Genetic predispositions are the earliest, most formidable, and continuous factors that shape the individual's adaptation to changing circumstance. The next, more encompassing system is at the level of the individual self, which represents the person's own integration of biological heritage and external social influences. Chapter 11 focuses on personal integration and corresponds in the life course paradigm to the *agency* factor. Immediate social ties and social convoys, such as the families and peer groups that are the subject of Chapter 12, represent *linked lives* in the life course paradigm. Finally, the institutional cultural and historical matrix treated in Chapter 13 indicates the most general life course factor, *location in time and place*.

Chapter 10, "Genetics and Behavior in the Life Course: A Promising Frontier" by Michael J. Shanahan and Jason D. Boardman, suggests the potential ongoing influence of genetic factors in shaping an individual's life. The authors analyze two main types of gene–environment interplay. First are G x Es, which represent gene–environment *interactions* and the various types of social environment that can either dampen or exacerbate a genetic vulnerability, such as a potential for addiction or antisocial behavior. Social environments (peers, laws, etc.) vary in their capacity to *trigger* a genetic vulnerability, *compensate* for that vulnerability (e. g., by neutralizing its effect), or *prevent* its expression through social control (e.g., antismoking laws). In the case of positive genetic predispositions, environmental factors can lead to *social enhancement*, such as an improvement in academic achievement over baseline performance that follows good parenting and cognitive training. The second major type of gene–environment interplay is found in rGEs, or gene–environment *correlations*. Passive correlations occur when persons are in an environment produced by some persistent genetic factor, such as having an antisocial genetic predisposition and being brought up by antisocial parents. Evocative or active correlations refer to cases in which the person selects an environment on the basis of an individual predisposition. One memorable example of gene–environment interaction is the correlation of a dopamine risk factor with low school performance and low rates of school completion. This factor is dampened when a boy comes from a family with high educational and socioeconomic status (SES); however, it has its biggest negative effect for those who come from lower SES families with less education.

In Chapter 11, "Life Stories to Understand Diversity: Variations by Class, Race, and Gender," Janet Z. Giele addresses three intertwined issues: the life story as a data collection tool, a theory of the major components of life stories, and a comparative method to analyze the impact of class, race, and gender. By asking questions about the person's expectations in young adulthood, memories of childhood, current experiences, and future hopes and expectations, the researcher elicits a story of the person's actions that contain the four main components of the life course paradigm. Then, having selected comparison groups with similar background characteristics but different role outcomes (e.g., homemaking or a career), Giele uses a comparative method based on Boolean sets to examine differences in the personal narratives of a sample of black and white college-educated women of similar age. She finds the *identity* (location in time and place) of career-oriented women to be more self-consciously different than that of homemakers, their *relational style* (linked lives) to be more egalitarian, their *goals and motiva-*

tion (agency) to be more ambitious for achievement in the public realm, and their *adaptive style* (timing) to be more flexible and innovative. Race differences show up among the black and white homemakers, but not among the black and white career women. Because life stories are comprehensive, subjective, and give an inside picture of change, they are especially well suited for understanding different ways of "doing" class, race, and gender.

Chapter 12, by Phyllis Moen and Elaine Hernandez, focuses on the interpersonal component of the life course paradigm. In "Social Convoys: Studying Linked Lives in Time, Context, and Motion," they consider examples of married couples, parents and children, and coworkers. They show how dynamic, ongoing relationships in any given social convoy affect the lives of the members. A major example of linked lives is the relationship of a married couple that shapes the decisions and actions of each partner. Key variables that affect couple behavior include changes in the economy, illness, job loss, job relocation, or retirement that affects one of the partners in particular. The chapter lists numerous examples of research on linked lives from the fields of education, medicine, health, and employment. The authors also note the wide range of analytical methods developed to examine effects of social ties, including qualitative approaches, event–history analyses, and hierarchical linear models. In addition to these quantitative methods that are typically based on longitudinal survey data, they suggest another possible strategy, which is to collect and assemble life histories of those whose lives are linked, and to examine the ways in which their calendars fit together. The central thesis of the chapter is that social convoys are dynamic systems that mediate between social forces and individual behavior across the life course. Thus, the study of social convoys involves investigation of social ties as causative factors, as well as the ways in which the life course is affected by them.

Chapter 13, "Comparative Life Course Research: A Cross-National and Longitudinal Perspective," by Hans Peter-Blossfeld, concludes the book with a focus on the macro social forces at the institutional and societal level. Blossfeld's main analytical strategy is to compare longitudinal and panel data for different countries. He attributes national differences in the life course to distinctive national institutions of education, employment. social welfare, and the family. Research suggests five universal sociological regularities: (1) the negative impact of lower social origins on educational attainment; (2) the association between women's continuing education and their delayed entry into marriage and motherhood; (3) the mixed effects of women's part-time work on their status in the workplace; (4) the existence of educational homogamy that not only promotes upward mobility but also contributes to growing income inequality; and (5) the continuing asymmetry in couples' allocation of household work despite the increased employment of married women. The chapter concludes with observations on the ways that globalization is affecting major life trajectories through a general delay in transition from youth to adulthood, a decrease in men's midlife job security, and an increase in women's education that promotes career commitment and lower family involvement. These observations are consistent with a theoretical perspective that sees changing environmental influences on the life course as being filtered through the distinctive culture and institutions of each society.

CHAPTER 10

Genetics and Behavior in the Life Course

A Promising Frontier

Michael J. Shanahan
Jason D. Boardman

Human development entails ongoing exchanges between person and context. Consequently, the fully informed study of biographical patterns encompasses longitudinal views of both the life course and biological processes. Indeed, the integration of life course sociology and genetic models of behavior represents an emerging and highly promising area of study that seeks to highlight these person–context exchanges.

This integration is facilitated by two considerations that perhaps are not widely appreciated by sociologists. First, many topics of interest to life course sociologists are linked in significant ways to biological processes. These topics include, for example, trajectories of physical and mental health; the stress process; age-graded patterns of aggression and deviance; life histories of sexual behavior, fertility, and parenting; and manifold dimensions of aging and mortality. Other topics are also likely to be associated with biological processes, albeit less conspicuously, including educational and occupational careers; close interpersonal relationships, both within and beyond the family; and one's involvement and status in organizations.

Second, a well-established consensus now holds that genetic factors, either specific genes or the sum total genetic material of an organism (called the "genotype"), by themselves do not cause complex behaviors.

215

Rather, the influence of genes depends on, among other things, the interplay between contextual and genetic factors. By "interplay" we refer to how contextual and genetic factors combine over time to change the likelihood of specific behaviors. This interplay between social and biological forces is complex and dynamic, ultimately defining ranges of likely behaviors. Thus, behavior cannot be fully understood without reference to prior experience nor can we realistically assume that human beings are blank slates who all respond and interpret their settings in the same way. Rather, behavior is likely to reflect the cumulative history of a person's social experiences as they combine with his or her genetic makeup. Indeed, there is widespread appreciation among behavioral geneticists that the links between genes and behavior are heavily conditioned by contextual factors.

At the same time, behavioral geneticists insufficiently appreciate that dynamic features of context often determine its meaning for a person. Put differently, the significance of social context for genetic expression will often depend on processes occurring in the life course as revealed, for example, by pathways, trajectories, transitions, turning points, durations, and cohorts. For example, persons with a high genetic propensity for alcoholism may or may not become alcoholics, depending on their *lifelong patterns* of stressors, social supports, sources of social control, and so on. In short, gene–environment interplay must surely reflect life course processes. Yet, to date, most studies of gene–environment interplay are cross-sectional or use longitudinal data without such life course distinctions in mind.

In this chapter, we seek to overcome this impasse by considering forms of gene–environment interplay and how life course research greatly enriches their study. We introduce basic processes of gene–environment interplay and ideas that serve as a meeting place between life course sociology and the genetic study of behavior. We then briefly examine an analytic strategy for studying gene–environment interplay, then suggest hypotheses that thus far have been neglected. Hence, the subtitle of this chapter refers to the many exciting ideas that we hope will animate future research on gene–environment interplay. Unlike many contributions to this volume, which draw on decades of relevant empirical work, this chapter focuses on a nascent topic; we therefore highlight more a body of conceptual ideas than an extensive body of empirical research.

Basic Forms of Gene–Environment Interplay

There are two prominent forms of gene–environment interplay: gene–environment interactions (commonly denoted G × Es) and gene–

environment correlations (rGEs). The field of behavioral genetics uses the term "environment," which actually refers to a broader range of phenomena than "social context." Both terms may refer to organized, enduring patterns of interaction among people, extending from interpersonal relationships to neighborhoods, to organizations (e.g., companies and schools), and to communities, societies, and institutions. This is the meaning sociologists typically assign to phrases such as "social structure" and "social context." But "environment," as used by behavioral geneticists, also refers to pollutants, toxins, diet and other ingested substances (e.g., medications), and also to intrauterine conditions. We use the terms "environment" and "context" interchangeably in this chapter, although our primary interest is in the narrower meaning of social context.

Gene–Environment Interactions

G × Es refer to processes by which the effects of genetic factors on a behavior are conditioned by environmental factors or vice versa. The term, somewhat unfortunately, connotes a multiplicative interaction term as conventionally tested in a general linear framework. The main point of the concept of G × E, however, is that the genetic effect is in some way dependent on environmental conditions (or vice versa), and this dependency (or conditioning) may be empirically expressed in any of a number of ways, including, but not limited to, a form consistent with a multiplicative interaction. Researchers presently use multiplicative interactions to test for G × Es, but this ubiquitous methodological practice is not at all dictated by the concept; indeed, it runs contrary to considerable empirical evidence from earlier animal studies (see, e.g., Gottlieb, 2003).

Another way to think about G × Es is to consider the effects of genes as averages that may differ across groups rather than as fixed values that apply to everyone. Consider Table 10.1, which shows the association between the dopamine D_2 receptor gene (*Taq1A*) and whether males continue their educations past high school.[1] Of course, there is no "college gene." Rather, the idea is that the risky form of *Taq1A* influences an individual's dopamine system to increase one's tendency to enact problematic and impulsive behaviors that interfere with success in the classroom. These behaviors, enacted on a fairly consistent basis over many years, would alter the likelihood of continuation.

The first row of Table 10.1 reports mean continuation rates by *Taq1A* risk status. For white boys in the study, those with the risky variant of the *Taq1A* gene are less likely to continue their education beyond high school. Nearly 60% of the boys without the risky variant of this gene continued their education, but only 44% of those with the risk variant did

TABLE 10.1. Percentage of White Males Continuing to College by *Taq1A* Risk Status and Configurations of Social Capital, National Longitudinal Study of Adolescent Health (Wave III)

	Taq1A risk	*Taq1A* non-risk
Base rate	44.4	59.3
High parental SES and high parental involvement and high-quality school	66.9	76.1
Low parental SES and low parental involvement and low-quality school (or parents do not talk about school)	30.1	42.1

so. These results suggest a strong association between *Taq1A* risk status and continuation rates. Indeed, the magnitude of the association rivals bivariate associations between continuation and its most potent predictors, including race and socioeconomic status (SES).

The next two rows reestimate the likelihood of continuing education by defining groups of white boys based on levels of social capital. The second row reports continuation rates for boys who are rich in social capital: Their parents report high SES; these same parents are highly involved in their child's high school, and the school is of high quality. Rates of continuation increase markedly within *Taq1A* groups. The highest rate of continuation is observed among the white boys without *Taq1A* risk and with high social capital (76.1%), but the continuation rate is also high for white boys with *Taq1A* risk and high social capital (66.9%). The third row shows rates of continuation for white boys who are low in social capital. Rates are quite depressed, and the lowest rate is observed among white boys with *Taq1A* risk and low social capital (30.1%). That is, the chances of continuing education are roughly 30% higher among those without the risky genotype, but this is an *average* effect of this particular gene. This influence is higher among students with lower social capital but very weak among students who are rich in social capital. In other words, *Taq1A* risk status differentiates people more in the less advantaged environments. This pattern of results speaks to the importance of social capital in the life course but also its interplay with genetic factors.

Beyond this specific example of a G × E, *how* would social context condition genetic effects (or vice versa)? Life course sociology is particularly well equipped to address this question. The next section provides an overview of a typology of G × E interactions, then considers how this typology is complicated by the nature of the environment, the outcome of interest, and the stage of the life course.

Typology of G × Es

Shanahan and Hofer (2005) proposed a typology of G × Es, suggesting four distinct ways that social context can condition genetic influences on complex behaviors. The first type, the "triggering interaction," refers to situations in which a person has a genetic vulnerability (or "diathesis") that is only expressed in the presence of a triggering agent ("strong triggering") or is expressed markedly more so in the presence of the agent ("weak triggering"). This idea builds on the stress paradigm, which holds that the experience of a stressor may result in some form of distress. That is, people with a genetic susceptibility are most likely to exhibit distress in the presence of the stressor or trigger.

A wide range of empirical examples of triggering interactions involve exposures to toxins and the ingestion of substances, particularly alcohol and tobacco products. However, there are also many examples of genetic vulnerabilities interacting with social context. As an example of weak triggering, Button and his colleagues (2007) report a relatively small influence of genetic factors with respect to conduct problems among those who do not associate with delinquent peers. However, the relative contribution of the additive genetic effect increases exponentially with increasing levels of delinquent peer affiliation. After adjusting for selection into delinquent groups, Button and his colleagues conclude that peers serve as a trigger, activating a genetic vulnerability to conduct problems. Strong triggering results also have been reported by Cadoret, Yates, Troughton, Woodworth, and Stewart (1995), who demonstrated that genetic risks for antisocial behavior were only observed when children are raised in adverse family environments.

Of special interest in a life course framework are those triggering agents that involve psychosocial stressors. One of the most highly cited examples involves Caspi and colleagues' (2002) G × E study of adult antisocial behavior. The authors begin by noting that maltreatment in childhood has a strong predictive relationship with antisocial behaviors in young adulthood, although this relationship is not entirely determinative. Caspi and colleagues observed that deficiencies in *monoamine oxidase A* (or *MAOA*), which metabolizes neurotransmitters, have been linked to antisocial behavior as well. Drawing on these bivariate patterns, the authors hypothesized (and found evidence) that severe childhood maltreatment leads to antisocial behavior in adulthood, but only among youth with a genetic polymorphism for low *MAOA* activity. Put differently, childhood maltreatment does not lead to antisocial behavior in the presence of high *MAOA* levels, which sufficiently metabolize high levels of neurotransmitters. In the framework of the triggering interaction, severe childhood maltreatment represents the trigger, but its effect depends on the low-activity *MAOA* gene, which is the genetic vulnerability (or diathesis). Although genetic factors are critical to the etiology of antisocial behavior, these genetic factors depend on the social environment to initiate the cascade of events called "genetic expression."

In addition to triggers that are typically considered "noxious," social forces of a more normative sort may also serve as triggers, a variant we refer to as "social expression," because the social environment may contain features that encourage otherwise latent genetic tendencies to manifest themselves. For example, Boardman, Saint Onge, Haberstick, Timberlake, and Hewitt (2008) demonstrate that the genetic factors responsible for smoking cigarettes are most predictive within schools in which the most popular students are also those who smoke cigarettes the most. They argue that social pressures to smoke have a stronger influence on students with a genetic vulnerability.

Whereas a "triggering interaction" refers to a detrimental context combining with a genetic vulnerability, the second G × E model, "social compensation," refers to a positive, possibly enriched social or environmental setting that *prevents* the expression of a genetic vulnerability. In some instances, compensation and triggering represent ends of a continuum: Absent significant stressors, people with a diathesis do not exhibit distress (i.e., "weak compensation"), but as the level of stressors increases, the likelihood of distress increases (i.e., "weak triggering"). In some cases, however, compensation may refer to situations in which only pronouncedly enriched settings can neutralize a genetic diathesis ("strong compensation"). In these cases, "compensation" refers not to the absence of a detrimental context (e.g., childhood maltreatment) but to the presence of a markedly positive feature in the environment. An example of a G × E compensation interaction involves Shanahan, Erickson, Vaisey, and Smolen's study (2007) of mentors and the likelihood of continuing education beyond high school. The authors observed that *TaqIA* risk significantly decreased the likelihood of continuing one's education past high school among both white and black boys. The authors found that this negative relationship was fully attenuated, however, by mentors who were teachers. That is, the negative association between the *TaqIA* risk allele and educational continuation could be totally compensated by having a teacher who was a mentor, the strong compensation variant.

"Social control," the third type of interaction, is similar to compensation in that both interactions involve a genetic diathesis in a context that squelches or completely prevents genetic expression. They differ, however, in their substantive meaning; "social control" refers to social norms and structural constraints that are placed on people to limit their behavior and their choices, whereas "compensation" refers to the avoidance of low levels of functioning because of the absence of a stressor ("weak variant") or an enriched environment ("strong variant"). Broadly conceived, "social control" refers to any social structure or process that maintains the social order (whether for the moral good or not).

Many studies show that in settings marked by high social control, the variance in behavior attributable to genetic variance decreases, whereas in context marked by low levels of social control, the proportion of variance in the behavior explained by genetic variance increases. Studies of alcohol use illustrate the social control interaction. For example, the gene *aldehyde dehydrigenase 2 (ALDH2)* is an enzyme that helps to metabolize alcohol. A large portion of people of Far East Asian descent (~ 40%) have a genetic variant (called the "homozygous form") that leads to a partially inactive form of the enzyme. This inactivation results in an increased level of response to alcohol (e.g., motor impairment and hangovers) and, consequently, lower rates of alcoholism in this population (see *www.aldh.org*); that is, such people are very likely to become drunk and ill when ingesting alcohol, whereas people with another variant (called the "heterozygous form") become less drunk and may or may not become ill.

Higuchi and his colleagues (1994) showed that although the suppressive effect of the homozygous form always inhibits alcoholism among Japanese people, the suppressive effect of the heterozygous genotype has waned through successive cohorts; that is, they report a birth cohort × gene interaction. The authors speculate that social controls on drunkenness have loosened in Japanese society throughout the 20th century.

There are many studies suggesting that as traditional markers of social control (e.g., religious involvements and parental monitoring) increase, the heritability of diverse forms of delinquent behaviors decrease as well. Boardman (2009) show that the heritability of regular smoking among adolescents is significantly *reduced* among sibling and twin pairs who reside in states with the highest taxes on cigarettes. The research cannot determine whether the real price of cigarettes controls genetic expression, or whether states with high cigarette taxes are also those with the strongest antismoking sentiment. However, both forms (normative and institutional) represent clear examples of control that limit the function of genes related to tobacco consumption.

Kendler, Thornton, and Pederson (2000) compared reported tobacco use among same-sex twin pairs across three birth cohorts (1910–1924, 1925–1939, and 1940–1958). They reported that genetic factors account for 50–60% of the variance in regular tobacco use for men, regardless of birth cohort. Among women, however, they demonstrated that none of the variance is due to genetic factors in the first cohort, but that there is a consistent convergence in these estimates such that, by the third cohort, there is no significant gender difference in the heritability of regular tobacco use. They argued that this is due to changes in social restrictions on women's tobacco use across these periods.

Among individuals without a genetic vulnerability, social context can also interact with genes to facilitate higher levels of developmental functioning. A "social enhancement" interaction refers to situations involving the accentuation of "positive" genetic predispositions. Although the triggering and enhancement interactions both refer to situations in which a genetic predisposition is expressed, their substantive meanings are different: A "trigger" involves the activation of a vulnerability or diathesis, and an "enhancement" refers to experiences that push behavior toward upper capacity for a given genotype. The concept of enhancement is similar to Baltes's (1987) idea of developmental reserve capacity. "Baseline capacity" refers to performance (e.g., physical, cognitive, emotional) under standardized conditions, and "developmental reserve capacity" is an improvement on baseline because of a developmentally sensitive intervention (e.g., cognitive training, good parenting, appropriate physical exercise). Developmental reserve capacity actually reflects a social enhancement process whereby an intervention pushes a person to her or his upper limit as defined by genotype.

Bronfenbrenner and Ceci's (1994) bioecological model suggests that proximal processes encourage the realization of genetic potential. They define a "proximal process" as one involving forms of social interactions characterized by progressive complexity, including, for example, those involving effective parents and teachers. As proximal processes improve, the genetic potential for positive development is increasingly actualized. Rowe, Jacobson, and Van den Oord (1999), for example, focused on how parental educational levels influence the heritability of vocabulary skills of their children. They found that the proportion of variance in vocabulary skills attributable to genetic factors increases substantially across households with less-educated parents, and households whose parents have more than a high school degree.

Evaluation

The four types of G × Es—triggering, compensation, control, and enhancement—refer to recognizable life course phenomena, because all four processes reflect dynamic patterns of social context. Psychosocial stressors that serve as triggers, for example, often refer to experiences with unique temporal properties: durations (e.g., poverty), experiences before and after transitions (e.g., life events), cumulations of experience (e.g., persistent work stressors), pathways (e.g., involving family and work), trajectories, and so on (for an empirical illustration involving life-events, see Caspi et al., 2003; Moffitt, Caspi, & Rutter, 2005). And these dynamic properties often reflect historical changes in communities. Without reference to their temporal qualities, psychosocial stressors are likely to be poorly understood and their importance to gene–environment interplay underappreciated.

The life course paradigm also encourages a highly interactive view of development. This proposition requires focusing on triggers—and compensators, controls, and enhancements—in multiple domains of a person's life, including work, family, and leisure. Thus, it is not possible to describe the genetic etiology of a form of distress unless an individual's cumulative trigger, compensation, control, and enhancement profile across domains is understood.

Similar observations may be made for environmental factors that constitute forms of compensation, control, and enhancement: Their meaning depends greatly on their temporal qualities, timing in a person's life, and their synchronization across domains. Thus, insights from life course sociology could prove especially helpful in "getting the E right in G × E." This is particularly important in developmental studies that focus on transitions across different stages of the life course. As Moffitt et al. (2005) observe, the impact of specific environmental influences is salient at different ages.

Gene–Environment Correlations

rGEs refer to processes by which genetic factors are associated with features of the environment (Jaffee & Price, 2007). The term is typically interpreted according to the mathematical formula used to compute rGEs in biometric studies (see Johnson, 2007, Equation 1) to mean the extent to which there are genetic influences common to both a behavior and an environmental component. In turn, this idea is often extended to cases wherein genetic factors associated with a behavior also lead to an environment that alters the likelihood of the behavior.

Like the G × E, the term "gene–environment correlation" is misleading. Although rGE suggests a Pearson correlation, the concept is not limited to one technique of gauging an association. Rather, an rGE simply refers to some form of meaningful pattern between genetic and environmental factors. Second, the idea of a correlation is inconsistent with the ultimate concern of any rGE: *causal* associations extending from gene to context to behavior, associations that are due to *dynamic processes.*

rGEs are important because their presence and nature may bear heavily on the interpretation of G × E effects; that is, the meaning of

G × E is only properly understood in light of the presence of rGE. As Jaffee and Price (2007) point out, the failure to consider rGE may artificially inflate G × E estimates in traditional epidemiological, behavioral genetic, or quantitative social scientific analyses. It is also possible that rGE may be so large that there is insufficient power to detect a G × E. For example (and hypothetically), if virtually all people with a genetic risk for high stress reactivity also lack social supports, then it would be difficult to test the hypothesis that social supports attenuate the effect of the genetic risk on forms of distress. Thus, rGEs are often considered a "statistical nuisance," but many times they are also phenomena of great substantive import.

Plomin, DeFries, and Loehlin (1977) proposed a typology of rGEs that has stood the test of time largely intact. First, "evocative (or reactive) correlations" refer to situations in which genetic factors evoke specific reactions that significantly define a person's context. For example, using an adoption design, Ge and his colleagues (1996) showed that psychiatric symptoms in biological parents are associated with harsh parenting of their children by the adoptive parents. Such an adoptive design supposes that genetic factors associated with the biological parents' difficulties are also associated with behavioral problems in the biological offspring, which, in turn, evoke negative parenting from the adoptive parents. In turn, this harsh parenting could exacerbate children's behavioral problems.

The "passive correlation" refers to situations in which a child inherits genetic factors from his or her parents and is also exposed to an environment that reflects these same genetic factors. For example, the antisocial behavior of parents has a genetic component, and these same parents may well create home environments that encourage antisocial behavior in their children. The children passively encounter both the genetic loading and the genetically inspired, deleterious environment. Finally, the "active (or selective) correlation" refers to situations in which a person's genetically influenced attributes are associated with selected environments. For example, an antisocial child may choose to associate with antisocial peers. This perspective is especially important to social demographers and sociologists, because these same processes emerge across important life course transitions. Active correlations are believed to be associated with marital satisfaction and duration (e.g., D'Onofrio et al., 2005).

Researchers generally acknowledge that there are actually only two types of rGEs in empirical settings: the passive and the nonpassive (which includes the evocative and active). In empirical settings, it is typically difficult to assess the extent to which someone chooses a setting and is chosen for that setting. For example, people apply to schools and for jobs, and they court potential mates, all of which reflect active mechanisms. Yet schools, employers, and potential mates respond affir-matively or negatively—reflecting reactive mechanisms.

Jaffee and Price (2007), in their review of rGE in the study of mental illness, note that many psychosocial stressors (e.g., life events) and distressful behaviors (e.g., risk taking) have shared heritable com-ponents that suggest rGEs. More broadly, it seems quite plausible that young people are subject to wide-ranging passive correlations and, as they disengage from the family of origin, it also seems likely that they try to select actively and shape their settings based on their behavioral predispositions. Drawing on the few extant empirical examples of rGEs, Jaffee and Price noted that individual differences in personality (and related constructs, e.g., temperament) and cognitive abilities appear to be major sources of rGEs. For example, biometric models suggest that roughly 30–80% of the variance attributable to heritability of marital status, marital quality, and divorce can be accounted for by such factors. At the same time, very little attention has been devoted to the social factors that may contribute to this mediation, including perhaps dimen-sions of values, self-conceptions, and social cognitions. These factors suggest ways in which personality and cognitive factors are related to differences in interpersonal relationships, but very little, if any, research, has examined whether such social-psychological factors play a role.

Once again, rGEs are recognizably life course phenomena. People's behavioral patterns are associated with (and often causally antecedent to) their environments. Yet these associations evolve over long periods of time in the context of age-graded opportunities and limitations. Fur-thermore, these associations likely cut across domains (work, school, family, leisure). Thus, rGEs are best studied with issues of aging, timing, and the multifaceted environment in mind. In fact, the real analytic task—both conceptually and methodologically—is to map the media-tional processes at work: how genetic factors are associated with envi-ronmental factors, which in turn are associated with behavior. In other words, rGEs direct attention to the possibility that genetic influences on behavior are partially or fully mediated by social context.

Gene–Environment Interplay: Interactions and Correlations Together

Viewed jointly, G × Es and rGEs map out the basic terrain of gene–environment interplay. Substantively, this interplay refers to two ongo-ing, potentially intersecting, processes: (1) the mechanisms by which social settings condition genetic effects on behavior by way of trigger-ing, compensation, social control, and enhancement, and (2) the mechanisms by which genetic propensities are passively and nonpassively associated with (and lead to) specific environments.

At present, there is very little empirical evidence on how this interplay—as two processes simultaneously—occurs. However, two studies suggest a possibility: Environmental factors may compensate for a genetic diathesis, but people with the vulnerability are least likely to experience compensatory settings. In other words, some people are most likely to benefit from help because of a genetic diathesis (a G × E), but these same people are least likely to get help (because of an rGE).

Shanahan, Vaisey, Erickson, and Smolen (2008) observed that the *Taq1A* risk allele has a large and negative relationship with educational continuation after secondary school among both white and black boys. The relationship is fully attenuated when accompanied by high levels of social capital (specifically, by educated parents who are highly involved in high-quality schools). But boys with the *Taq1A* risk allele are less likely to have such high social capital in the first place. The authors reasoned that *Taq1A* is related to behaviors that might discourage their parents from being highly involved in school. Furthermore, *Taq1A* boys with risk have a parent or parents with *Taq1A* risk, who may not have high levels of education.[2] In any event, studies of this nature bring to the fore the interrelated issues of how people get to specific social contexts and, once there, how they are affected. Presently, almost no existing simultaneously considers rGE and G × E at different stages of the life course.

Strategies for Studying Gene–Environment Interplay

Although the foregoing identifies the common conceptual ground between behavioral genetics and life course sociology, many behavioral scientists wonder how to proceed in terms of empirical research. Moffitt and her colleagues (2005) have articulated a very useful set of steps that may be taken when studying G × Es. Interestingly, although writing for a psychiatric audience, they emphasize the importance of social context and a life course perspective. We have revised their recommendations somewhat.

Identify an Entry Point for the Analysis

Identify Features of the Environment of Interest

Moffitt and her colleagues (2005) refer to "environmental pathogens" or "risks" (which we would call "triggers"), but we have suggested a broader interest in the environment that includes compensators, controls, and enhancers. They suggest three important criteria in evaluating "environmental candidates" (i.e., an environmental factor that is hypothesized to interact or correlate with a genetic factor in the prediction of a behavior). First, does the candidate have a truly causal relationship with the behavior to be predicted (i.e., causality)? If not, then any analyses will be plagued with problems of spuriousness. Second, do people respond in variable ways to the environmental candidate (i.e., variability)? This consideration reflects not only the practical matter of having variability to explain but also substantive importance: Variability in response to environmental factors is presumably subject to, in part, genetic factors. Third, is there a plausible link between the environmental condition and the biological system (i.e., plausibility)? In other words, is the variability in people's responses to the environment plausibly connected to human biology? Presently, the most popular way of thinking about this question is to draw on research in neuroscience, because this subfield concerns cognitive, emotional, and perceptual differences in how people perceive, interpret, and react to their surroundings.

Identify a Genetic Factor of Interest

Life course sociologists would quite naturally begin their study of gene–environment interplay with environmental factors—as suggested by Moffitt and her colleagues (2005)—but one could also begin with a genetic candidate. In that case, the same three considerations discussed earlier would apply, namely, causality, variability, and plausibility. "Causality" refers to a demonstrated association between the genetic factor and the behavior, and "functional significance," which means that the gene is directly involved in a relevant biological process. "Variability" refers to genetic factors that have common polymorphisms; that is, a reasonable percentage of the population carries different forms of the gene. "Plausibility" would then involve constructing links between genetic variability, differing genetic processes associated with the different polymorphisms, and the behavior of interest.

How are genetic candidates identified, and why would a sociologist start with genetics? Candidates can often be identified by consulting the interdisciplinary literatures in behavioral genetics (psychological; medical; and, increasingly, sociological), by learning about candidates that are included in available data sets, and by discussing interests with scholars working at the intersection between genetics and the behavioral sciences. The advantage to beginning with genetic factors is that such a starting point may actually enrich the sociological analyses that follow. For example, a life course sociologist might reasonably be interested in the stress process (or antisocial behavior or self-regulation).

What genetic factors are related to the stress process? Once identified and studied, one may then ask which stressors, social supports, and coping mechanisms are relevant to the link between the genetic candidate and the behavior of interest.

Identify a Behavior of Interest

Many life course sociologists organize their scholarly work around behavioral variables, either individual variables (smoking, educational attainment, depression) or categories of behavior (e.g., substance use, educational processes, mental health). This represents yet another legitimate entry point for the study of gene–environment interplay. In this case, questions of causality, variability, and plausibility once again apply. The advantage to this entry point is that it casts a wide genetic and environmental net. That is, many genetic and environmental factors will be relevant to the study of a given behavior, or set of behaviors. By acknowledging a high level of complexity at the outset, the scientist can then design a program of research that intelligently addresses it.

Our experience and working hypothesis ("the robust phenotype hypothesis") is that genetic factors are less likely to predict behaviors that are constrained in time and space, and they are more likely to predict behaviors that occur over long periods of time and that cut across multiple domains of life. For example, genetic factors are probably less likely to predict 10th-grade school attachment than grade point average in high school or educational continuation after high school. The rationale is that genetic factors influence behavioral tendencies that should be expressed on a fairly consistent basis across time and domains of life, but they could not be expected markedly to influence behavior in any specific narrow time frame or in any single domain of life. The robust phenotype hypothesis suggests "broad" conceptualizations and measures of behavior, as well as more specific measures.

Optimize Measurement to Capture Complexity

Moffit and her colleagues (2005) emphasize several distinctions when thinking about operationalizing environmental features, distinctions that are familiar to life course sociologists. First, social context can be classified as distal or proximal, a distinction that refers to how far removed in time, space, and causal mechanism a contextual factor is from the behavior of interest. Second, measures should be age-appropriate. For example, the specific attributes of peer groups that potentially matter are likely to differ between early childhood and adolescence. Another example: many life events (marriage, mortgages, illness or death of a spouse or child) become possible only in young adulthood. Third, measures should be capable of capturing the dynamic properties of social context. For example, there is now a considerable literature documenting the importance of the dynamic features of social stressors, marital histories, and social controls for understanding their behavioral implications. Probative concepts in the study of these and many other contextual features include durations, spells, transitions, pathways, trajectories, timing, turning points, and cumulation (see Shanahan & Macmillan, 2007). Finally, Moffit and her colleagues (2005) call for the improvement of retrospective measurement strategies. This strategy is potentially useful to capture dynamic features of social experiences that occur before one's data collection begins. The burden of accurate recall may be especially challenging when very early experiences are hypothesized to be of import. For example, Caspi and his colleagues' (2002) study of *MAOA* and antisocial behavior (discussed earlier) suggests the critical importance of parental abuse in early and perhaps middle childhood for understanding antisocial behaviors in young adulthood.

Many of these considerations also apply to genetic factors and the behavior of interest. The collection of DNA and the procedures by which genetic variation is described are highly specialized areas and beyond the scope of this chapter except to note that genetic information is currently considered in the form of single loci, haplotypes, and whole-genome scans. And as suggested by the "robust phenotype hypothesis," it may be strategic to study behaviors that capture behavioral tendencies over long periods of time and across multiple domains (i.e., work, family, school, leisure).

Consider a Variety of Statistical Approaches

As noted, G × E and rGE refer not to statistical tests but to conceptual ideas: the conditioning of a genetic influence by the environment (or vice versa) and a nonrandom pattern between genetic and environmental factors. Thus, the almost universal reliance on multiplicative interaction terms and analysis of variance (ANOVAs) to test for interactions and correlations (respectively) has quite possibly hindered discovery. Both concepts call for careful descriptive analyses and new and creative ways of thinking about data. In our view, a number of approaches thus far have been neglected, including various types of mixture models, combinatoric methods, data mining, and data visualization. Perhaps these suggestions surprise some readers, because their statistical foundations tend not to be as firm as those associated with generalized linear models. Nevertheless, when used prudently, they can be useful as methods of discovery.

Replicate and Extend Findings

Thus far, the genetically informed study of behavior has been plagued by nonreplication, with very few findings that have proven to be robust. A notable exception is the Caspi and colleagues (2002) study of *MAOA* and antisocial behavior discussed earlier (Kim-Cohen et al., 2006). The reasons for this nonreplication are not well understood, but Moffitt and her colleagues (2005) recommend heightened attention to replication and meta-analysis. Furthermore, do the initial findings extend to different measures and concepts? For example, Caspi and his colleagues (2002) examined diverse measures of antisocial behavior, showing that the *MAOA*–abuse interaction applied to a wide range of criteria for antisocial behavior. But one wonders whether parental abuse per se is necessary and sufficient, or whether other severe stressors may interact with *MAOA* to increase the likelihood of antisocial behavior.

Gene–Environment Interplay: Emerging Questions

Social context can modify the link between genetic factors and behaviors—by way of triggering, compensating, enhancing, and controlling mechanisms—and genetic predispositions can clearly become associated with social contexts. Most importantly for our purposes, there is substantial empirical evidence that environmental components of these interactive and correlational processes take place over time (i.e., they have important temporal qualities) and are multidimensional, consistent with life course sociology. Can these basic ideas be linked more closely with the concept of the life course? The question calls for a developmental view of behavioral genetics, but one that is firmly rooted in the idea of age-graded, socially based roles, opportunities, limitations, and institutional and organizational involvements. With the life course in mind, we discuss in preliminary fashion several ideas about behavioral genetics.

rGEs across the Life Course

It is commonly thought that passive and evocative correlations are dominant in early life and, as young people become more capable of taking agentic action (i.e., deliberate action based on choices), active correlations become increasingly important. These hypotheses are based on the premise that young children are highly subject to the passive processes in their family of origin but that, over time, they acquire more latitude in choosing and shaping their environments. These hypothesized patterns are shown in Figure 10.1. Yet evocative correlations may become important toward the end of the life as people become dependent on others for their care. And to the extent that one's caregivers include adult children, "*reverse passive correlations*" could emerge in the sense that the child's genes now contribute to the setting of the parent. Thus, a plausible variation of Figure 10.1 would involve an increase in passive correlations in late adulthood.

Transitions and Perturbations in rGEs

The age-graded roles of the life course are linked via transitions, and a key challenge has been identifying the factors that shape the quality and duration of these transitions and, in turn, the effects of these new experiences. Many of the transitions can be anticipated, suggesting that genetic factors associated with conscientiousness and, more broadly, planful competence, may be associated with transitions that "channel people" into their desired roles. "Conscientiousness," according to Costa and McCrae's formulation, encompasses competence, order, dutifulness, achievement-striving, self-discipline, and deliberation. "Planful competence," according to Clausen's (1991) formulation, includes the self-assertive, deliberative, and perseverative qualities that enable people to assess their situation, make a plan (which is subject to revision),

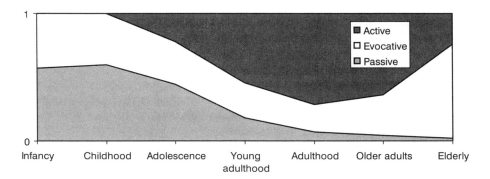

FIGURE 10.1. Hypothesized pattern of gene–environment correlations (rGE) across the life course.

and carry through with it. In contrast, qualities such as impulsivity and risk taking would obviously be detrimental. More broadly, Caspi and Moffitt (1993) have argued that transitions, because they are times of uncertainty, often result in behavior being more strongly informed by an individual's personality. This possibility in turn suggests that during transitions, active (and perhaps evocative) rGEs should strengthen, particularly when they are stressful and filled with uncertainty.[3] That is, perhaps during times of transitions Figure 10.1 will be punctuated with heightened correlations relative to the plotted baselines.

Life Course Patterns in G × Es

Biometric studies of heritability suggest the intriguing hypothesis that G × E processes are most common during childhood and adolescence. Kendler, Neale, Kessler, Heath, and Eaves (1993) showed that the heritability for major depression among women is roughly 40%, and most importantly, despite the fact that they sampled 18- to 55-year-olds, there was little evidence that this estimate changed over the life course. Similar age-related stability is also reported for personality (Johnson & Krueger, 2004; Pedersen & Reynolds, 1998), cognition (Plomin, Pedersen, Lichtenstein, & McClearn, 1994), and depression (McGue & Christensen, 2003). However, this same stability is *not* evident among adolescents and children, raising the possibility that the role of the environment changes during these periods, including how they interact with the genotype; that is, heritability studies suggest something like the pattern of age-grading of G × Es shown in Figure 10.2. This line of

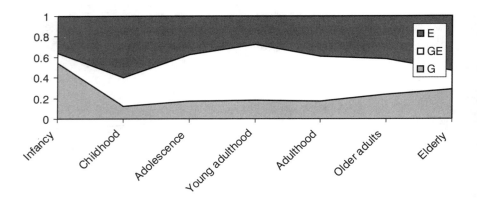

FIGURE 10.2. Gene–environment interactions across the life course.

reasoning depends on the assumption that estimates of the genetic and environmental variance components in heritability models are unbiased (but see Johnson, 2007).

A different perspective, emphasizing no age-grading of G × Es across the life course, is also plausible. According to this perspective, G × E processes occur over the entire life course, from conception to death, and their occurrence depends on the temporal properties of experiences in specific roles and settings. This expectation is based on the assumption that few environmental experiences are capable of instantaneously altering genetic processes. A very large body of evidence spanning diverse environmental factors and phenotypes now shows that temporal properties that describe the experiencing of environments over time are critical to understanding their implications for behavior (e.g., Elder & Shanahan, 2006). Even the effects of extreme environmental experiences—poverty, traumatic life events, experiences in armed conflicts—are known to depend on temporal distinctions, such as duration, timing, spells and intervals, sequences, and so forth; that is, the "E experience" has temporal properties that determine its meaning. Thus, G × Es may not be age-graded but they nevertheless depend on dynamic properties of context that are part and parcel of life course analysis. Of course both hypotheses may be true: Depending on the genetic and social factors at work, G × Es may be age-graded and subject to the life course's temporal distinctions.

Concluding Comments

As the 21st century commences, biology, especially genetics, has captivated both public and scientific imagination. Many fields of science have witnessed what may well be described as "explosive" interest in the role of genetic factors in explaining all manner of human behavior and well-being. And, concomitantly, public funding of research has increasingly depended on the inclusion of biological factors, as vividly illustrated by nationally representative, longitudinal data sets that include genetic variables (e.g., the National Longitudinal Study of Adolescent Health and the Health and Retirement Survey) and by recent large-scale Requests for Funding Applications by the National Institutes of Health and the National Institute of Aging. Yet these developments have scarcely registered in sociology when compared to many subfields of psychology, economics, and socially informed studies of medicine. Unfortunately, this lack of interest has the potential to undermine both the relevance of sociology in the broader intellectual landscape and advancement in understanding the role of genes in behavior.

The genetically informed analysis of behavior is clearly an inter-disciplinary task. From the vantage point of behavioral genetics, a wide range of empirical evidence strongly suggests that complex behaviors depend on the interplay between genetic and environmental factors. From the vantage point of sociology, the environment is best concep-tualized and measured by drawing on the life course paradigm. Join-ing these two fundamental insights defines the task that lies ahead: the study of gene–environment interplay in a life course framework that emphasizes age grading, timing, multiple dimensions and domains of context, and high levels of interaction. The central problem is to iden-tify the constellations of environmental factors that, through time, act in concert with genetic factors to make specific behaviors more or less likely. In this chapter we have identified some overarching themes that may usefully serve as points of departure and as lenses of interpretation for future empirical research. Increasingly, high-quality data sets will provide opportunities for exploration of themes that will surely enrich both behavioral genetics and life course sociology.

Acknowledgments

We wish to thank the editors for their helpful comments. Michael Shanahan's contribution to this chapter was supported, in part, by the Add Health Wave IV Program Project directed by Kathleen Mullan Harris (3P01 HDO31921), funded by the National Institute of Child Health and Human Development, with cooperative funding from 17 other agencies. Jason Boardman's contri-bution to this work was supported, in part, by the National Institute of Child Health and Human Development (Grant K01 HD 50336). Research funds were also provided by the National Institutes of Health and the National Institute of Child Health and Human Development–funded University of Colorado Popula-tion Center (Grant No. R21 HD 051146-01).

Note

1. Table 10.1 is based on data from Wave III of the National Longitudinal Study of Adolescent Health. A full description of this table can be found in Shana-han, Vaisey, Erikson, and Smolen (2008); for the sake of simplicity, results are reported for whites only.
2. Dick et al.'s (2006) study of *gamma-aminobutyric acid A receptor* gene (*GABRA2*), marital status and stability, and alcohol dependence provides a similar example.
3. From a predictive point of view, if all mediating factors could be measured, no genetic information would be needed for the purpose of prediction. For example, antisocial behaviors are predicted by *MAOA*, but *MAOA*'s asso-

ciation must be mediated by behaviors (e.g., possibly impulsivity, lack of executive control) to create these antisocial behaviors. That is, genes do not directly cause antisocial behavior; rather, they create behavioral tendencies that then make antisocial behaviors more or less likely. If all mediating factors were known and measured, then *MAOA* would add nothing to the prediction of antisocial behaviors. However, it seems likely that we can presently measure only some of this variance, and genetics findings could help fill in the missing pieces. And, in any event, *MAOA* status would always be necessary for explanatory purposes.

CHAPTER 11

Life Stories to Understand Diversity

Variations by Class, Race, and Gender

Janet Z. Giele

This chapter sets out to codify the use of biographical narratives and life stories for understanding differences in the life course that are linked to class, race, or gender identity. Over the past 30 years, qualitative methods, such as life stories, have gained increasing importance as a way to understand the meaning of life events to the individuals experiencing them. In addition, personal narratives have gained theoretical standing, because they are uniquely fitted for generating accounts that reveal identity, coherence, and direction in life. Both methodological and theoretical properties of life stories make them useful for comparing individuals and groups who differ in origin, experience of major life events, or life outcome.

At the same time that the life story has become a preferred method for documenting individual identity and agency, it has also been shown to be particularly well adapted to the study of reasons behind geographic and social mobility. Cross-sectional and quantitative demographic surveys show the magnitude and distribution of migration in entire populations, as well the effect of specific variables on these outcomes. But as Bertaux and Bertaux-Wiame (1981) and Bertaux and Thompson (1997) point out, only individual and family histories can explain fully why one individual moves and another stays put.

The use of life stories for the study of social mobility can be nicely adapted to the examination of those ascribed characteristics and "starting points" the individual cannot change, such as class of origin, race, or sex. The question to be framed is how some people arrive at a different social class destination than the one from which they started, or depart from the dominant racial or ethnic profile, or challenge the prevailing gender script. Stated in general terms: What are the life course factors that enable a "minority" individual with inferior *ascribed* status to *achieve* "majority" status? Or, to use the psychological language of identity, what enables an individual to depart from the master narrative of a given nation, class, race, or gender and construct a different narrative of the self (Hammack, 2008)?

In my own research on change in the lives of college-educated women, I had long relied on survey techniques, large samples, and cohort comparisons to account for change in the feminine role (Giele, 1987, 1998; Giele & Gilfus, 1990). But when I wanted to understand why married black and white college-educated mothers of similar age had variously become either homemakers or career women, I stumbled on the use of retrospective interviews to inquire about their life experience. I discovered certain themes over and over again that differentiated these women by role outcome. I also found thematic similarities between black and white career women, and thematic differences between black and white homemakers.

My research using life stories began as an accident because of limited research funds and the need to keep the sample small and use primarily my own labor for gathering data. However, the results proved so rich and rewarding that I found myself wanting to articulate some general principles that would enable others to replicate this approach. In addition, I wanted to lift the topic of diversity to greater visibility among life course researchers. Accordingly, this chapter has four main sections. The first reviews recent developments in uses of the life story method. The second raises the design question of how one structures a comparative study of life stories to examine minority status as a factor in shaping the life course. The third section is theoretical and addresses the question of what substantive differences to look for in a comparison of life stories. Finally, I illustrate the relevant methodological and theoretical principles by demonstrating how I used them in my own studies of the differences in women's lives related to race and gender.

Strengths of the Life Story Method

Life stories come in many forms—autobiography, memoir, biography, historical accounts, oral histories, qualitative interviews, and more. Bertaux and Kohli (1984) define "life stories" as oral or autobiographical narratives. What is common to all, and essential to a study of diversity, is a narrative that connects personal origins to individual outcomes. The subject passes through thick and thin to emerge as a distinctive individual, driven by a unique identity that is interactively shaped by the culture of origin and subsequent social forces. Although each life story is particular to one individual, certain crucial aspects of these experiences, which are related to starting position (e.g., class, race, gender) and to subsequent events correlated with that position, are also variously experienced by others. A number of scholars have noted that such narrative accounts are superior to quantitative survey methods for arriving at a deeper understanding of the dynamics that drive and shape the life course. Kohli (1981) finds that life stories are particularly useful because of their *comprehensiveness* that covers both social and individual life, their *subjectivity* that gives a view of life "from within," and their *narrative form* that adds the dimension of change over time.

Comprehensiveness That Conveys Coherence and Meaning

Sociologists who favor the life story method begin their recommendations of narrative with a critique of cross-sectional survey methodology. They note that large samples, "objective" questions, and causal analysis focused on variables cannot explain the individual circumstances that make some people change location, while others do not (Bertaux & Thompson, 1997). For example, the Bertaux and Bertaux-Wiame study of French bread makers discovered what could never be revealed by typical surveys. With a mere 30 life history interviews of master bakers in France, they found a common story: Bakers came from small villages, moved to even larger towns and cities, and by working long hours and enduring work-related health problems, rose into the middle class. Among those bakers working in Paris, not a single individual was born in Paris or its environs (Bertaux, 1981).

Life histories reveal patterns that surveys cannot, because surveys take a fragmented approach that examines the effects of *variables* on given outcomes in a population. As Mishler (1996) observed, cross-sectional data based on variables in a population can tell us about average group trends but not about individual cases. Any departure from the average tends to be treated as an error. The beauty of individual case studies is that they treat departures from the norm as interesting phenomena to be explored.

To understand individual variation, it is necessary to frame the research as a series of case studies and, in the process, gather any information that the respondent deems relevant. This has the effect of both incorporating the subject's perspective and reflecting the expectations of those in the surrounding social and cultural milieu. As McAdams (2001, p. 101) observes, the life story is "co-authored" by the person him- or herself, and the social and cultural context "within which that person's life is embedded and given meaning." Because the life story has a past, present, and future, it reveals the links between internal feelings and external situations, and shows the continuity and coherence of the person's life across time. The person as an entity is understood to be a living *system* that is adapting to the environment and taking one direction or another as a result of the integration of many internal and external forces.

The ultimate payoff of the life story method is that the observer can better understand why a person's life path took the twists and turns that it did. Although clues to explanation of a particular outcome can be found in descriptive group averages, understanding is much more complete when a person's story is available to suggest the meaning and purpose of his or her actions (McAdams, 2006).

Subjectivity That Depicts the "I"

In addition to being comprehensive, the life story puts the facts together from the subject's point of view and, in the process, constitutes a report on the self and a picture of the person's identity and sense of agency. As Kohli (1981, pp. 64–65) says, "The autobiographical form presupposes a developed individuality, a self-conscious 'I' being able to grasp itself as the organizer of its own life history and as distinct from its social world." This life story is not a collection of all the events of the individual's life but is a structured self-image which comes close to the concept of identity. It is this "I" as agent that mediates between the individual's conscious self and the demands of objective social identity. Thus, the personal life record is an ideal form of sociological material for understanding the interaction between self and other.

Psychologists in particular have adapted the life story method to create a new subdiscipline in personality psychology known as narrative identity research (Singer, 2004). They are concerned with how individuals employ narratives to develop and sustain a sense of personal unity and purpose across life, and they have further probed the question of what kind of personal narrative is typical of outstanding leaders or highly generative persons. In research on intellectuals, writers, and scientists, Howe (1982) discovered several distinctive features in their stories: high initial ability, childhood events that enabled achievement, desire and encouragement to achieve, and parental support. Csikszentmihalyi (1993) has described the "transcendent self" as characteristic of those individuals who contribute to progress in the world rather than to entropy. In *The Redemptive Self* McAdams (2006) outlines the characteristic life stories of highly generative individuals, which include an awareness of their advantage relative to the suffering of others, a steadfast sense of a moral imperative to help others, and a search for future growth and fulfillment. That it is possible to derive these generalizations from something as particular as life stories suggests that similar properties of identity and agency can be found in groups of individuals who arrived at similar outcomes.

Another potential for generalization comes from the social inputs into the life story. Compared with the psychologists' focus on identity development, there appears to be less research into generalizable patterns in life stories that are due to well-trodden social pathways. However, if one of the functions of a life narrative, as McAdams (2001) suggests, is to find and to fit into a niche in society, then the expectations and limitations surrounding a given class, racial/ethnic, or gender origin are good places to look for regularities.

For example, one ethnic pattern that has been a matter of public discussion is the expectation that Asian and Asian American students will do much better in mathematics than European Americans. In fact, there is a pattern related to family origin, but it is related to immigrant history rather than to a particular ethnic group. The winners of mathematical prizes are more likely to come from immigrant families, ethnic groups, and nationalities and family cultures in which mathematics is highly valued, children are expected to do well in math, and the students themselves strive to excel in their performance (Rimer, 2008).

Narrative Form That Accounts for Change

Because life stories are arranged as causal chains, they tell how the individual has integrated competing factors to arrive at a unique identity and to get from the past to the present in a certain way. As Bertaux and Thompson (1997) noted, the majority of people take their social status as a given and circulate within it to fill a space. But for those who are in search of a better life, one expects to find "the social and emotional launch pads for individual takeoff" (p. 2). The narrative form of a life story helps to uncover these social and emotional "launch pads." A story has the power to tie together the past, present, and future to answer the questions "Who am I?" and "How do I fit into the adult world?" (McAdams, 1985, pp. 17–18) At the same time, "Stories are structured such that events can be seen as 'causing' subsequent events, the action being arranged in causal chains" (McAdams, 1985, p. 67). Thus, the life story tells not only "who I am" but also how "I" got to be that way.

To the extent that individuals share a similar identity, occupation, or social location, it should be possible to find certain common themes or elements in their life stories. This is precisely what Daniel Bertaux and Isabelle Bertaux-Wiame discovered in their research on French bakers.

> One life story is only one life story. Thirty life stories of thirty men and women scattered in the whole social structure are only thirty life stories. But thirty life stories of thirty men who have lived their lives in one and the same sector of production (here bakery workers) represent more than thirty isolated life stories; taken together, they tell a different story, at a different level: the history of this sector of production at the level of its pattern of sociostructural relationships. (Bertaux, 1981, p. 187)

One concludes that it is the regularities, which come from similar sociostructural relationships, that constitute the parallel features in life stories of the bakers. One expects the same logic of similar social experience leading to similar outcomes to apply to those who are working class compared with professionals, blacks compared with whites, or women compared with men. Likewise, there must be some launch pads that enable *departure from one's ascribed status* to seek a better life. Singer (2004, p. 438) suggests that there will be similarities in narrative identity that reveal "how individuals understand themselves as unique individuals and as social beings who are multiply defined by life stage, gender, ethnicity, class, and culture." On the other hand, Hammack (2008) notes that some personal narratives depart from the master narrative, whereas others do not, and this variability is highly contingent on the cultural context of development. Thus, if we find some working-class individuals whose personal narratives are at odds with a master working-class narrative; or a black person's narrative that is atypical, or a woman's story that is more like that of a man, it should be possible, through the narrative, to relate these patterns to the particular sociocultural contexts in which the storytellers have constructed their identity. A preliminary literature review in fact suggests some of the differences between persons who stay within their ascribed social roles and those who challenge expectations about their class, race, or gender.

Class Mobility

The personal narratives of those who experience upward mobility show a lack of acceptance of their original status and a search for something better. In an early comparison of 15 white working-class men and 15 white professional men, ranging in age from 35 to 75, Csikszentmihalyi and Beattie (1979) discovered several broad differences in life stories. Although an equal number from each group had faced hardship as children, the professionals looked beyond their own situation and were working to help others to attain better health, escape from poverty, and go to school. The blue-collar men, however, thought primarily in terms of their own situation and of solutions to their own problems. In addition, the professionals had a much higher level of ambition. Their parents had read to them as children and held higher hopes and expectations for them. Hogan (1981) found that college-educated men from blue-collar and farm backgrounds were more likely to have followed an atypical sequence in finishing their education, getting a job, and getting married than those from urban and higher-status origins. Dumais (2002), using the National Educational Longitudinal Study, found that working-class students who finished high school or college had fewer adversities and parents with more involvement in their education than those who dropped out early. Atwood (2007), who analyzed the memoirs of 30 writers who grew up in poor or working-class families (e.g., Maya Angelou, Russell Baker, Vivian Gornick, and Richard Wright), also found that almost all were recognized by a teacher or other mentor who provided support for moving up and out.

Transcendence of Racial or Ethnic Stereotypes

It is a theorem of social psychology that greater experience and familiarity with the outgroup will reduce racial prejudice if the contact is between persons *of equal social status* (Allport, 1954), and if they are *not in conflict or competition* with each other (Pettigrew 1998). Hammack's (2008) findings on the evolving identities of Israeli and Palestinian youth support this principle. After participating in peace-oriented summer coexistence programs, the only students who were able to transcend their separatist identities were those who had sufficient security beforehand and positive experience with collaboration across the Israeli–Palestinian divide to be able to take a more inclusive view.

A similar history of security and positive reinforcement appears to enable members of a racial minority to resist stereotyping and to express self-confidence and pride. Coard and Sellers (2005) showed how black parents instill both respect for their culture and coping skills and self-esteem to help their children be able to resist the effects of disrespect and low expectations. Higginbotham (2001) found that many female "racial pioneers" were black women who had attended predominantly white colleges in the 1960s. Slevin and Wingrove (1998) discovered that successful black women professionals typically received strong support and were a source of pride to their local churches and communities.

Their families highly valued education. The women themselves persisted as professionals by adapting to limited opportunities and working as teachers, nurses, and social workers.

"Doing Gender" Differently

Just as transcendence of class and race is made possible by coming from an atypical background, receiving family encouragement, and having positive outside contacts with the majority group, so also being an atypical man or an atypical woman is associated with analogous types of life experience. West and Zimmerman (1987), in their famous paper on "doing gender," held that male and female roles are more the enactment of cultural expectations than of innate propensities. Bertaux-Wiame (1981), in her research on the wives of French bakers, discovered a 90-year-old woman who talked "like a man"—speaking more in terms of herself as the central actor than in terms of relationships to others. What was special about her life was that she had been independent, making choices and charting her own course. Up to age 30, when she was widowed, her story sounded like that of other women. But her narrative after that reflected her entrepreneurial and independent status as a head of household. This structural location, similar to that of a man and requiring similar actions, was presumably what made her talk "like a man."

Women and men who rebel against sex stereotypes and create new alternatives have often been marginal in some way. Many come from humble beginnings, are the smartest in the class or minority group members, and are surrounded by like-minded people in their church, community, or family. High-achieving black women are encouraged to get higher education and to aim for professional and public responsibilities (Slevin & Wingrove, 1998). Coltrane (1996) found that egalitarian men had a history of admiring and respecting women as much or more than men. Men who are nurturant come from families and have peers and partners who are supportive of their less "macho" life style (Coltrane & Adams, 2001; Connell, 1995).

These clues about the factors leading to the wide internal variation in identity and life stories within any one class, race, or gender invite a more systematic examination of life stories to understand diversity. The task is to design a comparison of cases in such a way that the explanatory factors behind different outcomes become apparent. To do this, one has to choose cases for comparison and collect relevant data so that one can see differences and similarities in the factors that lead to a given life outcome. Choice of methods and a research design is the first step in using life stories to understand diversity.

Life Stories and the Comparative Method

Both to investigate the effect of diverse origins on the life course and to explain why some lives take one direction rather than another, it is necessary to view each life story as a case study and to use the logic of the comparative method to understand the reasons for similarities and differences. Several steps are involved: (1) selection of cases; (2) collection of data; (3) description of key attributes of the cases; and (4) comparative analysis to identify similarities and differences. I have used these methods in a qualitative study of 48 college-educated women to understand why some combine careers with families, while others become full-time homemakers. This example illustrates the use of a comparative method, life history interviews, and the theory of action to understand diversity in ascribed roles (Giele, 2008).

Selection of Cases

The starting point of the comparative method is selection of cases. The most frequent examples used by Ragin (1987) are whole societies, such as "rich" countries, those that experienced a revolution or contain territories with linguistic minorities. In such comparisons there are relatively few cases, and the focus is on what characteristics are sufficient to account for a given outcome. Rather than variable attributes, it is the whole case that is examined to determine what key factors account for a revolution, an ethnic conflict, or being a rich country. In life course research the comparative method is also appropriate, because life stories are also case studies at the level of the individual. To explain a particular role pattern, political bent, or ideological position, one examines the person's life as a whole, not just specific events, attributes, or variables. For the comparative method to work, however, cases must be selected in such a way that they can be analyzed using John Stuart Mill's classic method of agreement and indirect method of difference (Ragin, 1987).

In my research on homemakers and career women, I ruled out easy explanations based on differences in age, education, marital and parental status, income, and social class by attempting to "control" the effect of these obvious background factors through a selection of only married women who had children, a college education, and were roughly the same age. In comparing career women and homemakers who were similar in these respects, I approximated the logic of the experimental method. I could then look for differences in life experience of the career women and homemakers.

By selecting an equal number of whites and blacks in the career and homemaker groups who were similar in major background factors except for race, I was able to investigate the variability of outcomes within the gender group, as well as the two racial groups. Thus, the study made possible an identification of possible race differences in the way whites and blacks arrived at a career or homemaker destination. Ragin (2000, p. 126) affirms that "the examination of outcomes is a central part of constructing a property space and generating configurations, especially when it comes to the selection of causally relevant aspects of cases."

Collection of Retrospective and Qualitative Data

Having selected the cases, the investigator's next task is to assemble relevant data that describe not only the outcome to be explained but also contain the most likely precursors to that outcome. Such material can come from a set of biographies, a collection of memoirs, or case records and qualitative interviews. Alternatively, the investigator might prospectively gather specific information on major life transitions, such as that contained in a life history calendar, supplemented by contemporaneous diaries or other records.

I used retrospective life stories covering four time periods to elicit major themes in each woman's life. The first question focused on *young adulthood* and asked the respondent's major in college and her vision at that time of her future occupation and family situation. The second question asked the woman to look back to *childhood* and think about her family's attitudes toward women's education, similarities and differences with brothers and sisters, family finances, and general expectations. The third question brought the respondent up to her present situation *as an adult in midlife* and asked her to reflect on the kind of achievement and frustration, and rewards and problems she had experienced since college, in both work and family life. The last question invited the respondent to project her *expectations for the future* and articulate problems to be solved and goals to be realized. The resulting transcripts were 30–40 pages long, and were remarkably rich and varied in the clues they gave to the formative factors underlying each woman's life course.

A Theory of Action to Interpret Life Stories

Implicit in existing studies of life stories are the recurrent factors that shape a person's life. Family background, social pressure, individual traits, and economic conditions all play a part. The theoretical challenge is to identify the key variables that lead to one kind of outcome or another; for example, what distinguishes pioneers and the upwardly mobile from more typical exemplars of a specific class, race, or gender?

Life course scholars have over the years developed an implicit theory of action that sees the person's life path as shaped by several key factors. Some of these factors, such as culture and social relationships, are external to the individual; others, such as self-concept or adaptive style, reflect characteristics of the person. In the theory of action each person is understood to be a living behavioral system in which personal values, social expectations, and motives are all brought to bear on any given opportunity or challenge. According to the reinforcement axiom of psychology, successful resolution of a problem is likely to strengthen the beliefs and behaviors that bring about good results, whereas failure or frustration brings discouragement, anger, withdrawal, or change in that behavior. Thus, to understand a particular life course, one must look to the key factors that make up an individual's behavioral system.

In the life course field, the emerging paradigm for describing the individual's behavioral system includes four main factors: (1) historical and cultural location, (2) social relationships, (3) personal motives, and (4) timing and adaptation to major life events (Giele & Elder, 1998a). This formulation is consistent with both Parsons, Bales, and Shils's (1953) general theory of action (L–latent pattern maintenance, I–integration, G–goal attainment, and A–adaptation) and Burke's (1945) "grammar of motives," which identifies the key elements of any drama or story (purpose, setting, agent and agency, and action). The paradigm is also latent in the "Listener's Guide," a method developed by Brown and Gilligan (1992) for interpreting the life stories of teenage girls (plot, relationships, voice of the "I," and reality testing and learning; Giele, 2002). I have used these several congruent conceptual frameworks to look for similarities and differences in the life patterns of college-educated career women and homemakers (Giele, 2004, 2008). The synthesis yields four familiar concepts that are also theoretically grounded: identity, relational style, motivation, and adaptive style (as shown in Table 11.1).

This four-factor theory is not only parsimonious but sufficiently generalizable for explaining various life patterns. Each component is derived from a major research tradition within the social sciences. The idealistic tradition, here exemplified by Max Weber and anthropologists Benedict and Mead, emphasizes the power of culture, values, and purpose in shaping action. The strong influence of social relationships on individual action that is mediated through family ties and community membership is documented in Polish peasants by Thomas and Znaniecki (1918–1920) and in children of the Great Depression by Elder (1974).

TABLE 11.1. Four Factors That Shape the Life Course and Life Stories

Theory of action (Parsons et al., 1953)	Life course framework (Elder, 1998b; Giele & Elder, 1998b)	Life course factors (classic theoretical foundations)	Life story themes (Giele, 2002, 2004, 2008)
Latent pattern maintenance (L)	Historical and cultural location	Values, beliefs, purpose (Weber, 1930; Benedict, 1946; Mead, 1963)	Identity (e.g., different or conventional)
Integration (I)	Linked lives	Social networks, context (Thomas & Znaniecki, 1918/1920; Elder, 1974, 1998a)	Relational style (e.g., equal or hierarchical)
Goal attainment (G)	Agency	Needs, desires (Allport, 1937; Murray, 1938; McClelland, 1967, 1975)	Motivation, drives (e.g., achievement, power, affiliation)
Adaptation (A)	Timing of events	Competence (White, 1952/1966; Clausen, 1993)	Adaptive style (e.g., innovative or traditional)

To explain the nature and uniqueness of individual lives over time, psychologists Allport (1937) and Murray (1938), beginning in the 1930s, conceived of personality as the dynamic system that organizes goals and action throughout the life course. Finally, at the level of specific events and transitions, White (1952/1966) and Clausen (1993) focused on the adaptive behavior of individuals, particularly the development of competence, which enables one to negotiate changing situations successfully.

Influence of Values on Identity and Action: Weber, Benedict, and Mead

Max Weber (1930) not only illuminated the importance of major world religions in shaping the economy and polity of their regions, but he also traced the influence of Protestantism on entrepreneurs who promoted the growth of capitalism. Because Calvinists could not know whether they were predestined to heaven or hell, they looked for a sign that they were among the elect rather than the reprobate and began to rely on worldly success as evidence that they had been chosen. Such beliefs fueled their passion for entrepreneurship and risk taking, and defined their achievements as the glorification of God in this world. Similar beliefs appear also to have motivated the scientific revolution of that period, as Merton (1949/1957) discovered in the significant number of Puritans among early members of the Royal Academy of Science.

Researchers in the personality-and-culture field found analogous connections between cultural values and "modal personality." In *The Chrysanthemum and the Sword,* Ruth Benedict (1946) described distinctive themes in Japanese culture and character. In *Sex and Temperament in Three Primitive Societies,* Margaret Mead (1963) likewise showed how life patterns of men and women differed across three cultures in New Guinea.

Social Relations and Life Course Outcomes: Thomas, Znaniecki, and Elder

The distinct new contribution of W. I. Thomas and Florian Znaniecki (1927/1984) was to examine the social relationships of Polish peasants who moved to America. By analyzing their letters and the shared expectations of the family members left behind, they illuminated the enormous and continuing importance of obligations and responsibilities that were carried over from an earlier stage in life to a later stage. A husband in America continued to hear from his wife and children in Poland—about their loneliness, their poverty, and their hope that he would send them another remittance or even return home. At the same time, life for the immigrant to the New World also brought a new set of obligations and expectations that competed with the old. Each individual had to reconcile in his or her own life the competing obligations to the extended family that were established in the past with the new obligations and social relationships of the present. In the process of coping with these competing claims, individuals had to adjust their life patterns to adapt to the new circumstances.

Glen Elder (1998a) uses the term "linked lives" to capture the matrix of social institutions and group memberships that enfold and shape an individual's path over the course of a lifetime. In his classic *Children of the Great Depression,* Elder (1974) shows how family expectations shaped the subsequent lives of boys and girls as they became adult men and women. The girls who grew up in deprived families and had to help at home, because their mothers were working in place of the unemployed father, turned out in the 1950s to be more likely to become full-time homemakers themselves. But the girls from less deprived families were more likely to get further education, and combine work and family when they were adults. Thus, the way social relationships affect the life course is partly a function of life history. But it is also true that social expectations from an earlier period are not just directly imprinted on later action; rather, they set in motion selective processes that limit the range of future opportunities and experience.

Personality, Motives, and Lives in Progress: Allport, Murray, and McClelland

At the same time that culture and social ties influence individual behavior, each person has the power of individual action which is never altogether certain or predictable. Through the new psychology of personality that emerged in the 1930s, both Gordon W. Allport (1937) and Henry A. Murray (1938) established the study of the person as not just a bundle of attitudes, traits, or unconscious desires but as an integrated system (Hall & Lindzey, 1957). "Personality," according to Allport (1937, p. 48) "is the dynamic organization within the individual of those psycho-physical systems that determine his unique adjustments to his environment." Allport was interested in the ways that individuals make rational attempts to meet their needs by combining their attitudes and intentions with their particular traits, capacities, and motives to reach a goal. Allport's ideographic emphasis was quite different from that of the stimulus–response psychologists who, in looking for general laws, examined short-term segments of behavior that could be compared across individuals. Allport, in focusing on the ego and on conscious rational and forward-looking behavior, also challenged the psychoanalytically oriented psychologists who drew heavily on insights from abnormal psychology and early childhood experience to understand adult behavior.

Henry Murray (1938), who came into psychology from medicine, also saw personality as the organizing or governing agent of the individual. Like Allport, he rejected a fragmented study of individual behavior and thought it important to study persons longitudinally and as living wholes by observing their lives in progress. With a team of psychologists at the Harvard Psychological Clinic, he studied 50 young men from different aspects—their needs, desires, fears, characteristic perceptions of social structure, strategies for problem solving, childhood experience, fantasy life, and the like. Key to his conceptual framework was a carefully specified classification of needs and motives such as the Need for Achievement (N Ach), Need for Affiliation (N Aff), Nurturance, Dominance, and many others.

What is perhaps most useful for the study of the life course in both Allport's and Murray's work is their focus on individual life history and the many kinds of motivation. They both asked the question that is still vital today for students of the life course: "What are the fundamental variables in terms of which a personality may be comprehensively and adequately described?" (Murray, 1938, p. x). This important question was taken up by David McClelland (1967, 1975) in his careful experimental studies of the need for achievement that showed the importance of early independence training and, later, the need for power.

Competence and Adaptation: White and Clausen

Whereas Allport and Murray laid the foundation for the study of lives over time, their colleague Robert White particularly pressed forward the project of studying "lives in progress." White (1952/1966, p. 22) observed that the most neglected area in personality psychology was continuous development over time. What interested him was the process of growth and development through which the individual learns to deal successfully and creatively with new and changing circumstances. He emphasized that "personality does not stand still.... The person... is not always a passive victim of the forces that influence him. He is himself a center of energy and an active agent in changing his material and human surroundings" (White, 1952/1966, p. iv).

Like Allport, White eschewed controlled scientific experiments as a way of studying personality, as well as inferences based on abnormal behavior and any overemphasis on social influence. He gravitated instead to the ways that people actively and playfully test their surroundings, and derive gratification and reinforcement from successfully handling new challenges. Thus, he attached special importance to *competence* in dealing with the environment, by which he intended to restore to the person "what we all experience as initiative and efficacy in leading our lives" (White, 1952/1966, p. 25).

Forty years after White's first edition of *Lives in Progress,* John Clausen (1993), in *American Lives,* provided strong support for the significance of varying degrees of competence as a mode of adaptation that continues throughout the life course. Using data collected from a sample of children born in 1928–1931 who were studied during childhood, adolescence, and adulthood by the Berkeley Institute of Child Welfare, Clausen compared adaptive styles early in life with outcomes later on. He was particularly interested in differences between those who scored high and low on "planful competence" during adolescence, and whether their adult lives turned out differently. Those who scored high in planful competence exhibited qualities related to (1) *knowledge* (including skill and intelligence); (2) *dependability* (self-control and taking responsibility); and (3) *self-confidence* (self-direction, ego resilience, and friendliness). Clausen hypothesized that these qualities are particularly useful for effective functioning. Comparisons of the same children as adults in fact showed that those who had exhibited planful competence in adolescence were more likely to have reached a higher level of education, to be married to the same spouse, and to have avoided a severe discontinuity or crisis.

Works by White and Clausen are particularly useful to life course researchers for their specification of competence as an indicator of successful growth and development. Despite very different identities, social relationships, and motives, people can so organize their behavior that they are more or less efficacious. Being competent—knowledgeable, dependable, and self-confident—is a style of adaptation to changing situations that augurs well for healthy growth and development.

Synthesis: Identity, Social Relations, Agency, and Adaptation

The life course scholar who puts these four elements together—a person's values, social networks, motivation, and adaptive style—has a conceptual framework and an implicit theory for explaining differences in life course outcomes, as well as differences associated with origins or "starting position." Such a framework meets the tests of coherence, parsimony, and generalizability that are required of any theory. Moreover, such a framework is consistent with the reigning paradigm of systems theory, in which the key elements are understood to intertwine and mutually affect each other in shaping the life course of the person.

Using this theoretical framework to analyze the data, the next step is to apply it both inductively and deductively to identify similarities and differences in life stories.

Descriptive and Causal Analysis of Life Stories

With the biographies, life history records, or interview transcripts for the selected cases, the next task is to identify what appear to be the major antecedents or causal influences leading to one outcome or another. The theory of action comes into play with codification of the data that proceeds both inductively and deductively. Strauss and Corbin (1990) describe "induction" as grounded theory. Miles and Huberman (1994) give extensive pointers on how to list major themes, aggregate them chronologically or by level of generality, and diagram their relationship to each other and to an outcome. Willie (1988) gives an example of how induction works in his discussion of common themes in the lives of eight prominent sociologists. He finds a recurring theme of moral and ethical concern, coupled with a desire to end racial, ethnic, class, or gender discrimination. He then reflects on the common antidiscrimination theme that comes from each person's feeling of being oppressed in some way as a member of one or another type of "subdominant" group.

In my study of homemakers and career women, I began to notice that the career women always seemed to be struggling against what was considered normal for women, whereas the homemakers were doing what most people expected. I then linked this central insight to my four-factor framework and discovered that feeling "different" in one's identity was a master theme accompanied by a feminist (egalitarian) relational style, a pattern of motivation focused on achievement, and an innovative mode of adaptation to life transitions that sometimes challenges convention.

Two coders (myself and a student assistant) read through the interviews and identified passages that pertained to each of these dimensions. We used the following guidelines (Giele, 2008):

- *Identity:* How does R (respondent) see herself? With whom does she identify as being like herself? Does she mention her race, ethnicity, social class, or how she is different or similar to her family? What qualities does she mention that distinguish her (intelligence, being quiet, likable, innovative, outstanding, a good mother, lawyer, wife, etc.)?
- *Relational style*: What is R's typical way of relating to others? As a leader, follower, negotiator, equal colleague? Does she take charge? Is she independent or very reliant on others for company and support? Does she have a lot of friends or is she lonely? What is the nature of her relationship with her husband?
- *Drive and motivation*: What is R's need for achievement, affiliation, power? Is R ambitious and driven or relaxed and easygoing? Is she concerned about making a name for herself? Is she focused more on helping her husband and children than on her own needs (nurturance vs. personal achievement)? Does she mention enjoying life and wanting to have time for other things besides work? Does she enjoy being with children, doing volunteer work, seeing friends? Does she have a desire to be in control of her own schedule, to be in charge rather than to take orders?
- *Adaptive style:* What is her energy level? Is R an innovator and a risk taker or is she conventional and uncomfortable with change and new experience? Does R like to manage change, to think of new ways of doing things? Is she self-confident or cautious? Is she used to a slow or fast pace, to routine and having plenty of time, or to doing several things at once?

Comparative Analysis

The underlying logic of the comparative method is built on Boolean algebra and the comparison of sets (Ragin, 1987, 2000). Ideally, the outcome variable is unambiguously dichotomous, and the presumed causes can be neatly associated with different outcomes. Thus, in distinguishing between middle-class, educated women who are homemakers and those who have careers, the antecedents of being a homemaker or career woman are expected to be different. In contrast with career women, homemakers' identities are expected to involve thinking of themselves as similar to other women, with relational styles that are more accepting of role and status differences between the sexes, drive that is more oriented to affiliation than to independent achievements, and adaptation to transitions that is more conventional than innovative.

There are two main axes of comparison among members of my sample, which was deliberately constructed to comprise 24 white and 24 black women, two-thirds of whom were combining careers and families, and one-third of whom were homemakers at the time they were interviewed between 2001 and 2006 (Giele, 2008). The first line of analysis, rather than drawing contrasts between the sexes or middle-class and working-class women, focused on occupational variation within this middle class, educated group, comparing differences in the stories of homemakers and career women. The second comparison contrasts these two types by race.

Variation in Occupational Role Outcomes among Middle-Class Women

Holding constant gender and class, it turns out there is a wide variety in the work role choices of middle-class women. The employed mothers who are professionals and managers see their roles as dual (encompassing both work and family) and try to share both types of responsibility as equally as possible with their partners. Homemakers focus on motherhood as their primary role and accept a sex-differentiated division of labor between the breadwinner and themselves.

Racial Similarities

The distinction in life patterns between career women and homemakers also holds up within each racial group. The career women of both races work with a dual-earner model of work and family life, in which they believe paid work can be combined with having a family. Although educated black homemakers are harder to find than educated white homemakers, they do exist. Black and white homemakers are similar in accepting a more sex-differentiated division of labor in family work and paid work.

Racial Differences

The career women had somewhat different stories depending on their race. They had all been told they were exceptional—bright, talented, and destined for something special. But for the black women, this sense of difference was more often associated with feeling a special responsibility to overcome racial discrimination. The white career women, on the other hand, had fought to overcome other kinds of obstacles— discrimination because of their religion, coming from a poor or dysfunctional family, or having to live with a disability.

Life stories of black and white homemakers also revealed several subtle differences by race. The black homemakers, who typically had once had successful careers, explicitly viewed their time at home as temporary. Some were actually criticized by their mothers for trying to do the "white woman thing" by staying at home. They persisted, however, supported by evangelical teachings to honor the man of the family, and affirm his authority and dignity by relying on him as the breadwinner for sole support, at least for a time. A second motive was to protect their children by strategies such as home-schooling and intensive monitoring to keep them from doing badly in school or getting into trouble. White homemakers, on the other hand, tended to be married to husbands with much higher earning power than their own, and to see their opportunity for leisure, volunteer activities, and time with their children as an entitlement that was not time-limited.

Ambiguous Outcomes, Antecedents, and the Use of Fuzzy Sets

Sometimes it is difficult to draw dichotomous distinctions between types of cases, descriptive categories, and outcomes. For example, regarding selection of cases in my study, if a long-time homemaker had returned to the work force part-time, or if a career woman had decided to stay at home for a period, I excluded them, because it was not obvious how each case should be classified, thus presenting a complication in the comparison and contrast of mutually exclusive Boolean sets. A similar challenge arises when coding any quality or state that involves gradation rather than a clear-cut dichotomy. Fortunately, in cases of gradation between 0 and 1, the methodology of fuzzy sets provide a means to include "in-between" cases in the selection of outcome sets and in the coding of graded properties of those sets. A "fuzzy set" is a property space that registers degrees of membership in a given set, in which 1 represents totally "in," 0 stands for totally "out," and 0.5 means "neither in nor out."

Ragin (2000) demonstrates how one can construct a "fuzzy set" by assigning a value between 0 and 1 (e.g., 0.3 or 0.7) to qualitative attributes that are not strictly dichotomous. Such a notation, by accommodating gradation, expands "crisp" Boolean sets into "fuzzy" sets. Ragin considers this method to be particularly well suited to the study of any kind of diversity, where group membership is better viewed on a continuum rather than as a rigid set of mutually exclusive categories. In my analysis of women's life course patterns, for example, being a part-time worker, having an interrupted career, or having few or many children could be handled by using fuzzy sets and coding these states as somewhere between 0 and 1. The analytic task would then become a search for the distinguishing features associated with different degrees of membership in the category of homemaker or career woman.

Ragin has two principal strategies for using fuzzy sets: The first is to identify those qualities that are *necessary* to a given outcome, and the second is to identify the combination of qualities that is *sufficient* to produce the outcome. "Necessary conditions" are identified as the set of cases that is *positive* on a given quality and larger than the outcome set. For example, I might find that the number of college-educated, married women with children who also had high motivation for achievement was larger than the set of career women alone; this would be an indicator that desire for achievement is a *necessary* condition for pursuing a career. But if I found that those in high-powered persistent careers all had a *combination* of a special identity, an egalitarian marriage, achievement drive, and innovativeness, and those who worked part-time did not, I would have screened out some *negative cases*, and in the process would have identified a smaller subset than the larger, inclusive "fuzzy set" of all the women working either part-time or full-time. Using this strategy, I would be able to pinpoint the *sufficient causes* for membership in the most committed career group.

Summary and Conclusion

To answer the question of how class, race, or gender origin affects the life course, it is necessary to have a method and a theory capable of linking starting position to life outcome. This chapter is concerned with how to understand the differences between those individuals from an ascribed "minority" status who, in some sense, become part of the "majority"—the person from working-class origins who becomes middle class, the person of color who is accepted into the ranks of power, the woman who enters what was once thought a "male" role.

Life stories are an important method for uncovering the features that distinguish such persons from peers who fit a more conventional or stereotypical role. Life stories, unlike quantitative methods that rely on surveys and large samples, get at individuals' inner identity and purpose and thus help to distinguish between those who are mobile and those who are not. In addition, life stories reveal the distinctive social and cultural experience that helped to form the self; they also provide a narrative of change over time.

The first step to using life stories to understand diversity is careful selection of cases based on similar and contrasting outcomes. The object of selection is to compare the antecedents leading up to different outcomes and at the same time "control for" as many background differences as possible (other than the ascribed characteristics under study). For my own research on black and white middle-class women, I chose persons who were similar in age, education, and marital and parental status but who differed in role outcome—being a homemaker or having a career.

To collect the life stories of these comparison groups, the questions should cover major stages of life and elicit memories of respondents' plans in early adulthood, how they were treated as children, their current life and its rewards and frustrations, and finally their challenges and hopes for the future. Then begins the critical discernment of major themes that link these persons' origins to their life outcomes. These can be derived from the basic theory of action and the life course framework. "Identity" is associated with a person's location in time and space and cultural milieu. "Relational style" is shaped by social networks and loyalties. "Personal agency" reflects the individual's goals and motivation. "Adaptive style" sums up the accommodations and changes a person has learned to negotiate while living through changing conditions and life transitions.

In my study, the *identity* of the career women was "different" from an early age. These women also deliberately looked for an egalitarian *relationship* in their marriage. They showed strong *motivation* to achieve in their work and to gain public recognition. Their *adaptation* to change was to seek innovative rather than conventional solutions. Black and white women were similar in the career-oriented group. But black homemakers differed from white homemakers in seeing their time at home as more temporary and in pursuing a moral purpose: They withdrew from the workforce to elevate their husbands' authority and at the same time, through strategies such as home-schooling, sought to shield their children from harm and promote their academic and social development.

By using the comparative method of agreement and the indirect method of difference, along with the logic of "crisp" and "fuzzy" sets, one can look for precursors associated with each outcome and at the same time discern both the necessary and sufficient causal factors that contribute to a given life outcome. In the end, as a result of such analysis, one sees that there are many ways of "doing" class, race, and gender. Life stories demonstrate the ways in which stereotypes can be exploded. To understand these mechanisms, it is necessary to examine not only the constraints imposed by starting position but also the life course factors that can loosen those constraints. A clear-eyed examination of ways that minorities break the bonds of ascription reveals the potential for even greater diversity in life course outcomes than in origins.

Acknowledgments

The research reported here was supported with grants from the Murray Center for the Study of Lives of the Radcliffe Institute for Advanced Study, Harvard University, and the Mazer Fund of Brandeis University. I thank Meg Lovejoy for her help with interviewing. I also thank Meg Lovejoy, Dan P. McAdams, and Elliot Mishler for their helpful comments on an earlier version of this chapter.

CHAPTER 12

Social Convoys

Studying Linked Lives in Time,
Context, and Motion

Phyllis Moen
Elaine Hernandez

Social research is, by definition, about relationships, but most scholars study individuals. Why this methodological individualism? First, individuals are much easier (and cheaper) to survey than families, groups, networks, or organizations. Second, most methods of quantitative analysis assume independence across analytic units, discouraging research designs that incorporate connections between respondents. Third, individuals seem somehow more "permanent"; families, friendship networks, and teams change over time as members join or leave. Scholars undertaking longitudinal studies find it far easier to follow individuals, because group memberships shift with each passing year.

For example, the *Panel Study of Income Dynamics* (PSID) began as a study of 5,000 family households in 1968. Each subsequent survey year documented people's movement in and out of the core families/ households with remarkable frequency: starting new households (and families), dissolving existing arrangements, and/or moving into others. These changes made it difficult to continue to identify and to collect data over time on the "original" families in the 1968 study. The PSID founders decided the solution was to follow *all* individual family members *and* their emergent households, not only expanding the sample exponentially over time but also creating a national treasure of data on lives in time. The PSID has now collected information on over 7,000 families and more than 65,000 individuals, spanning multiple decades of people's lives.

Linked Lives as Convoys and Contexts

Life course scholars (e.g., Elder, 1974; Mortimer & Shanahan, 2003; Shanahan & Macmillan, 2007) highlight the embeddedness of individuals within the social fabric of evolving, overlapping networks of close and distal ties. For example, early scholarship on status attainment charted the career paths of individuals (men) but showed the links between fathers' and sons' occupational prestige. However, this influential body of theoretical and empirical analysis of men's occupational attainment did not take into account the fact that men in the mid-20th century could focus on their jobs precisely because they had wives taking care of everything else. Life course scholars Pavalko and Elder (1993) demonstrated the importance of wives as partners in their husbands' careers.

In this chapter we underscore how individual lives are always *linked lives* (Elder, 1985a); one person's resources, resource deficits, successes, failures, chronic strains, and (expected or unexpected) transitions can become focal conditions, even turning points, in the lives of others, especially other family members. For example, when scholars began investigating women's status attainment and gender inequality in the 1980s and 1990s, they captured a range of career paths that did not follow the conventional (male) lockstep career progression. Women's status attainment and wages continue to be shaped by their transitions into and out of jobs, the workforce, and schooling, often accommodating the careers of husbands and the care needs of children and aging relatives (Blossfeld & Hofmeister, 2006; Moen & Roehling, 2005).

Men's lives are also embedded in the matrix of others' lives. For example, a father may forgo a promotion requiring relocation because his oldest son is a high school junior and wants to graduate from his current school with his friends. Both these examples capture what we mean by "social convoys": the dynamics of linked lives over time. The father moves through his own occupational career even as his son grows up and moves through schooling. Both fathers and children, and husbands and wives are part of each other's social convoy, along with other family and social network members (e.g., Bengtson, 2001; Mortimer, 2003).

We use the term "social convoys" to connote linked lives that play out as dynamic *ongoing relationships of two or more people over time*. Kahn and Antonucci (1980) first introduced the concept of social convoys to capture networks of kin and friends. We build on their original formulation of these convoys as supportive by also considering these (and other) ties as potentially fostering conflicts and strains, as well as adaptive strategies, at different points in the life course.

Note that although we focus in this chapter on social convoys, lives and relationships are also molded by "time convoys": the taken-for-granted institutionalized bundles of time- and age-related rules, resources, and expectations "attached" to particular roles, relationships, and network memberships (see also Moen & Chesley, 2008). We imagine time convoys as invisible tugboats, channeling people into or out of activities and experiences (and locations) based on the legitimated norms around time (e.g., going to one's job on Mondays, using weekends for fun and domestic work, leaving at noon for lunch). Time convoys include expectations about time to be "spent" in relationships such as parenting, being a neighbor, and caring for aging parents. They also operate to construct and constrain age-graded life course paths (e.g., occupational career paths) and relationships (e.g., marriage and parenting).

Plan of the Chapter

In this chapter we suggest techniques and strategies for capturing the embeddedness of individuals within the lives of others as linked lives at any one point in time and as social convoys over time. First, we encourage researchers to bring social contexts back into their studies of individuals, embedding individual respondents within the contexts of the people in their lives. Second, we encourage use of social groupings as units of analysis when it makes theoretical sense, and a move from studying individuals' beliefs and behaviors to studying relational units—the beliefs and behaviors of married couples, family members, social networks, or work groups.

We draw on research on couples as our primary case example to illustrate how researchers can profit from theorizing and operationalizing the concept of individuals in relational contexts, as well as using higher-level units of two or more people as their focus of analysis. Changing the analytic unit from the individual man or woman, husband or wife, to the couple (husband *and* wife) captures a couple's joint resources, status, and circumstances, as well as the within-couple division of resources, power, decision making, and behavior. We also touch briefly on other types of linked lives: the intergenerational experiences of parents and children, and the role of coworkers as shapers of employees' experiences and expectations.

Data Sources and Analytic Approaches

To study couples and families/households requires creation of couple-level (or family-level) variables: concepts and measures that cannot be reduced to, or created from, information on just one person. Examples include household income, household composition, age dispersion, degree of educational homogamy within the household, frequency of family conflict, styles of couples' decision making, and ranges of social network ties common to all household members. Armed with such variables, the researcher can then compare and contrast households of various types, in various locations, in different historical periods, across cultures, and/or at different points in the life course. Alternatively, the researcher can investigate within-couple variables, such as couples' agreement about the household division of paid and unpaid labor, or couples' conjoint descriptions of their decision-making processes.

Couple or Higher-Level Variables

Sometimes couple-level variables are dependent variables, the outcomes of interest. For example, Altobelli and Moen (2007) used latent class analysis to identify couple patterns of "work–family spillover" (the degree to which each spouse sees work as "spilling over" into their home lives and vice versa. They investigated the positive and negative work-to-family and family-to-work spillover of both spouses, and found three distinct couple spillover constellations: *conjointly negative, enriched,* and *husband (only) negative.* This provides far more insight, and potentially more explanatory power, than knowing, for example, only husbands' level of work–family conflict. Using data from a second survey wave 2 years later, Altobelli and Moen analyzed the conditions at work and at home that increased the likelihood of couples moving from one constellation to another.

Couple-level measures are also useful as independent variables in predicting outcomes related to individuals. For example, in their study of "coworking couples" (both partners working for the same employer), Moen and Sweet (2002; Sweet & Moen, 2007) created a typology of dual earners based on whether both spouses have professional occupations, the husband only, the wife only, or neither partner has a professional-level job. They found that wives report more negative spillover from work to family in coworking couples in which only the wives are professionals (their husbands hold nonprofessional, lower-status jobs), compared to the reported spillover by wives when both partners are in nonprofessional jobs.

A life course perspective on linked lives encourages analysis of similarities and differences between couples at different ages and stages. Clarkberg and Moen (2001) drew on couple-level data from the National Study of Families and Households to assess the gap between actual and preferred working hours of men and women in couples, examining the size of this gap at different ages and life stages.

Another life course approach is to look for changes when one or both spouses undergo a major life course transition or life event, such as having a baby, moving, being laid off, being diagnosed with an illness, or retiring.

Given that most researchers only have access to data on individuals, what is the best way to capture lives as linked at one point in time or as social convoys over time? Let us say that a survey of employees (as individuals) includes some information obtained from the employee respondents about their spouses. Typically, independent variables for each spouse (e.g., working hours) are included in regression equations separately, with the researcher looking for additive or interaction effects between them. But we find it instructive to construct *couple-level measures*. Stolzenberg (2001), for example, used *constructed-pair data*, created from the Americans' Changing Lives (ACL) survey of individuals, to bring in dyadic relationships. The constructed-pair data allowed Stolzenberg to assess dyadic work–health effects within each couple. Van de Rijt and Buskens (2006) followed a similar strategy and created couple-level measures, such as "couple education."

Of course, there are other types of linked lives. Table 12.1 provides examples of the levels of data used in various studies, and the availability of dyad, organizational, and network data linked to individuals as well as larger social units. Bennett and Lehman (1999) studied work groups, investigating whether coworkers influence employees' substance use (see Table 12.1). Their study exemplifies the interconnectedness of employees in workplace settings, showing that work groups can influence individual behavior. Neighborhoods provide an example of lives that are linked in distal ways. Wheaton and Clarke (2003) drew on data from the National Survey of Children to construct neighborhood-level variables; they then assessed the relationship between a neighborhood's socioeconomic status while children were growing up and children's subsequent mental health in adulthood (see Table 12.1).

Data from Couples

The "gold standard" in studying couples is to collect data from both partners, as well as other members of the household, especially when rating subjective appraisals (e.g., job or marital satisfaction, or mental health). For instance, Northouse, Mood, Templin, Mellon, and George (2000) examined couple role adjustment after a health diagnosis by interviewing both spouses separately about their respective adjustments. Gager and Sanchez (2003) used couple-level measures from the National Survey of Families and Households to capture the level of concordance or discordance between husbands' and wives' subjective perceptions of marital quality, time spent together, and risk of divorce. Using these couple-level measures, they were better able to understand the association between couples' perceptions and their actual risk of divorce, which, they found, varies by gender. Schoen, Rogers, and Amato (2006) used couple-level measures to assess the influence of marital happiness on wives' employment. Moen and Sweet (2003) used data from both spouses to create a couple work–hour variable. Using cluster analytic techniques, they found five patterned couple work–hour arrangements in their dual-earner, middle-class sample, the most common of which was the *neotraditional* pattern, with husbands putting in long hours and wives working far less. Additional examples in Table 12.1 show the multiplicity of research topics that can be addressed from the vantage point of linked lives.

Often surveys of individual respondents inquire about husbands or wives, or other family members. Having one person report about spousal characteristics makes sense, *provided* that respondents can be expected to offer reasonably accurate information about their spouses. We feel comfortable using one person as the reporter of concrete characteristics, such as a spouse's employment, work hours, educational level, or life stage, but not about the assessment by the persons interviewed about the quality of their spouses' personal or marital lives, or their plans and expectations about the future.

Methods of Analysis

Most social science is variable-oriented, analyzing relationships between two or more variables at one point in time, with variations in one or more measure "explaining" variations in another measure. Such statistical techniques also permit researchers to "control" for the effects of other factors that are extraneous to the variables of interest. But lives are linked as *interdependent social systems*, not as isolated variables. A life course approach points to the importance of asking the "right" questions, in this case, questions that lead to ways of theorizing and analyzing linked lives. One key question is: In what social-relational systems are the studied individuals embedded?

TABLE 12.1. Examples of Research Linking Lives

Outcome of interest	Citation	Theoretical unit of analysis	Operational unit of analysis	Data set	Measurement
Education	Sweet & Moen (2007)	Couple level	Husband–wife dyad	Ecology of Careers Study April 1998–March 2000	• Dependent variable: entry and departure to/from school • Independent variables (e.g., family satisfaction) assessed by both wife and husband
Marriage	Gager & Sanchez (2003)	Couple level	Individual and spouse or partner dyad	National Survey of Families and Households 1987–1988 and 1992–1994	• Dependent variable: marital dissolution, measured as separation or divorce • Independent variables (e.g., marital happiness) constructed with separate partner evaluations
Marriage	Schoen, Rogers, & Amato (2006)	Couple level	Individual and spouse or partner dyad	National Survey of Families and Households 1987–1988 and 1992–1994	• Dependent variable: marital happiness and wives' employment • Independent variables (e.g., marital quality and marital stability) using separate evaluations from partners
Marriage	Van de Rijt & Buskens (2006)	Couple level	Individual	Chicago Health and Social Life Survey 1995–1997	• Dependent variable: marital status • Independent variables (e.g., age, education, trying to become pregnant) as reported by one partner in the relationship
Health and illness	Northouse et al. (2000)	Couple level	Husband–wife dyad and patient–caregiver dyad	Sample of colon cancer patients and their spouses	• Dependent variable: spousal role adjustment measured separately for patient and spouse • Independent variables (e.g., psychosocial adjustment) assessment scales given to patient and spouse
Health and illness	Bennett & Lehman	Work-group level	Work groups	Sample of employees in two cities in	• Dependent variable: negative consequences of coworkers' alcohol and substance use

Topic	Author (year)	Level	Unit	Data source	Variables
	(1999)			southwestern U.S.	• Independent variables (e.g., job stress) asked of each group member
Health and illness	Stolzenberg (2001)	Couple level	Individual	Americans' Changing Lives (ACL) survey 1986 and 1989	• Dependent variable: husband's–wife's health • Independent variables (e.g., employment, educational attainment, family income) as reported by husband or wife
Health and illness	Christakis & Fowler (2007)	Social-network level	Social network	Framingham Heart Study 1971–2003	• Dependent variable: weight gain • Independent variable: weight gain among social ties
Health and illness	Wheaton & Clarke (2003)	Neighborhood level	Neighborhood	National Survey of Children 1976, 1981, 1987	• Dependent variable: adult mental health • Independent variables: neighborhood socioeconomic status, and individual exposure to stressful events
Employment	Singley & Hynes (2005)	Couple level	Husband–wife dyad	New Parents Study: in-depth interviews with new-parent couples from Cornell Couples and Careers Study	• Dependent variable: new parents' decision about paid work • Other varying factors: effect work–family policies on decision making, parents' joint negotiation of new roles
Employment	Raley, Mattingly, & Bianchi (2006)	Couple level	Individual	Current Population Survey (March Supplement) 1970, 1980, 1990, 2001	• Dependent variable: percentage of income contributed by husband and wife, as reported by spouse responding to survey • Independent variable: spousal employment reported by spouse responding to survey
Employment	Dahlin, Kelly, & Moen (2008)	Social-network level	Individual	Ecology of Careers Study April 1998–March 2000	• Dependent variable: social ties to person with whom respondent discussed important matters • Independent variables: family satisfaction, work hours, job tenure, firm size, and total network size

Impact of Relational Context

Life course scholars theorize about *lives in context,* examining histori-cal, cultural, and structural risks, resources, and constraints shaping life chances and life quality. Social convoys are a key part of the contexts in which individuals' beliefs, behaviors, and strategic adaptations play out. Two popular quantitative methods facilitate locating individuals within larger social groups: hierarchical linear modeling (HLM; also known as "multilevel modeling") and network analysis (Bennett & Lehman, 1999; Straits, 1996; Wheaton & Clarke, 2003). HLM allows researchers to consider group-level *and* individual-level effects simultaneously. An important aspect of HLM is its capacity to identify the impact of various contexts (families, cohorts, work groups) on individual behavior. For example, Bennett and Lehman (1999) used HLM to understand the effect of coworker substance use on employees' behaviors.

Network analysis is another way of locating individuals within rela-tional contexts and identifying characteristics of their relationship. Straits (1996), for example, used General Social Survey network data to investigate whether coworker ties are gendered. Dahlin, Kelly, and Moen (2008) have drawn on similar types of network data in the Ecol-ogy of Careers Study, and finding that dual-earner employees tend to have close relationships with kin and coworkers but not neighbors.

Both HLM and network analysis can capture social networks at one point in time, providing a "snapshot" of linked lives. Ethnography, in-depth interviews, life histories, and historical trend data can capture the dynamics of social convoys as they shift in composition and influ-ence over time. For example, in her study of the gendered division of housework and family care among couples, Hochschild (1989) used interview and observational data to investigate how relationships play out as processes over time. Another strategy is to collect, graph, and analyze *life histories.* Life history data can be collected either retrospec-tively, by asking about past experiences, or prospectively, by following people over a period of months or years.

Dynamics of Higher-Level Units

A second key question is: Do couples, families, networks, or work groups operate as systems or as loose configurations of individuals? This ques-tion of how *couples, families, networks, or work groups operate* in making decisions, dividing up tasks, or allocating resources, as well as the degree to which they hold similar beliefs and values, moves the focus of interest from individuals to higher-level units. These groups can be analyzed in a variety of ways. Table 12.2 provides an overview of studies

TABLE 12.2. Examples of Alternative Data Sources and Methods for Analyzing Linked Lives

Data sets	Highest level	Date of collection	Study design	Examples of methods
Ecology of Careers Study Subsets	Couple level	1998–2000	Mixed method	Ordinary least squares and general linear models (Sweet & Moen, 2007)
Cornell Couples and Careers Study	Couple level	1997–1998	Mixed method	Qualitative analysis (Becker & Moen, 1999)
New Parents Study	Couple level	2000–2001	In-depth interviews	Qualitative analysis (Singley & Hynes, 2005)
National Survey of Families and Households	Couple level	1987–1988 and 1992–1994	Longitudinal survey	Event–history analysis (Gager & Sanchez, 2003; Schoen, Rogers, & Amato, 2006)
Qualitative interviews	Couple level		In-depth interviews	Qualitative analysis (Gerstel, 2000)
National Survey of Children	Neighborhood level	1976, 1981, 1987	Longitudinal survey	Hierarchical linear models (Wheaton & Clarke, 2003)
General Social Survey	Network level	1985	Cross-sectional survey	Negative binomial regression analysis (Straits, 1996)

using a range of types of data and methods, including in-depth interviews, cross-sectional surveys, longitudinal surveys, and mixed methods to study couples, families, workgroups, or other units of interest.

One potential methodological difficulty, however, is that information from two or more people in relationships is not statistically independent (Maguire, 1999; Thompson & Walker, 1982). This issue can be avoided by creating variables that are truly relational, such as difference scores (e.g., in couples, his age minus hers), ratios (her salary divided by his), or typologies based on both spouses' circumstances, behavior, or values (e.g., whether both partners are religious, the husband only, the wife only, or neither partner is religious). Maguire (1999) suggests the use of intraclass correlations of both partners' values as an index of within-couple similarity or difference. She also points to the utility of repeated-measures analysis of variance if the research question relates to within-dyad levels and directions of difference among diverse subgroups of couples.

Ethnographic and in-depth qualitative data are especially useful in the study of relationships as processes and social systems (cf. Becker & Moen, 1999; Cowan & Cowan, 1999; Gerstel, 2000). Drawing on existing long-term panel studies can provide the data necessary to reconstruct the life courses of respondents as they intersect over time. Putting together the life histories of spouses can reveal the ways their paths converge, intertwine, and diverge at different points in the life course of each. Collecting life histories from members of couples in different cohorts, cultures, or settings can illuminate both similarities and differences over historical time, as well as subcultural similarities and differences in social relationships. For example, Moen and Roehling (2005) used life history vignettes of individuals and couples to illustrate the (gendered) processes of combining work and family career paths. Han and Moen (1999, 2001) used job histories (collected separately from husbands and wives with the use of life history calendars) to capture the career pathways of husbands and wives. Figure 12.1 provides an example of a life history calendar.

Other Questions

Glen Elder always tells colleagues and students that the key to life course research is asking the right questions. Even when life history data are absent, it may prove useful before launching a study of linked lives to undertake a basic armchair description of the phenomenon of interest and to examine the larger context in which it is occurring. For example, what is the nature of the sample? How is the focus of study embedded in and affected by the historical times, as well as by biographical and

Respondent's ID _____   Date of birth _____

| | AGE | e.g., 18–28 | 29–39 | 40–49 | 50–60 | 61–69 |
	YEAR	e.g., 1990				
EMPLOYMENT HISTORY Occupation Title/part time or full time or more Unemployed/not in labor force Reason for change						
EDUCATION HISTORY Type, date, degree						
GEOGRAPHICAL MOVES						
MARITAL/PARTNERSHIP HISTORY Date/changes						
FAMILY CHANGE/ HOUSEHOLD COMPOSITION Birth of child/gender Leaving home, returning Relationship to respondent, changes						
PARTNER'S EMPLOYMENT Occupation, title, part time or full time						
RESPONDENT'S HEALTH HISTORY Illnesses, disabilities/severity, duration Hospital stays, surgery						
SPOUSE'S/CHILDREN'S HEALTH HISTORY Illnesses, disabilities/severity						
VOLUNTEER WORK Type, days, amount of time Reasons for change						
CAREGIVING Amount of time, for whom, why						

ADDITIONAL NOTES /QUOTES HERE:

FIGURE 12.1. Sample life history calendar (collapsed).

institutional clocks? Who else is affected? This "thought experiment" can uncover new questions and unexpected patterns. For example, in a study of adult students, Sweet and Moen (2007) investigated how a husband's or wife's return to school affects not just the returnee but also his or her spouse. In an analysis of social networks, Dahlin et al. (2008) examined whether most nonfamily social ties are now work- rather than neighborhood-related. In a study of family time pressures, Clarkberg and Moen (2001) asked why couples confronting a time squeeze do not opt to have both partners work part time.

Asking such counterintuitive questions, even if they cannot always be answered, can illuminate the hidden cultures and structures shaping virtually every "choice" and every social relationship. For example, couples rarely "choose" to have both spouses work part time because part-time jobs do not offer sufficient income, much less the medical care, pensions, security, and prospects traditionally associated with full-time employment. Consequently, as Becker and Moen (1999) and Moen and Orrange (2002) found, when couples want or need to scale back at work because of family responsibilities, the most common strategy is to have the wife reduce her hours or else leave the workforce for a time. Why is this strategy gendered, with the wife being the one to scale back? To answer such questions requires knowledge of the historical, structural, cultural, and biographical embeddedness of lives and relationships.

To be sure, researchers often have scant contextual data and little knowledge of respondents' relationships or circumstances prior to data collection. But imagination, a review of existing literature, and some evidence gleaned from available data can illuminate the contexts and pathways by which respondents arrive and remain in the particular sample you plan to use. This process matters, because there are almost always issues of sample selection, that is, skewing based on who is not included in the sample, leading to sample selection bias, which we discuss next.

Data Limitations

It is always important to consider the possibility of "selection bias" (the absence within a study sample of values on a particular variable of interest). Often selection bias reflects self-selection of people into or out of the group being investigated. For example, individuals "select" themselves into or out of certain couple dyads: They enter into relationships, cohabit, get married, and/or get divorced. Or they are selected out by events, such as becoming widowed.

Consider a study of spousal or child abuse drawing on data from a random sample of families. Families with especially high levels of spousal or child abuse may not even be in a community sample of households, since these families have either dissolved themselves (divorce, separation) or been dissolved by social service agencies (foster care, no visitation rights). Similarly, couples with high levels of work–family conflict may no longer be in a dual-earner sample, because one partner might have left the workforce (Stone, 2007).

Selection bias may well affect research results. A study of couple marital satisfaction may find that older couples tend to be more satisfied than younger couples with their marriages. Is this an age, cohort, or marital duration effect? Or is it simply because the most conflicted couples got divorced years ago, excluding themselves from the "older married couple" sample?

Panel data following individuals, couples, or other groupings over time may also be subject to selection bias, depending on who drops out and who is apt to stay in the sample. For instance, Han and Moen (2001) found that women who follow continuous, full-time career paths are more apt to divorce than are women with other career trajectories. Since these women would not be included in samples of couples, this career strategy (opting out of a marriage) is overlooked.

Consider how the people being studied have come to be where they are at the historical point in time they are surveyed, observed, or interviewed. Ask why families in a study have specific members employed for certain hours in certain jobs; why they have no, one, two, or more children; why they spend little, a moderate amount, or a lot of time together; and why they live in the neighborhoods, houses, or cities they do.

As a case in point, recall that Moen and Sweet (2002; Sweet & Moen, 2007) drew on a subsample from the Ecology of Careers Study to investigate the phenomenon of "coworking couples," in which both spouses work for the same employer. There are a number of pathways to being part of a coworking couple: Partners may meet because they are students in the same field—such as law or engineering—and thereafter pursue the same type of occupation, seeking jobs together. Or couples may have met on the job, which means that they were coworkers before they were in a relationship. Or an employer wanting to retain a valued employee might find a job for that employee's spouse. Moen and Sweet (2002) found that coworking husbands typically have longer tenure in the organization than do their wives, suggesting that most couples working for the same employer may have met on the job, or that the employer offered the wife a job when it appeared the husband might follow her as she sought employment elsewhere.

Selection bias is often dealt with as a methodological issue. But it is also a descriptive and theoretical issue, a way of thinking and theorizing

about the predictors or outcomes being investigated. Always ask who is/
is not in a sample and why. Does this represent selection as a result of
individual choice or systematic exclusion?

Linked Lives and Convoys as the Object of Study

Scholars can study linked lives from a number of vantage points. Even
though most available social science information (data) is about individuals, life course researchers can bring relationships into their theoretical and analytic models by (1) looking at demographic and historical
trends in relationships over time, (2) investigating crossover from one
person to another, (3) theorizing and examining group-level adaptive
strategies, and (4) considering trajectories and transitions, the ways
relationships both shape and are shaped by the time and timing of experiences and insights of individuals. Each of these four approaches offers
considerable payoff.

Studying the Demography of Linked Lives over Time

One way of studying linked lives is as *trends over time*, drawing on census
or other time series data to chart marriage or fertility rates for different
subgroups of the population. Topics that can be examined in this way
are household-related relationships—the average age of marriage or
parenthood, the incidence of divorce and remarriage, the percentages
of dual-earner or single-parent households—as they increase or decline
over time. There are also time use data that permit the study of trends
in men's and women's division of paid and unpaid labor, as well as the
amount and distribution of leisure time. Life course researchers also
study how individual and couple strategies shift over time (Elder & Shanahan, 2006; Heinz, 1996, 2002). For example, Raley, Mattingly, and
Bianchi (2006) use repeated cross-sectional individual-level data—the
Current Population Survey—to create a range of couple-level measures,
such as couples' educational attainment, number of children, and life
stage, to capture trends in dual-earner couple status.

Moving the focus from individual to group characteristics is yet
another strategy for capturing trends. For example, Jacobs and Gerson
(2004) charted trends in couples' working hours over time, showing
that work hours have increased at the family level. Researchers can theorize and investigate a number of group-level outcomes, such as rates,
differences, similarities, and/or totals. These are concepts about relationships, not individuals—such as *age difference* (i.e., between spouses),
homogamy (i.e., similarity in religion, social class, fertility plans, or politi-

cal attitudes), or the *degree of inequality* (i.e., division of household labor between spouses; differences in salaries, status, power, or couple-level decision-making strategies).

Capturing trends in relationships and behavior over time reveals that the human impacts of large-scale social transformations—technological, demographic, economic, and cultural—are invariably filtered through networks of close and distal ties of obligation, expectation, and interpretation (cf. Heinz, 1996, 2002), in other words, lives that are linked together.

Studying Dynamic Crossover Effects in Real Time and Motion

The mechanisms by which lives are linked are especially apparent when viewed from the perspective of *crossover* effects. For example, Almeida and colleagues (Almeida, Chandler, & Wethington, 1999; Larson & Almeida, 1999; Yorgason, Almeida, Neupert, Spiro, & Hoffman, 2006) used daily diary methods to examine whether a husband's experience of conflict on the job affects his wife's experience of stress, and vice versa, as well as stress crossover from one generation (parents) to the next (children).

Researchers can also study crossover effects using survey data. For example, one study found that when one member of a couple is involved in caring for an aging relative, this "crosses over" to affect the well-being of the spouse, but it does so differently depending on whether the husband or the wife is the caregiver (see Chesley & Moen, 2006).

Studying Strategies of Adaptation

A particularly fruitful approach incorporates the concept of *family-level adaptive strategies*. When something happens to one person, such as job loss, or to the household, such as the birth of a child, how do relationships and roles change? Decisions about employment provide one example of various couple-level adaptive strategies. Women and men as members of couples, as parents, as adult children of aging parents, and as employees make *strategic selections* about whether and how to combine work and family roles within the context of their relationships. Couples make strategic (and often gendered) selections about who will work for pay, and for how many hours, as well as who will care for infants or aging family members. These choices in turn produce and reproduce gender differentiation and inequality in roles and resources (Blossfeld & Drobnič, 2001; Chesley, 2005; Clarkberg & Moen, 2001; Dentinger & Clarkberg, 2002; Drobnič & Blossfeld, 2004; Elder, Johnson, & Crosnoe, 2003).

One potentially fruitful way of theorizing and studying adaptive strategies is to consider a spouse's behavior as predictive of the respondent's own behavior. In families raising children, a mother or father who travels a lot on the job may well predict limited job-related travel by the other parent. Such strategies are *compensatory*, in that one person is compensating (by limiting his or her own travel) for the other's absence.

Or strategies might reflect *competing choices*—such as by professional couples who may have the same education and training but find they must prioritize one person's jobs over that of the other partner (e.g., deciding to move for one person's advancement). Over time such couple-level decisions produce (within couples and across gender) disparities in earnings and status that widen with age (see Pixley, 2008).

Some couples may follow *parallel paths,* taking turns in child care and allotting equal time to each person's job. Or each member might operate *independently,* making decisions and following paths that are not interdependent. Cohabiting couples, for example, may be more apt to have separate bank accounts and to keep purchases separate, something that might change with marriage or the birth of a child. Couples who live apart may also pursue independent tracks.

The very nature of the linkage between members of a couple can vary over the life course and may also differ depending on the question of interest. Young marrieds may be similar in some ways because of assortative mating: People tend to marry others very much like themselves. Or else one or both members of the couple may "adapt" to the other in ways that foster homogamy. Still another possibility is that similar couples could become different by strategically selecting different behaviors—such as differences in their work hours or job travel—to allow one person to compensate at home for the long absences of the other.

It is important to recognize that couple patterns can only be understood within the multilayered contexts of relationships, norms, and opportunities/constraints. Life course scholars can contribute to greater understanding of linked lives by identifying the number and frequency of patterns, as well as the factors predicting them. Scholars can also show how choices earlier in the life course can contribute to differences and inequalities within and among couples over time.

Couples can also accommodate to prior decisions over time. In their study of marital happiness and wives' employment, Schoen et al. (2006) found that over about a 5-year time span, couples were able to adopt adaptive or protective strategies to compensate for any negative effects associated with the wives' moving back into employment.

Life course researchers can capture the human meaning of large-scale social changes by studying the strategic adaptations of couples or other units in particular times and places. The value of Pavalko and Elder's (1993) study of women's involvement in and support of their husbands' careers is that it locates linked lives in historical time (early 20th century) and place (United States). Today more couples are dual earners, but jobs and career paths remain constructed as if workers have no family responsibilities (see Moen & Roehling, 2005). Many couples who start out with similar occupational goals, and who strongly believe in gender equality, often find themselves following neotraditional strategies. Gendered career paths become especially prominent around the transition to parenthood (Stone, 2007) and the transition to caring for impaired parents and other relatives (Gerstel, 2000).

Lives as Trajectories and Transitions, Evolving in and over Time

The life course theme of linked lives invariably incorporates and plays out over *time*. As Bronfenbrenner and Crouter (1983, p. 360) remind us, "Not only the person, but also the context, undergoes a course of development."

Early experiences and choices of couples may well set the course of each partner's life, as well as the trajectory of the relationship. Consider the transition to adulthood (Moen & Orrange, 2002; Mortimer, 2003), the transition of two people moving in together (Brines & Joyner, 1999; Clarkberg, 1999), the transition to or timing of parenthood (Altucher & Williams, 2003; Hynes & Clarkberg, 2005; Reichart, Chesley, & Moen, 2007), and the transition to retirement (Han & Moen, 1999; Moen, Sweet, & Swisher, 2005)—all of which tend to recalibrate the nature and direction of both work and family ties for couples, as well as for men and women as individuals.

A life course focus on linked lives can illuminate the ways that gender plays out in a wide range of venues. Family care arrangements, spousal interactions, and power relationships, work–home conflicts and enhancements, couples' conjoint retirement plans and transitions, caring for sick and infirm relatives (often adult children caring for older parents) are examples of the ways lives are linked over time in distinctive ways for women and men (cf. Chesley & Moen, 2006; Gerstel, 2000; Northouse et al., 2000; Pavalko & Woodbury, 2000). For example, one study found that older women who care for their ailing husbands are more likely to exit the workforce as a response to these care responsibilities, whereas older men who care for ailing wives are unlikely to leave their jobs and hire care providers rather than taking on that role themselves (Dentinger & Clarkberg, 2002).

Methodological advances and the availability of longitudinal data are allowing life course scholars to operationalize and analyze interdependent trajectories and transitions—of couples, of family members in different generations, and of members of different cohorts.

Broadening the Focus

We conclude where we began: Most social scientists study individuals, not groups. More precisely, most social scientists study *variables about* individuals. When relationships are brought into the analysis, it is often as "controls" (i.e., controlling for marital status). In this chapter we have pointed to the value of theorizing (and suggested methods for studying) individuals' lives as linked lives, embedded in social convoys of ongoing relationships over the life course. Broadening the focus beyond individuals can reveal the effects of social ties on the economic security, occupational status, health, and behavior of individuals, families, and members of organizations, as well as of different cohorts.

We have also emphasized social convoys as key to understanding the ways macro-level social structures and forces play out in the micro-level experiences and perceptions of individuals. The impacts of large-scale forces on individuals and groups—in terms of both social stability and social change—are filtered through networks of close and distal ties (convoys) of obligation, expectation, and interpretation. For example, changing gender norms and a globalizing information economy have transformed the lives of women and, thereby, also have transformed men's and children's experiences. Greater longevity and economic downsizing are affecting couples' deliberations about when either partner should retire and couples' actual experiences of the retirement status passage.

We have used couples to illustrate the interdependence of lives moving through time. Couples provide a good case example of fairly stable units of individuals who move in tandem along various family and employment trajectories and transitions. But the concepts and methods we describe are equally useful for other forms of linked lives, those spanning generations, such as the ongoing social convoys of parents and children, and the far looser but important links among coworkers or cohorts of high school or college graduates.

Generational Convoys

Families as institutionalized relational arrangements evolve and are transformed as children are born, enter school, then graduate from elementary school, high school, college—at some point leaving (as well as returning to) the family nest. At each stage, families operate within the context of legitimated regimens reinforcing traditional within-household distributions and divisions of resources and labor, along with bundles of intergenerational, interpersonal, and intimate relationships (Bianchi, Robinson, & Milkie, 2006; Daly, 2003). Studying linked lives across generations allows life course scholars to consider relationships between family members at different ages and life stages. In their review of marital interaction, Gottman and Notarius (2000) described research on child outcomes leading to the following questions: How do parents' relationships while children are young affect children later on during *their* adult course? Are parents' marital problems replicated in the adult children's own marriages? Using longitudinal data on parents and their offspring, Amato and Booth (2001) found that marital problems of parents predict their adult children's marital problems. Orbuch, Thornton, and Cancio (2000) also showed that marital disruption affect the parent–child bond. And Zarit and Eggebeen (2002) categorized the parent–child relationship as a life-span issue, noting that these intergenerational linkages have become progressively more important as life expectancy has increased.

Another example of lives linked across generations is the multigenerational relationship between grandparents, parents, and children, the importance of which life course scholar Vern Bengtson recognized early (1975). Over the last several decades, life course researchers have highlighted the diversity of these relationships (Rossi & Rossi, 1990; Silverstein, Bengtson, & Lawton, 1997). For example, Giarrusso, Feng, Silverstein, and Bengtson (2001) underscored variations within and across gender and ethnic groups in cross-generational relationships by drawing on data collected separately from grandparents and adult children.

Who is the best reporter of generational relationships? Feng, Silverstein, Giarrusso, McArdle, and Bengtson (2006) found that adult children are better at reporting "more objective aspects of their intergenerational relationship" (p. S327) than the older parents themselves. But no one is guaranteed as the "best" reporter: They also found that whereas older parents *under*estimate their dependency on their adult children, the adult children *over*estimate their parents' dependency on them.

Lives More Loosely Linked

Much social connectedness consists of weak ties among individuals who are not related to one another, such as coworkers, friends, club members, or other social networks. Studying such relations through hierarchical models permits analysis of group and individual effects simultaneously. Research on workgroups using HLM examines effects on employees working in teams of numerous different variables, such as employment policies (Blair-Loy & Wharton, 2002), supervisor support (Griffin, Patterson, & West, 2001), and group cohesiveness and behavior (Kidwell, Mossholder, & Bennett, 1997). Analyzing work groups permits focus on the culture, policies, and practices characterizing particular subgroups within organizations. For instance, in their analysis of work groups, Blair-Loy and Wharton (2002) showed that employees working with powerful colleagues and supervisors are more likely to use work–family policies. In a study of group absenteeism among employee work-groups, Mason and Griffin (2003) examined group effects over time using HLM. Though not yet common, longitudinal group-level data provide a promising window into the dynamics of the social organization of coworkers, as well as neighborhood and other social relations over time.

Another fruitful area of inquiry is the use of catch-up samples of cohorts of individuals graduating from the same high school or college the same year and interviewing them years later (Komarovsky, 1985; Strober & Chan, 1999; Warren & Halpern-Manners, 2007). Griffith (2002), who used multilevel techniques to study military groups, found that soldiers within combat units reported enhanced combat readiness if they had supportive leaders and cooperative peer relations.

Next Steps: Theorizing and Measuring Context and Process

A life course theoretical approach is increasingly popular among social scientists (sociologists, economists, psychologists, anthropologists), in large part because of the confluence of social changes now transforming lives and rendering existing blueprints obsolete. Previously taken-for-granted transitions into and out of social relationships are becoming more contingent and more varied, with widespread implications for individuals, groups, and society. Contemporary adults are (1) returning to school at all ages, or young adults are staying in school longer; (2) delaying marriage or not marrying at all; (3) delaying childbearing or having no (or fewer) children; and (4) retiring early, late, not at all, or several times. Traditionally, each of these topics has been studied in isolation, and frequently only in the cross section, either as choices of individuals or as societal trends, not as linked choices and convoys.

In this chapter we have argued that a life course focus on social convoys can promote understanding of continuity and change in lives, families, communities, networks, and organizations—as well as how they intersect with one another. Married women's occupational paths and work hours cannot be understood apart from the parallel occupational paths and work hours of their husbands. Even retirement is increasingly a couple transition. These examples point to the way social transformations (in gender ideologies, families, and labor markets), change social relationships and how relationships in turn shape individuals' beliefs, behavior, and decision making.

One way to capture the dynamics of linked lives is to collect panel data over a span of time. But because most of us cannot do so, another strategy is to collect life histories, ask each of those whose lives are linked about their transitions and trajectories, and record them in life history calendars, then put the calendars together.

Life course scholars have a real opportunity to contribute to the mapping of the 21st-century life course, as well as the effects of large-scale historical events and cultural, demographic, technological or economic transformations on people's lives. Doing so requires studying social convoys as dynamic systems and as mediators between social forces and individuals' life chances and life quality across the life course.

Acknowledgments

This chapter was developed with support provided by the Alfred P. Sloan Foundation (No. 2002-6-8), and as part of the Work, Family and Health Network funded by a cooperative agreement through the National Institutes of Health and the Centers for Disease Control and Prevention: National Institute of Child Health and Human Development (Grant Nos. U01HD051217, U01HD051218, U01HD051256, and U01HD051276), National Institute on Aging (Grant No. U01AG027669), Office of Behavioral and Science Sciences Research, and National Institute for Occupational Safety and Health (Grant No. U01OH008788). The contents of this publication are solely our responsibility and do not necessarily represent the official views of these institutes and offices. Persons interested in learning more about the Network should go to *www.kpchr.org/workplacenetwork*. We are especially grateful for the assistance of Jane Peterson in manuscript preparation.

CHAPTER 13

Comparative Life Course Research

A Cross-National and Longitudinal Perspective

Hans-Peter Blossfeld

In recent decades, study of the life course has become one of the most active research fields in the social sciences. Retrospective life course and prospective panel studies have become available during this period in most modern societies, especially in North America and in Western Europe. Well-known examples are the Oakland Life History Study (Elder, 1999) and the Panel Study of Income Dynamics (PSID) in the United States of America, the German Life History Study (Mayer, 1990) and the Socio-Economic Panel Study (SOEP) in Germany, and the National Cohort Studies (Ferri, Bynner, & Wadsworth, 2002) and the British Household Panel Study (BHPS) in the United Kingdom. Most of these data sets are nationally representative longitudinal studies that explicitly recognize the dynamic nature of social roles and circumstances as men and women move through their life paths, the interdependence of lives and life choices, the situational imperatives confronting actors in various countries, and the cumulation of advantages and disadvantages experienced by the individual within national settings (Elder, Johnson, & Crosnoe 2003).

Today, most of the life course analyses have been studies of, and in, single societies. Based on such limited work, some life course researchers have interpreted their findings by contrasting what they have learned about the country they actually studied and what is known or is believed to be true about some other country or countries. Melvin Kohn (1987) has classified such interpretations and comparisons as *implicitly* cross-national. The increasing availability of life history and panel studies for many countries provides the extraordinary opportunity for more *explicit* cross-national life course analysis (1) to establish the generality of findings about the life course found in one particular society, and (2) to study the specific impact of variations in institutional settings and social structures, historically developed and country-specific, on specific phases of the life course or the life course as a whole (Kohn, 1987).

Thus, cross-national life course studies can greatly extend the scope of sociological knowledge by answering the question of whether a specific life course mechanism established in one country also applies outside the particular context of this country. They also tend to deepen our understanding of cross-national differences when we give a convincing explanation of the impact of institutional and social-structural conditions on the life course in various nations. In other words, cross-national life course research helps us escape cultural one-sidedness or ethnocentrism, because we, as life course researchers, often wear cultural blinders of some sort that are connected to the society in which we are socialized: "When we see other ways of doing things, we then approach our own culture with new eyes, and new questions emerge" (Janoski & Hicks, 1994, p. 7).

Major types of cross-national life course studies are often classified as *quantitative–longitudinal, ethnographic,* or *a mixture of both.* In this chapter, I focus on the value of quantitative cross-national research on the life course and address some of its limitations. I argue that research based on longitudinal data from diverse countries provides a promising way to generate, test, and further develop causal theory (Kohn, 1987). This is the case because quantitative longitudinal data provide a much better handle for "internal analysis"—the analysis of variations within each country in a cross-national study (Janoski & Hicks, 1994). The analysis of cross-national studies of the life course is also made possible by statistical methods, such as event–history techniques or panel analyses that stress the sensitivity to time, as well as place, and offer new opportunities for causal analysis (Blossfeld, Golsch, & Rohwer, 2007).

Cross-national research on the life course can be classified further in terms of whether it is based on retrospective or prospective panel studies, or both. "Retrospective studies" collect the life histories at one particular point in time. The German Life History Study is an example (Brückner & Mayer, 1998). By contrast, "prospective panel studies" collect states of life histories in successive sweeps. However, it is unclear what happened before the first wave or between waves of a panel. There-fore, modern panel studies combine both designs and collect not only the retrospective histories of the past but also the changes from one panel wave to the next. In this chapter, my examples utilize data from both life course studies and modern panel studies.

Finally, cross-national studies of the life course often entail differ-ent levels of analysis, some of which concentrate on the social life course in historical context; others investigate the interplay between the social life course and individual behavior or psychological outcomes. Another possible focus is on intrasocietal variations, such as those between devel-oped and less-developed sectors of society. In this chapter, I demon-strate the extent to which specific life course mechanisms are affected by differences in institutional contexts, and how changes in historical macro-contexts, such as globalization, affect individual life courses in various societies. I use my own research as a source to discuss these issues more concretely.

Because life course research is closely connected to methodologi-cal innovations in longitudinal research, I first describe the strength of longitudinal methods compared to cross-sectional analysis in doing cross-national research. Second, using selected research examples, I show how the generality of life course mechanisms can be established in cross-national research. Of course, this is not an easy task, because life courses in modern societies still vary greatly. Third, I suggest analyti-cal instruments for the classification of national institutions that signifi-cantly affect life courses in modern societies. These are educational sys-tems, patterns of employment relations, national welfare state regimes, and the various family traditions in modern societies. The usefulness of these comparative concepts is illustrated by recent studies (see Bloss-feld, Buchholz, & Hofäcker, 2006; Blossfeld & Hofmeister, 2006; Bloss-feld, Mills, & Bernardi, 2006; Blossfeld, Mills, Klijzing, & Kurtz, 2005) that ask how the macro-level globalization process is "institutionally fil-tered" and channeled by domestic institutions toward the individual life courses of specific social groups in modern societies.

Advantages of Longitudinal Data for Cross-National Research

Today, most cross-national research is still based on cross-sectional data. However, Coleman (1981) has argued that one must be cautious in drawing causal inferences about explanatory processes on the basis of cross-sectional data, because, implicitly or explicitly, social research-ers must assume that the social process under study is in some kind of "statistical equilibrium." This equilibrium or "stability of the process" means that the state probabilities relative to nations at particular points in time are trendless or stable. Yet we know that modern societies and the life course of particular social groups in these societies are marked by rapid structural changes.

Life history and panel studies from single societies demonstrate that change across age, cohort, and historical period is an important feature in all domains of modern individuals' lives (cf. family systems, job and employment structures, and educational systems; see, e.g., Blossfeld & Hakim, 1997; Mayer, 1990; Shavit & Blossfeld, 1993). Thus, if modern societies are characterized by dynamic processes, cross-national comparative research should be based on longitudinal data. In other words, a major advantage of retrospective and prospective life course data in cross-national comparative research is that they provide an opportunity to compare complex histories over long stretches of time across several societies, and to trace often diverse pathways to common ends.

Limits of Cross-Sectional Data for Causal Analysis

Beyond the crucial assumption of process stability, cross-sectional data have a series of inferential limitations for causal analysis in a cross-national domain. These limitations make it difficult to determine direction of causality, the relative strength of reciprocal effects, the relative importance of different causal factors, the historical process that led to a given outcome, and the origin of the causal influence.

Indeterminate Direction of Causality

In cross-national research, the direction of causality can seldom be established from cross-sectional data. Consider the strong positive association between parental socioeconomic characteristics and the educational attainment of sons and daughters in many modern societies, once researchers control for other important influences (Erikson & Jonsson, 1996; Shavit & Blossfeld, 1993). A convincing interpretation of this effect might be that being born into a middle-class family increases the likelihood of attaining a university degree, because one is unable to think of any other plausible explanation for the statistical association. However, such "recursive relationships," in which all the causal linkages run "one way" and have no "feedback" effects, are rare in modern social life.

For example, in comparative studies there is very often a complex association between the age of the youngest child and female labor force participation (Blossfeld & Hakim, 1997; Blossfeld & Drobnič, 2001). The common interpretation is that the care of young children tends to keep mothers at home in modern societies. However, it is also plausible that the lack of jobs encourages women to enter into a stay-at-home marriage and motherhood, suggesting a "reversed causal relationship" (Blossfeld et al., 2005). Thus, issues of reversed causation in cross-national research can only be solved with longitudinal data.

Unknown Strength of Reciprocal Effects

Cross-sectional survey data cannot be used to discover which one of two correlated factors is of greater importance. For example, many cross-national demographic studies have shown that first marriage and first motherhood are highly correlated (e.g., Blossfeld, 1995; Blossfeld & Mills, 2001). To understand what has been happening to family formation in modern societies, it would be of interest to know the effect of marriage on birthrates, and also the effect of pregnancy or first birth on getting married (Blossfeld, 1995; Blossfeld & Huinink, 1991; Blossfeld & Mills, 2001); as well as, perhaps, how these effects have changed over historical time in various countries (see, e.g., Manting, 1996). This kind of cross-national analysis can only be carried out with longitudinal data.

Unknown Relative Importance of Causal Factors

Compared to cross-sectional surveys, retrospective life history data or prospective panel data offer much better opportunities to disentangle from other forces operating at the same time the effects of the causal factors of interest on the outcome, because these data are more informative about the process of change. Cross-national research is normally based on nonexperimental observations of social processes, which are complex and selective. For example, Lieberson (1985) has distinguished at least three types of nonrandom processes or selectivity among schools: (1) *self-selectivity*, in which the units of analysis, such as individuals, sort themselves out by choice (e.g., a cross-societal variation in the extent to which particular students choose specific types of schools); (2) *selective assignment* by the independent variable itself, which determines, say, which members of a population are exposed to specific levels of the independent variable (e.g., in some countries, schools select students based on their past achievement; in other countries, this is not the case); and (3) *selectivity due to forces exogenous to variables under consideration* (e.g., socioeconomic background, ethnicity, gender, previous school career, development of competences over the life course are normally distributed very differently across countries). Of course, no cross-national comparative study is able to overcome all problems of identification of these effects, but longitudinal data provide much better opportunities to identify these effects.

Lack of Historical Record

Cross-national analysis based on cross-sectional data may be performed with some proxy-variables and with assumptions of the causal order, as well as interdependencies between the explanatory variables. However, it is seldom possible to trace back appropriately the time-related selective processes operating in the previous history, because these data are simply not available. In particular, life course research has demonstrated that the past of an individual is an indispensable factor for understanding his or her actions at present (Buchmann, 1989; Mayer, 1990; Weymann, Heinz, & Alheit, 1996). Longitudinal data normally provide histories on various domains of life; therefore, they significantly improve the implementation of statistical controls in cross-national comparisons.

Inherent Ambiguity of Level of Observation—Individual or Group

Suppose we know that 30% of employed women in West Germany were working part time in 1970 (Blossfeld & Hakim, 1997). At the one extreme, this might imply that each employed woman in West Germany had a 30% chance of being employed part time in that year, but at the other, one could infer that 30% of employed West German women always worked part time and 70 % were full-timers only. In other words, cross-sectional data do not convey information about the time women have spent in different forms of employment. Therefore, they are open to various substantive interpretations in cross-national research (Blossfeld & Hakim, 1997; Blossfeld & Drobnič, 2001). In the first case, each woman would be expected to move back and forth between part-time and full-time employment. This is typically the case in open, liberal, competitive economies, such as the United States. In the second, there is no mobility between part-time and full-time work, and the estimated percentages describe the proportions of two completely different groups of employed women. This is typically the case in so-called insider–outsider mobility regimes, in which the employed people are highly protected and outsiders struggle to get into the employment system, as in Italy and Spain. Therefore, from an analytical point of view, it is important to have longitudinal data about durations in a state in cross-national comparative studies. Also, repeated cross-sectional studies using comparable samples of the same population (e.g., a series of micro-censuses or cross-sectional surveys) can only show net change, not the flow of individuals (see, e.g., DiPrete, deGraaf, Luijkx, Tåhlin, & Blossfeld, 1997).

Strengths of Longitudinal Data for Causal Analysis

Longitudinal data are no panacea for all problems of cross-national comparative research, but they are obviously much stronger and more effective, and have fewer inferential limitations than cross-sectional data (Mayer & Tuma, 1990). They are indispensable for the cross-national study of life course processes and their relation to historical changes in different countries. Therefore, cross-national designs aimed at a causal understanding of social processes should be based on longitudinal data at the micro-level of individuals as the units of analysis (Mayer, 1997). They allow a much better "internal analysis" (Janoski & Hicks, 1994) of variations within each country in a cross-national comparison. In particular, longitudinal data can illuminate age and cohort effects, specific historical processes, varying national "clocks" for the timing of life events, and contextual effects.

Distinction among Age, Cohort, and Period Effects

Distinguishing between age and cohort effects in cross-national comparative studies (Mayer & Huinink, 1990) is important, because it is often of substantive importance to know whether the behavior of people (e.g., their tendency to vote for a political party) is different because they belong to a given age group (e.g., young or old) or to a particular birth cohort (e. g., the Depression or the Baby Boom). Longitudinal data offer a better opportunity to separate these two effects. Longitudinal data also take into account the effect of a given economic or social phenomenon on the life course of a specific group of individuals (Elder et al., 2003). For example, in addition to individual resources (age, education, labor force experience, etc.), there are at least two ways in which a changing labor market might affect career opportunities. The first is that people in various countries start their careers in different structural contexts. It has often been assumed that specific historical conditions in a particular country at the point of entry into the labor market have a substantial impact on people's subsequent careers. This kind of influence is generally called a "cohort effect" (Glenn, 1977).

The second way a changing labor market influences career opportunities is that it improves or worsens the career prospects of all people within the labor market at a given time (Blossfeld, 1986). For example, in a favorable economic situation with low unemployment, there will be a relatively wide range of opportunities. These influences are generally called a "period effect" (Mason & Fienberg, 1985). Blossfeld (1986) has shown that life course, cohort, and period effects can be identified in terms of substantively developed measures of these concepts (see, e.g., Rodgers, 1982), and that these effects represent central mechanisms of career mobility that must be analytically distinguished. Cross-national life course research can apply such methodological advancements in the study of time-related similarities and differences among countries.

Illumination of Different National "Clocks"

Longitudinal data can be used to study the importance of *various national cultures and norms* for the timing of major life events in different countries (Blossfeld et al., 2007). From a theoretical point of view, very often multiple clocks, historical eras, and current events influence the typical life course in any given nation (Mayer & Tuma, 1990). For example, in demographic studies of divorce, types of clocks, such as age of respondent, time of cohabitation, duration of marriage, ages of children, as well as different phases in the state of the business cycle or changes in national (divorce) laws, are of importance. In a cross-national study of divorce, Blossfeld, De Rose, Hoem, and Rohwer (1995) demonstrated that the divorce risks in Germany and Sweden change differently relative to duration of marriage, ages of children, changes in divorce laws, and the economic business cycle.

Distinction among Contextual Processes at Individual, Group, or National Levels

Cross-national comparative researchers are very often interested in how changes in an individual's or group's context affects a given outcome (Huinink, 1989). For example, the career mobility of an individual in a specific country may be conceived of as being dependent on changes at the individual level (e.g., in social background, educational attainment, experience), in the success of a firm in which he or she is employed (e.g., expansion or contraction of the organization) at the intermediate level, and changes in the business cycle at the national macro-level (Blossfeld, 1986; DiPrete et al., 1997). Longitudinal data can be used to trace processes at various aggregation levels in cross-national studies.

In summary, from a causal-analytical point of view, the dynamic study of parallel and interdependent processes is one of the most important advances of cross-national life course research (Blossfeld et al., 2007; Elder, 1999; Elder et al., 2003; Mayer & Tuma, 1990). These parallel and interdependent processes can operate at an individual, group, institutional, or national level, or a combination of all of these.

At the level of *the individual*, a person's upward and downward job moves are presumed to influence his or her family trajectory and vice versa, in various countries (e.g., Blossfeld, 1995). At the level of *group* or *linked lives* (Elder, 1987a), one might study the effect of the career of the husband on his wife's labor force participation in various countries (Blossfeld & Drobnič, 2001), or how the migration of the head of the household impacts other family members (Courgeau & Lelièvre, 1992). At the level of *intermediate organizations,* one might examine how the changing household or organizational structure of a business firm determines women's labor force participation in different countries (Blossfeld & Hakim, 1997). At the *macro-level,* the researcher may be interested, for instance, in the effect of changes in the business cycle on family formation in various countries (e.g., Blossfeld & Huinink, 1991), or how the globalization process affects entry into the labor market and career process of men and women (Blossfeld et al., 2005). It is also possible to examine any simultaneous combination of the aforementioned levels. For example, in the study of life course, cohort, and period effects, time-dependent covariates measured at different levels must be included simultaneously in cross-national comparative analyses (Blossfeld, 1986; Mayer & Huinink, 1990). Such studies combine processes at the individual level (life course change) and two kinds of processes at the macro-level: (1) country-specific variations in structural conditions across successive (birth, marriage, etc.) cohorts; and (2) country-specific changes in particular historical conditions affecting all cohorts in the same way.

Generality versus Variation in Life Course Mechanisms

I have used cross-national comparative life course studies in several instances to establish the generality of findings and the validity of my interpretations based on the German Life History Study (Mayer, 1990) and the German SOEP. In principle, cross-national research is no more different than any other comparative research, although in practice it allows a much broader range of comparisons and is normally much more complex (see Kohn, 1987). My choice of countries for cross-national comparisons has been determined by the availability of nationally representative longitudinal data (a secondary analysis) and by asking whether including a particular country sheds additional light on the theoretical issue at hand. I regularly have included about nine to 15 countries in cross-national comparisons. Of course, these comparisons require identical or highly similar meanings of survey questions in each country. Also the concepts have to be at least functionally equivalent, which means that they may take different forms in different countries (e.g., different legal definitions of part-time work in various countries; see Blossfeld & Hakim, 1997), but they should refer to the same conceptual framework (e.g., a concept that differentiates the main types of part-time work).

In cross-national studies that involve nine to 15 countries, one researcher cannot possibly know all the intimate details of each country's history. Therefore, the comparisons I have conducted are based on a series of country case studies carried out by national experts who are familiar with the data sets available within each country and are able to analyze them to the fullest advantage. International workshops provided the setting for developing the comparative perspective and method. This work includes specification of theory and hypotheses, research design, the question of how countries can be compared over time, the application of statistical controls, the comparability of concepts, and measurement of dependent and independent variables. In what follows, I describe five examples of cross-national comparative research, with the aim of establishing the generality and limitations of findings, and the validity of interpretations that were initially found through pilot studies for Germany.

Methods and Examples of Establishing Generality

Two areas of the life course in which it has been possible to establish some generality of patterns are the impact of social origins on children's educational attainment and women's timing of entry into marriage and parenthood. In both instances, there appear to be cross-national similarities.

Impact of Social Origins on Educational Attainment

A first example of my cross-national life course research can be found in a book edited by Yossi Shavit and Hans-Peter Blossfeld (1993). This book is based on a pilot study (with complex statistical controls) of the impact of social origin (parent's education and social class position) on successive educational transitions of children in the life course, as conducted for Germany, then systematically replicated in 12 other countries by a group of life course researchers who knew these countries well. The countries varied considerably on (1) level and timing of industrialization, (2) political system, (3) structure of the distributive system, (4) organizational form of the school system, (5) degree of "tracking," (6) educational attendance rates, and (7) formal public commitment to equality of opportunity. Thus, we could demonstrate that in almost all of these heterogeneous industrialized countries (with the exception of the Netherlands and Sweden), inequalities in educational opportunity among students from different social strata have been remarkably stable since the early 20th century—even during the period of massive educational expansion.

The proportion of all social strata that attain higher educational levels has increased, but the relative advantage associated with privileged origins has persisted in most countries. The study showed that educational expansion may even account for the stable patterns of educational stratification. It is a well-known fact that the larger the pie, the less the conflict relative to the size of the slices. As long as the educational attainment of lower social strata is increasing rapidly in modern societies, political attention can neglect any parallel increases among the privileged classes. Therefore, educational expansion can alleviate political pressure to reduce inequalities. The modernization theorist's hypothesis that educational expansion results in greater equality of educational opportunity must therefore be turned on its head: In modern societies, educational expansion actually facilitates to a large extent the persistence of inequalities in educational opportunity.

Impact of Continuing Education on Women's Entry into Marriage and Parenthood

A second example of my cross-national life course research is a study of women's entry into marriage and motherhood in the life course (Blossfeld, 1995). An international group of researchers examined the impact of women's increasing levels of educational attainment and career resources on marriage and motherhood decisions. The starting point of this comparative research, a pilot analysis, showed that entry of West German women into marriage and motherhood was less dependent on their level of educational attainment (as commonly assumed by the economic theory of the family; Becker, 1981), than on whether they extended their participation in the educational system. Nine countries in the project possessed marked differences in the distribution of household types (single, married, divorced), the age when children leave the parental home, the proportion and significance of consensual unions, the fertility rate, the stability of marriage, and the rate of entry into remarriage. These differences were analyzed in detail and compared cross-nationally. The results indicated huge changes in the timing of marriage and motherhood that have stemmed mainly from women's extended enrollment in the educational system. But in most countries, level of education had little or no effect on marital timing. Thus, in most modern societies, the more educated women marry later. Hence, the decline of marriage in Europe and the United States seems not to be due to an improvement in women's educational status.

However, because women still take primary responsibility for child care, they are still disadvantaged when they interrupt their careers for the birth of a child. Therefore, women who have accumulated a high stock of human capital in their life course tend to postpone or avoid the birth of a first child. This effect, and the economically based conflict between a woman's accumulation of human capital and society's expectations of her role as mother, is especially pronounced in traditional family systems, such as those in Italy.

Methods and Examples for Testing the Limits of Generality

Unlike the impact of social origin on children's education, or the impact of continuing education on women's changing role patterns, other dimensions of life course experience appear to vary considerably by national context. Three known examples come from research on women's part-time work, marital equality, and married couples' allocation of household work.

Women's Part-Time Work

A third example of my cross-national life course research focuses on women's work and family roles in Europe and in the United States (Blossfeld & Hakim, 1997). The main research question of the German pilot study was whether, and to what extent, the expansion of part-time work disadvantages or marginalizes women in the labor market and the family. The study looked at a series of conflicting perspectives on women's part-time employment, ranging from equalization to marginalization hypotheses. Using longitudinal data on the labor force participation of women from 12 different modern countries, the researchers described the patterns of part-time work and reassessed competing theories on the impact of part-time work among women. This comparative study concluded that part-time work clearly does not equalize women's position vis-à-vis full-time workers, nor does it leave women in part-time jobs wholly marginalized. This result clearly could be generalized across all countries. In addition, however, the study revealed the limits of this generalization: In some countries, part-time jobs provide new opportunities for secondary earners and play a special role in the context of the nation-specific and gendered division of labor in the family. In other countries, this clearly was not the case.

Educational Homogamy, Upward Mobility, and Growing Income Inequality

In a fourth example, our cross-national study of the life course explored the role of the educational system as a marriage market and investigated changes in marriage patterns induced by the educational expansion of modern societies. Educational expansion increases the chance to meet people of the opposite sex with the same educational level, at an age when individuals typically begin to form couples. Therefore, educational expansion could quite unintentionally increase the likelihood of educational homogamy across cohorts and, as a consequence, not only reinforce social inequality among married couples from one birth cohort to the next but also lead to a growing divergence of social opportunities for the next generation of children.

A pilot study of educational homogamy was conducted in West Germany, then replicated in 12 other countries (see Blossfeld & Timm, 2003). All country-specific case studies showed that observed homogamy rates have always been higher than rates estimated under the assumption of a random process of marital matching. In other words, in all countries we found a strong preference for an equally educated partner. This finding supports Becker's (1981) hypothesis that men and women receive the greatest mutual benefit if they resemble each other as much as possible, or Blau's (1994) thesis that "like likes like." This study found that in most modern societies a combination of at least three factors promote educational homogamy: (1) People often prefer to associate with equally educated partners; (2) educational expansion increases contact opportunities for equally educated men and women at an age when young people start to look for partners and form couples; and (3) women's changing economic role in dual-earner societies increases the importance of women's education and labor force attachment. The main driving forces behind this development involve the increasing role of the educational system as a marriage market in the course of educational expansion, and the fact that wives' employment and income have become a significant determinant of family income and the "lifestyle" of the family in modern societies. Because increasing rates of homogamy reflect the degree to which individuals with the same characteristics, such as educational level, marry each other, they also indicate a rising degree of exclusion through the social structure and an increasing extent to which social networks are closed to outsiders. Therefore, educational expansion has quite unintentionally increased the degree of educational homogamy across cohorts and, as a consequence, has not only reinforced social inequality among households in modern societies but also engendered a growing divergence of economic and educational resources across families for the next generation of children. However, the degree of homogamy varied strongly among the countries studied. It was clear that the greater the importance of educational tracking in a country, the greater the trend toward educational homogamy. Thus, tracking differences among countries clearly limits generalization of the homogamy hypothesis.

Couples' Allocation of Household Work

My fifth example of a cross-national life course study suggests that participation of married women and men in household work responds quite differently to the increasing employment of wives. Wives respond in ways that are consistent with the logic of the gender-neutral theoretical approaches: They do less housework and spend less time on child care when they do more paid work. But the same is not true for husbands: Their participation in housework has hardly changed. Thus, gender role change has been asymmetrical in modern societies, with a greater movement of women into the traditional male sphere than vice versa. This means that, in most modern countries, where the role performance of women has changed considerably, the dimensions of role specialization among dual-earner couples have not been transformed to the same extent. Thus, the findings of this cross-national comparative study clearly support "doing gender" approaches (Brines, 1994) or the gender-specific identity formation model (Bielby & Bielby, 1988). These theories locate gender itself at the heart of the division of labor between women and men, and also predict asymmetrical processes of change for husbands and wives. They suggest the general conclusion that the equalization of gender roles is a much slower process than assumed by economic and bargaining approaches, and—at least in the initial stages—leads to only a modest reduction of gender segregation in the workplace and even less change in the household division of labor.

However, when the impact of partners' resources on women's work careers is examined in more detail in different countries, significant diversity across countries can be detected (Blossfeld & Drobnič, 2001). This example again demonstrates the limits of generalization. Gender role specialization, as predicted by economic theory of the family, seems to be very common in conservative and Mediterranean welfare states in which the middle-class male breadwinner is still able to earn a family wage and husbands' resources have a negative impact on their wives' labor force participation. This can be observed particularly in Germany, where the tax system directly penalizes wives' full-time employment and protects the male-breadwinner family. This, of course, dampens the speed of diffusion of dual-earner families in these countries.

In general, however, the increasing influx of women into the workforce diminishes the role of men as sole breadwinners in all countries and leads to a point at which the whole system shifts from a family wage economy to an individual wage economy. For the individual wage economy, the socioeconomic status of the family is increasingly determined by two income sources. The combined income of the two-earner family then becomes a sort of social standard. The wife's employment and income is also in the interests of the husband. This can be seen in the positive effects of husbands' resources on their wives' labor force participation, particularly in social democratic and (former) socialist countries. In countries associated with the social democratic welfare state regime, the spread of the dual-earner model was especially rapid because of a steeply progressive individualized tax system and public sector provision of family services. Also, in the former socialist countries, the dual-earner family was a social norm, supported by the official gender equality ideology and economic necessity. In the liberal welfare state regimes, no clear effect of husbands' resources on wives' labor force participation was detected. It seems that these countries, particularly the United States, have experienced a very fast transition from the family wage economy to the individual wage economy, accompanied by a stagnation or actual decline of real male wages and an increase of job instability.

Advantages and Difficulties
of Establishing General Life Course Mechanisms

These five examples of cross-national research on the life course demonstrate that *cross-national similarities* greatly extend the scope of our knowledge about life course mechanisms in modern societies (see also Kohn, 1987). Based on comparisons of diverse societies that vary widely in important characteristics, our sociological interpretations have gained considerable generality. Relevant factors include industrial development and culture; the political system and its history; differentiation of educational, employment, and family systems; the role of the state; and the extent to which the roles of men and women have undergone a progressive transformation. In the absence of cross-national evidence, there is no way to know whether our interpretations of life course mechanisms apply outside the particular historical, institutional, and cultural contexts of a specific country. By using an *explicit cross-national comparison*, researchers have shown that there is empirical evidence for more universal sociological regularities.

Of course, such regularities are far from being sociological laws. They can only be generalized to the nations actually studied. Nevertheless, our *theoretical explanations* need not focus on the particular histories, cultures, politics, or economic circumstances of each of the countries, but can instead *focus on more general life course mechanisms common to them all* (Kohn, 1987, p. 719). Of course, apparent similarities can always mask profound societal differences, but this danger is reduced significantly when the studies in one particular country are replicated by competent social scientists from other countries using comparable measurements and concepts, as well as systematic techniques of longitudinal analyses (event–history and panel methods) with extensive time-related statistical controls.

However, I should also mention that several of the five examples of cross-national comparative life course studies also produced some *cross-national differences*. For example, in the fifth example, the impact of partners' resources on women's work careers is different across countries (Blossfeld & Drobnič, 2001). When observed relationships differ from country to country, these inconsistencies have to be interpreted in terms of how the country-specific case studies or the countries differ. If we can rule out methodological differences between case studies as an explanation, then we must take into account what is idiosyncratic about the particular countries for our interpretation.

The social scientist, then, must often resolve the tension between sociological regularities and idiographic explanations. As Melvin Kohn (1987) has noted, in interpreting differences, things become much less certain and more difficult, because we often do not have a convincing clue as to which of the many differences between countries lies at the heart of the differences in results. Kohn proposed two solutions to the problem: The first is that the researcher curtails the scope of an interpretation by limiting the generalizations to *exclude* certain relationships or types of countries. Of course, this procedure is often unsatisfactory. The second is that the cross-national differences are addressed by a reformulation of the substantive interpretation, which provides a new understanding of the discrepant findings. This was the solution we used in the fifth example (Blossfeld & Drobnič, 2001). The problem with this procedure is that such interpretations often seem to be quite ad hoc and arbitrary. From an analytical point of view, it would be better if cross-national life course differences could be interpreted as instances of lawful regularities. This, however, requires a more explicit consideration of historical, cultural, political, and economic characteristics of modern societies.

Analytical Perspectives for More Systematic Comparisons of Life Courses across Countries

Comparative social research inevitably deals with a small number of nations. Modern nations are large units with complex histories and often unique structures. If social scientists compare characteristics between countries or types of countries more systematically, they are engaged in external analysis (Janoski & Hicks, 1994). The question, therefore, is: Which characteristics should be used in cross-national life course research? Over the last 10 years, several fruitful classifications of highly industrialized countries, based on historically developed institutional differences, have resulted. I have discussed the role of differences in educational systems, industrial relations systems, welfare state regimes, and family traditions. At the level of individual (or collective) actors, nationally distinct combinations of such institutional structures manifest themselves as incentives or disincentives for particular organizational or individual adjustments during the life course; therefore, they systematically influence life courses in various countries differently.

Consequences of Differences in Educational Systems

In modern societies, general and vocational training systems, as well as institutions of higher education, are organized in different ways, with life course consequences for (1) the timing of entry into the labor force, (2) the way in which workers are matched to jobs at entry into the labor force and during their later career, and (3) the capacity of workers and organizations to adjust themselves in a flexible way to structural changes of the occupational structure (Blossfeld & Stockmann, 1998/1999).

Vocational training systems in different countries can be compared with respect to the way they combine theoretical learning and practical work experience (Blossfeld & Stockmann, 1998/1999). Here, it is important to make a distinction between countries that organize vocational training (1) mostly in vocational schools (e.g., France, Luxembourg, the Netherlands, or Belgium), (2) mainly by on-the-job training at the workplace (e.g., the United States of America, the United Kingdom, or Italy), or (3) through the so-called dual system, a pragmatic combination of theoretical learning at school and job experience at the workplace (e.g., as in Germany, Austria, Switzerland, Denmark, or Spain).

Theoretical learning in vocational schools is likely to promote a broad theoretical understanding of occupational activities and to foster general education. People in school learn to learn (i.e., to adjust themselves in a learning society). However, vocational schools also have the disadvantage that they do not confront people with real work situations, and they neglect the learning environments of firms and working places. The acquisition of practical experience, therefore, necessarily is shifted to the period after the phase of vocational training, normally with high youth unemployment rates in the transition from school to work (Blossfeld & Stockmann, 1998/1999).

The German "dual system" has the comparative advantage of allowing a large number of young adults to make a smooth transition from the general educational school system to the employment system, because this vocational training system feeds directly into the job system, with comparatively low youth unemployment (Blossfeld & Stockmann, 1998/1999). In addition, the dual system is characterized by a highly standardized set of job qualifications with recognized certificates. Therefore, employers can use these certificates as indications of particular employment possibilities for workers, and workers can use them as reference points in defining their social status in collective and individual negotiations with employers. Thus, the dual system fosters between-firm mobility, mainly among small and medium-size firms. However, the disadvantage of the "dual system" in a world of growing change in the occupational structure is that it leads to a close coupling of vocational certificates and occupational opportunities, with a high degree of rigidity and a low level of job mobility in the labor force.

On-the-job training, on the other hand, has the advantage that workers are not so much restricted to narrowly defined occupational fields in their later career, and that new generations of entrants can be flexibly directed to new and future-oriented occupational fields. Thus, countries with on-the-job training generally are connected with a high rate of job mobility in the life course. The disadvantage, however, is that the quality of training is normally very heterogeneous, because training conditions are not controlled and standardized across firms. Furthermore, if workers move from one job to the next between firms, neither workers nor employers can rely on shared definitions and standards with respect to skills, income, and job requirements. This increases the risk for individual workers (in terms of income, job standards, etc.) if they move between firms, and makes it more likely that employers recruit the wrong person for a specific job. Thus, such a vocational training system fosters intrafirm mobility, mainly in large companies with large internal labor markets, and reduces between-firm mobility.

Finally, vocational training systems differ with regard to the extent in which they differentiate between unskilled and semiskilled workers on the one hand, and occupationally trained workers on the other, and in which they give trained workers the opportunity to climb up the job ladder (Blossfeld & Mayer, 1988). In the more or less "open" system of on-the-job training, there are only a few structural barriers in terms of recognized certificates between unskilled, semiskilled, and skilled work-ers. The career perspectives of trained workers are also strongly depen-dent on the quality of on-the-job training in a specific company. In labor markets based on the "dual system," however, there is a clear division of job opportunities between the unskilled and the trained in the labor force, and only the trained have a common basis for further qualifica-tions as master craftsmen or technicians, and also often as technical, college-educated engineers.

Impact of Different Industrial Relations Systems

Modern countries also differ with respect to the nature of their indus-trial relations between employers and workers (e.g., types of work coun-cils, collective bargaining systems, strength of unions vs. employer organizations, labor legislation or administrative regulations). These differences produce distinct national variations of occupational struc-tures and industries; patterns of labor–capital negotiations; strike fre-quencies; and collective agreements on wages, job security, labor condi-tions, and work hours (Soskice, 1991).

The United States and also the United Kingdom (after Margaret Thatcher) are often cited in literature as examples of industrial rela-tions systems that are decentralized, dualistic and based on free mar-ket forces; in short, as systems in which so-called "open" employment relationships dominate. Labor unions are quite weak, so that workers are relatively unprotected against the flexibility demands of firms. The consequence of relatively unconstrained competition is that (1) wages for most jobs are comparatively low; (2) entry into the labor force by young workers proceeds rather smoothly; (3) the rate of job mobility is relatively high; (4) unemployment is of short duration (principle of "hire and fire"); and (5) precarious employment forms are more evenly spread among various social groups. It is characteristic of these "individ-ualistic" mobility regimes that an individual's resources (social origin, education, labor force experience, etc.) play a dominant role in labor market outcomes over the life course (DiPrete et al., 1997).

Western European countries, on the other hand, are often classi-fied as having labor markets with relatively "closed" employment rela-tionships and centralized mechanisms for negotiating wages (DiPrete et al., 1997). Sweden and Germany are known as countries with par-ticularly strong labor unions, whereas Southern European countries such as Spain and Italy are taken as extreme cases of so-called "insider–outsider" labor markets. In such "closed" systems, most workers within companies are relatively shielded against the growing uncertainty and flexibility demands of the world market. Therefore, increasing economic and social risks are largely channeled to groups outside the labor force (young workers who want to enter the labor force, women who want to reenter the labor force after a family-related employment interruption, or unemployed midcareer workers who are looking for work). This means that whereas the global innovation process in these countries tends to create a new kind of underclass of the socially excluded, the employed have high levels of job security with relatively high wages (Esping-Andersen, 1990).

The main consequences of "closed" employment systems are that (1) entry into the labor force by young workers is problematic, particularly under conditions of high general unemployment; (2) the rate of job mobility is relatively low; (3) unemployment is usually of a long duration; and (4) precarious employment forms (fixed-term contracts, part-time work, seasonal labor) are highly concentrated among specific groups seeking access to the labor market. In these "collective" employment systems, individual resources (e.g., social origin, education, labor force experience) of the already employed play a minor role for market outcomes such as income and career opportunities (DiPrete et al., 1997).

Influences of Welfare State Regimes

Modern countries have also developed different welfare states, which implies diverse national ideologies about social solidarity, as well as gender and social equality (Esping-Andersen, 1990). As far as job mobility is concerned, these differences between welfare states manifest themselves in the priority of (1) active, employment-sustaining labor market policies (i.e., the commitment to full employment); (2) welfare-sustaining employment exit policies, that is, welfare support for those who are outside the labor market (e.g., the youth, unemployed, ill, poor, women taking care of the family, pensioners); and (3) the share of the public sector in the labor force.

The United States and, to a lesser extent, Canada, as well as the United Kingdom, are generally seen as "liberal" welfare states characterized by passive labor market policies, moderate support for the underprivileged, and relatively small public sector employment. In contrast, Norway, Denmark, and Sweden are often considered examples of the so-called "social-democratic" welfare state model. Active labor market and taxation policies in these countries aim at full employment; gender equality in the workplace, as well as at home; and "fair" income distribution, with a high degree of wage compression. Achieving full employment is mostly attempted by a combination of Keynesian demand policies and mobility-stimulating measures, such as retraining, mobility grants, and temporary jobs. The large participation of (married) women in full-time employment in these welfare states rests on both (1) the rapid expansion of job opportunities in the service and public sector, engendered in particular by the demands of social services (kindergartens, schools, hospitals, day care centers and homes for the elderly) and (2) the highly progressive individual income tax that makes a second household income necessary for most families, if they want to enjoy the products of a technologically advanced service society.

Germany and the Netherlands are often cited in the literature as examples of "conservative" welfare state regimes. Social policies in these countries are not so much designed to promote job mobility, employment opportunities, and full employment by Keynesian demand policy measures as to ensure that those workers who leave employment because of job loss, disability or, in some cases, as part of an early retirement program, are protected against serious declines in living standards. Therefore, countries like the Netherlands and Germany support the unemployed for relatively long durations and have generous arrangements for early retirement. This type of welfare state is strongly transfer oriented, with decommodifying effects for those who are economically inactive. The conservative welfare state is also committed to the traditional division of labor in the family that makes wives economically dependent on their husbands. In particular, it supports wives and mothers who give priority to family activities (taking care of children and the elderly) and seek to work part time. Correspondingly, welfare state provisions (e.g., kindergartens, day care centers, homes for the elderly) are far less developed than those in the social democratic model, and female economic activity rates are considerably lower and restricted mostly to part-time jobs (see Blossfeld & Hakim, 1997).

With regard to the welfare state institutions, Southern European countries, such as Italy, Greece, and Spain, also share common features. They have developed a welfare state model that might be called "family-oriented" (Guerrero & Naldini, 1996). In terms of labor market policy, support for the less privileged, and the importance of public sector employment, this welfare state is very similar to the "liberal" one. Unlike the latter, however, it is characterized by a strong ideological and indeed practical involvement of family and kinship networks in protecting its members against economic and social risks. This model is based on the deeply rooted cultural view that family and kinship represent an important institution of reciprocal help, and that family members should support each other. In everyday life, however, this support is mostly provided by women, with two important results: (1) Their labor force participation (including part-time work) is extremely low by international standards; and (2) especially if young women want to make their own career in the labor force, there is a particularly severe conflict between family tasks and (mostly full-time) job requirements, leading to very low fertility levels in Spain or Italy, for example.

Impact of Different Family Systems

The educational and industrial relations systems, as well as the various welfare state regimes, are closely connected to specific family and fertility traditions (Blossfeld, 1995). Family systems regulate the degree of pluralization of private living arrangements. "Pluralization" refers to lifestyles beyond the traditional marital couple or nuclear family to include nonmarital cohabitation, remaining single, or postponement or forgoing of fertility. A north–south divide in the pluralization of private living arrangements emerges due to not only institutional but also cultural differences (Blossfeld, 1995). Scandinavian countries such as Sweden and Norway seem to have a pioneering role, and countries such as Germany, France, the Netherlands, the United Kingdom, the United States, and Canada appear to follow this trend. Familistic countries, such as Italy, Spain, Ireland, and Mexico, are less affected. The strong institutionalization of marriage in Southern Europe and Mexico translates into small numbers of nonmarital unions and one-person households among youth, low divorce, low extramarital birthrates, and an asymmetrical relationship between the sexes within the family.

The Changing Life Course in Modern Societies: How Globalization Is Differently Filtered by Domestic Institutions

Finally, I would like to illustrate the usefulness of these more systematic analytical concepts of comparative life course research. For this purpose, I draw on the results of a recent cross-national study that asked how the globalization process is "institutionally filtered" and channeled by domestic institutions to shape the individual life course in modern societies. This complex study analyzes in detail the changes for the most important life course transitions in different countries: (1) the transition from youth to adulthood (e.g., entry into the labor market and family formation; Blossfeld et al., 2005); (2) men's midlife career mobility patterns (Blossfeld, Mills, & Bernardi, 2006); (3) women's midlife transitions between employment and family (Blossfeld & Hofmeister, 2006); and (4) late job careers of men and women and their transition into retirement (Blossfeld, Buchholz, & Hofäcker, 2006).

Globalization as a Macroprocess Affecting All Modern Societies

Nowadays, most social scientists agree that the globalization process is characterized by the simultaneous coaction of four macrostructural trends that have become increasingly dominant, particularly since the 1980s:

1. The increasing internationalization of markets and the associated growth in competition between countries with very different wage and productivity levels, as well as different social and environmental standards (particularly since the fall of the Iron Curtain and the integration of East European and Asian nations into the global market).

2. The intensification of competition between nation–states and the resulting tendency for modern states to reduce business taxes and to engage in deregulation, privatization, and liberalization, while also strengthening the market as a coordinating mechanism.

3. The rapid, worldwide networking of persons, companies, and states through new information and communication technologies, and, as a result, the increasing global interdependence of actors, along with the increasing acceleration of social and economic interaction.

4. The fast growth in the importance of globally networked markets and the accompanying increase in the interdependence and volatility of local markets that are ever more vulnerable to unpredictable social, political, and economic "external shocks" and events throughout the world (e.g., wars, economic crises, subprime mortgage turbulences, oil price shocks, consumer fashions, technological innovations).

Thus, globalization is accompanied by a growth in unexpected market trends in an increasingly changing global economy, by more rapid processes of social and economic change, by an ever-stronger decline in the predictability of economic and social trends, and, as a result of this, by a general increase in uncertainty.

As a consequence, globalization has led to a significant shift in power relations on the labor market. Employers increasingly try to shift their own greater market risks due to the globalization process and their resulting needs for flexibility on to their employees. So far, there is no consensus in sociological research with regard to how these changes in the labor market and the rise in uncertainty have influenced the development of social inequalities in modern societies. Currently, two opposite interpretations of the effects of globalization on the development of social inequality structures can be found (Blossfeld et al., 2005). The first perspective argues that present-day societies can no longer be characterized as "class societies," but need to be understood as "risk societies" (Beck, 1992). In the course of the globalization process, new forms of risks and uncertainty have emerged and have become generalized across all social strata, thereby breaking down the logic of the traditional class structure. The second perspective suggests the opposite, namely, the strengthening of existing social inequalities in the globalization process (Breen, 1997).

Globalization Effects on Life Transitions of the Young Generation

Because of space, I limit the discussion of results only to the cross-national comparative analysis of globalization's impact on the early life course of youth in 14 countries (Blossfeld et al., 2005). How are the changed labor market entry patterns in young persons' lives affecting familial decisions, such as marrying or having a baby? The results show that young persons face greater uncertainties when entering the labor market (Blossfeld et al., 2005). These uncertainties are manifested particularly in the form of a major increase in precarious, atypical forms of employment (e.g., short-term jobs; part-time jobs; precarious forms of self-employment; and, compared with older cohorts, lower income). Such developments tend to make young people "losers" in the globalization process. At first glance, this seems to be counterintuitive, because the young generation is far more educated than older ones, and many of these young people have spent a longer part of their lives abroad. However, they are affected particularly strongly, because they frequently lack job experience and strong ties to business networks, particularly to those jobs that are more secure. Often they are unable to fall back on established contacts, and they do not possess the negotiating powers to demand stable and continuous employment. Thus, it is comparatively easy for employers and unions to adjust young people's work contracts and make them more flexible and less advantageous at the workers' expense.

However, the concrete effects of the globalization process on the labor market positions of young adults vary according to the specific welfare state and labor market regime. The strong insider–outsider markets of Southern Europe (but, in part, also Germany) reveal increasing phases of unemployment and/or short-term work contracts (Blossfeld et al., 2005). Particularly in Southern Europe, various forms of precarious self-employment can be found. In the Netherlands, there is a massive increase in part-time jobs for young women and men, and in the open employment systems of the liberal countries (United States, Great Britain), effects of the globalization process are manifested across the generations, but particularly as increasing income losses for young persons (Blossfeld et al., 2005).

Independent of the national context, education is clearly becoming more and more important in the globalization process (Blossfeld et al., 2005). Poorly qualified labor market entrants are hit particularly hard by the global changes. This is how globalization generally reinforces the social inequalities within the younger generation, because individual (human capital) resources gain in importance through the growing relevance of the market and individual competition.

The increasing experience of employment uncertainties in young adulthood has consequences for familial decision processes. Growing economic and temporal uncertainties lead young people more and more to postpone or even to forgo family formation (Blossfeld et al., 2005). On the societal level, this leads to a dilemma, because not only improved conditions for labor market flexibility, in the sense of greater competitiveness, but also rising birthrates are viewed as desirable.

Young adults have developed four behavioral and adaptive strategies as a reaction to growing uncertainties in the life course (Blossfeld et al., 2005):

1. They increasingly postpone decisions requiring a long-term commitment; the youth phase becomes more and more a "moratorium," and transitions to gainful employment often take a chaotic course.
2. They switch increasingly to alternative roles instead of employment (e.g., they spend longer in the education system instead of letting themselves be defined as "unemployed").
3. They are increasingly forming more flexible forms of partnership (e.g., consensual unions) that permit an adaptation to rising uncertainty, without having to make long-term commitments (Nazio & Blossfeld, 2003).
4. Particularly in the family-oriented welfare states of Central and Southern Europe, they have developed gender-specific strategies to deal with uncertainty: Men are increasingly less able to guarantee any long-term income security as the "breadwinner" for a household, often leading to delay in family formation. In contrast, many unqualified women who "have nothing to lose" react to the growing uncertainties in the labor market by turning to the security of the family and the traditional roles of mother and housewife (as a strategy to reduce uncertainty).

On the contrary, the tendency for highly qualified women to have children in increasingly uncertain labor markets depends on whether they can protect their careers by making family and career compatible. When child care facilities are underdeveloped, as is particularly the case in Southern Europe, many qualified women decide in favor of their careers rather than for children.

Hence, a paradoxical outcome of the globalization process is that precisely in traditional, family-oriented societies the birthrate is declining markedly because of the growing experience of employment uncertainties for young men, and the incompatibility of family and career for qualified women. Similar restrained fertility behavior can also be found in the transformation countries of Eastern Europe, in which uncertainties have grown enormously since the collapse of socialism (Blossfeld et al., 2005).

It is important to point out in this context that it is not the *absolute* level of uncertainty that is decisive for the structuring of decisions on family formation, but the subjectively perceived *relative* level of uncertainty in the specific country's labor force (Blossfeld et al., 2005). In each country, young adults compare themselves in daily life with "significant others" (e.g., friends, relatives, acquaintances) when judging their individual labor market situation. In the United States, for example, the absolute level of uncertainty for the younger generation is higher as a whole than that in many European countries. People lose their jobs more frequently, but the unemployed can rely on soon finding another job, that is, becoming an "insider" again, because of the low mobility barriers in the labor market. This is why labor market uncertainty, career mobility, and flexibility possess a different social significance in the United States. Subjectively, they are perceived differently than in the insider–outsider markets of Europe, where "being an outsider" often means identity-threatening, long-term exclusion from work, in a climate in which flexible work arrangements are generally viewed as only a stopgap solution on the way toward a permanent job. Therefore, young persons in flexible forms of employment in the European insider–outsider markets experience their fate as being far more negative than that of their peers in the United States.

Summary

Cross-national research on the life course is connected with methodological innovations, such as the collection of retrospective or prospective panel data, and the application of event–history and panel methods. Therefore, I have described the strength of longitudinal methods compared to cross-sectional analysis for this kind of research. Using some examples from my research, I have shown how the generality of life course mechanisms can be established through cross-national life course research. This is a complex project, because life course patterns in modern societies are still molded to a large extent by domestic institutions and social structures. In a third step, therefore, I have presented analytical strategies to identify the variation in institutions that significantly affects the characteristic life course patterns of modern societies. These are classifications of educational systems, patterns of employment relations, national welfare state regimes, and the various family traditions of each society. The usefulness of these comparative concepts is illustrated by a recent study that demonstrated how globalization on the macro-level is "institutionally filtered" and channeled by domestic institutions toward the lives of individuals, particularly the life course transitions of young people in modern societies.

References

Abbott, A., & Hrycak, A. (1990). Measuring resemblance in sequence data. *American Journal of Sociology, 96*(1), 144–185.

Agar, M. H. (1996). *The professional stranger: An informal introduction to ethnography.* San Diego: Academic Press.

Allport, G. (1937). *Personality: A psychological interpretation.* New York: Holt.

Allport, G. W. (1954). *The nature of prejudice.* Reading, MA: Perseus.

Almeida, D. M. (2005). Resilience and vulnerability to daily stressors assessed via diary methods. *Current Directions in Psychological Science, 14*(2), 64–68.

Almeida, D. M., Chandler, A. L., & Wethington, E. (1999). Daily transmission of tensions between marital dyads and parent–child dyads. *Journal of Marriage and the Family, 61*(1), 49–61.

Almeida, D. M., & Horn, M. C. (2004). Is daily life more stressful during middle adulthood? In O. G. Brim, C. D. Ryff, & R. C. Kessler (Eds.), *How healthy are we?: A national study of well-being at midlife* (pp. 425–451). Chicago: University of Chicago Press.

Almeida, D. M., & Kessler, R. C. (1998). Everyday stressors and gender differences in daily distress. *Journal of Personality and Social Psychology, 75*(3), 670–680.

Almeida, D. M., Serido, J., & McDonald, D. (2006). Daily life stressors of early and late Baby Boomers. In S. K. Whitbourne & S. L. Willis (Eds.), *The Baby Boomers grow up: Contemporary perspectives on midlife* (pp. 165–184). Mahwah, NJ: Erlbaum.

Almeida, D. M., Wethington, E., & Kessler, R. C. (2002). The Daily Inventory of Stressful Experiences (DISE): An interview-based approach for measuring daily stressors. *Assessment, 9*(1), 41–55.

Alter, G., & Oris, M. (2001). The family and mortality: A case study from rural Belgium. *Annales de Dèmographie Historique, 101*, 11–31.

Altobelli, J., & Moen, P. (2007). Work–family spillover among dual-earner couples. In J. J. Suitor & T. J. Owens (Eds.), *Advances in life course research: Interpersonal relations across the life course* (Vol. 12, pp. 361–382). Oxford, England: Elsevier Science.

Altucher, K., & Williams, L. B. (2003). Family clocks: Timing parenthood. In P. Moen (Ed.), *It's about time: Couples and careers* (pp. 49–59). Ithaca, NY: Cornell University Press.

Amato, P. R., & Booth, A. (2001). The legacy of parents' marital discord: Consequences for children's marital quality. *Journal of Personality and Social Psychology, 81*(4), 627–638.

Anderson, C. A., Bowman, M. J., & Tinto, V. (1972). *Where colleges are and who attends: Effects of accessibility on college attendance.* New York: McGraw-Hill.

Andersson, F., Holzer, H. J., & Lane, J. I. (2005). *Moving up or moving on: Who advances in the low-wage labor market?* New York: Russell Sage Foundation.

Andrew, M., & Hauser, R. M. (2008, August). *Evaluating the "strategic center": Race–ethnic differences in updating and applying educational expectations.* Paper presented at the annual meeting of the American Sociological Association, Boston, MA.

Aneshensel, C. S., Botticello, A. L., & Yamamoto-Mitani, N. (2004). When caregiving ends: The course of depressive symptoms after bereavement. *Journal of Health and Social Behavior, 45*(3), 422–440.

Antonucci, T. C., & Akiyama, H. (1995). Convoys of social relations: Family and friendships within a life span context. In R. Blieszner & V. H. Bedford (Eds.), *Handbook of aging and the family* (pp. 355–371). Westport, CT: Greenwood Press.

Asher, R. M., & Fine, G. A. (1991). Fragile ties: Shaping relationships with women married to alcoholics. In W. B. Shaffir & R. A. Stebbins (Eds.), *Experiencing fieldwork: An inside view of qualitative research* (pp. 196–205). Newbury Park, CA: Sage.

Atwood, N. C. (2007). *Growing up bookish in a working class world.* Manuscript under review.

Bachman, R., & Saltzman, L. E. (1995). *Violence against women: Estimates from the redesigned survey.* Washington, DC: Bureau of Justice Statistics.

Baltes, P. B. (1987). Theoretical propositions of life-span developmental psychology: On the dynamics between growth and decline. *Developmental Psychology, 23*(5), 611–626.

Baltes, P. B., & Baltes, M. M. (1990). Psychological perspectives on successful aging: The model of selective optimization with compensation. In *Successful aging: Perspectives from the behavioral sciences* (pp. 1–34). Cambridge, England: Cambridge University Press.

Baltrus, P. T., Lynch, J. W., Everson-Rose, S., Raghunathan, T. E., & Kaplan, G. A. (2005). Race/ethnicity, life course socioeconomic position, and body weight trajectories over 34 years: The Alameda County Study. *American Journal of Public Health, 95*(9), 1595–1601.

Barker, D. J. P. (2001). *Fetal origins of cardiovascular and lung disease.* New York: Dekker.

Barrett, A. E. (2000). Marital trajectories and mental health. *Journal of Health and Social Behavior, 41*, 451–464.

Bauer, D., & Curran, P. J. (2003). Distributional assumptions of growth mixture models: Implications for over-extraction of latent trajectory classes. *Psychological Methods, 8*(3), 338–363.

Beck, U. (1992). *Risk society: Towards a new modernity.* London: Sage.

Becker, G. S. (1981). *A treatise on the family.* Cambridge, MA: Harvard University Press.

Becker, H. S. (1960). Notes on the concept of commitment. *American Journal of Sociology, 66*(1), 32–40.

Becker, H. S. (1996). The epistemology of qualitative research. In R. Jessor, A. Colby, & R. A. Shweder (Eds.), *Ethnography and human development: Context and meaning in social inquiry* (pp. 53–71). Chicago: University of Chicago Press.

Becker, P. E., & Moen, P. (1999). Scaling back: Dual-career couples' work–family strategies. *Journal of Marriage and the Family, 61*(3), 995–1007.

Becker-Blease, K. A., & Freyd, J. J. (2006). Research participants telling the truth about their lives: The ethics of asking and not asking about abuse. *American Psychologist, 61*(3), 218–226.

Benedict, R. (1946). *The chrysanthemum and the sword: Patterns of Japanese culture.* Boston: Houghton Mifflin.

Bengston, V. L. (1975). Generation and family effects in value socialization. *American Sociological Review, 40*(3), 358–371.

Bengston, V. L. (2001). Beyond the nuclear family: The increasing importance of multigenerational bonds. *Journal of Marriage and the Family, 63*(1), 1–16.

Bennett, J. B., & Lehman, W. E. (1999). Employee exposure to coworker substance use and negative consequences: The moderating effects of work group membership. *Journal of Health and Social Behavior, 40*(2), 307–322.

Bernhardt, A., Morris, M., Handcock, M. S., & Scott, M. A. (2001). *Divergent paths: Economic mobility in the new American labor market.* New York: Sage.

Bertaux, D. (1981). Life stories in the bakers' trade. In D. Bertaux & I. Bertaux-Wiame (Eds.), *Biography and society: The life history approach in the social sciences* (pp. 169–189). Beverly Hills, CA: Sage.

Bertaux, D., & Bertaux-Wiame, I. (Eds.). *Biography and society: The life history approach in the social sciences.* Beverly Hills, CA: Sage.

Bertaux, D., & Kohli, M. (1984). The life story approach: A continental view. *Annual Review of Sociology, 10,* 215–237.

Bertaux, D., & Thompson, P. (1997). *Pathways to social class: A qualitative approach to social mobility.* New York: Oxford University Press.

Bertaux-Wiame, I. (1981). The life history approach to the study of internal migration. In D. Bertaux & I. Bertaux-Wiame (Eds.), *Biography and society: The life history approach in the social sciences* (pp. 249–265). Beverly Hills, CA: Sage.

Bianchi, S. M., Robinson, J. P., & Milkie, M. A. (2006). *Changing rhythms of American family life.* New York: Russell Sage Foundation.

Bielby, D. D., & Bielby, W. T. (1988). She works hard for the money: Household responsibilities and the allocation of work effort. *American Journal of Sociology, 93*(5), 1031–1059.

Bielby, W. T., & Hauser, R. M. (1977). Response error in earnings functions for nonblack males. *Sociological Methods and Research, 6*(2), 241–280.

Bielby, W. T., Hauser, R. M., & Featherman, D. L. (1977). Response errors of black and nonblack males in models of the intergenerational transmission of socioeconomic status. *American Journal of Sociology, 82*(6), 1242–1288.

Bilgrad, R. (1990). *National Death Index user's manual.* Hyattsville, MD: U.S. Department of Health and Human Services, Public Health Service, Centers for Disease Control, National Center for Health Statistics.

Birch, M., & Miller, T. (2000). Inviting intimacy: The interview as therapeutic opportunity. *International Journal of Social Research Methodology, 3*(3), 189–202.

Birdett, K. S., Fingerman, K. L., & Almeida, D. M. (2005). Age differences in exposure and reactions to interpersonal tensions: A daily diary study. *Psychology and Aging, 20*(2), 330–340.

Blair-Loy, M. (1999). Career patterns of executive women in finance: An optimal matching analysis. *American Journal of Sociology, 104*(4), 1346–1397.

Blair-Loy, M., & Wharton, A. S. (2002). Employees' use of work–family policies and the workplace social context. *Social Forces, 80*(3), 813–845.

Blanchard-Fields, F., & Cooper, C. (2004). Social cognition and social relationships. In F. R. Lang & K. L. Fingerman (Eds.), *Growing together: Personal relationships across the lifespan* (pp. 268–289). New York: Cambridge University Press.

Blatter, C. W., & Jacobsen, J. J. (1993). Older women coping with divorce: Peer support groups. *Women and Therapy, 14*(1/2), 141–155.

Blau, P. M. (1994). *Structural contexts of opportunities.* Chicago: University of Chicago Press.

Blau, P. M., & Duncan, O. D. (1967). *The American occupational structure.* New York: Wiley.

Blossfeld, H.-P. (1986). Career opportunities in the Federal Republic of Germany: A dynamic approach to the study of life course, cohort, and period effects. *European Sociological Review, 2*(3), 208–225.

Blossfeld, H.-P. (1995). *The new role of women. Family formation in modern societies.* Boulder, CO: Westview Press.

Blossfeld, H.-P., Buchholz, S., & Hofäcker, D. (2006). *Globalization, uncertainty and late careers in society.* New York: Routledge.

Blossfeld, H.-P., DeRose, A., Hoem, J. M., & Rohwer, G. (1995). Education, modernization, and the risk of marriage disruption: Differences in the effect of women's educational attainment in Sweden, West Germany, and Italy. In K. O. Mason & A.-M. Jenson (Eds.), *Gender and family change in industrialized countries* (pp. 200–222). Oxford, England: Clarendon.

Blossfeld, H.-P., & Drobnič, S. (2001). *Careers of couples in contemporary societies. From male breadwinner to dual-earner families.* Oxford, England: Oxford University Press.

Blossfeld, H.-P., Golsch, K., & Rohwer, G. (2007). *Event history analysis with Stata.* Mahwah, NJ: Erlbaum.

Blossfeld, H.-P., & Hakim, C. (1997). *Between equalization and marginalization: Women working part-time in Europe and the United States of America.* Oxford, England: Oxford University Press.

Blossfeld, H.-P., & Hofmeister, H. A. E. (2006). *Globalization, uncertainty and women's careers in international comparison.* Cheltenham, England: Edward Elgar.

Blossfeld, H.-P., & Huinink, J. (1991). Human capital investments or norms of role transition?: How women's schooling and career affect the process of family formation. *American Journal of Sociology, 97*(1), 143–168.

Blossfeld, H.-P., & Mayer, K. U. (1988). Labor market segmentation in the FRG: An empirical study of segmentation theories from a life course perspective. *European Sociological Review, 4*(2), 123–140.

Blossfeld, H.-P., & Mills, M. (2001). A causal approach to interrelated family events: A cross-national comparison of cohabitation, nonmarital conception, and marriage. *Canadian Journal of Population, 28*(2), 409–437.

Blossfeld, H.-P., Mills, M., & Bernardi, F. E. (2006). *Globalization, uncertainty and men's careers in international comparison.* Cheltenham, England: Edward Elgar.

Blossfeld, H.-P., Mills, M., Klijzing, E., & Kurz, K. E. (2005). *Globalization, uncertainty and youth in society.* London: Routledge.

Blossfeld, H.-P., & Stockmann, R. (1998/1999). Globalization and changes in vocational training systems in developing and advanced industrialized societies, Vol. I–III. *International Journal of Sociology, 28*(4), 29(1, 2).

Blossfeld, H.-P., & Timm, A. (2003). *Who marries whom?: Educational systems as marriage markets in modern societies.* Dordrecht: Kluwer Academic.

Blumer, H. (1955). Attitudes and the social act. *Social Problems, 3*(2), 59–65.

Blumstein, A., Cohen, J., & Farrington, D. P. (1988a). Criminal career research: Its value for criminology. *Criminology, 26*(1), 1–35.

Blumstein, A., Cohen, J., & Farrington, D. P. (1988b). Longitudinal and criminal career research: Further clarifications. *Criminology, 26*(1), 57–74.

Blumstein, A., Cohen, J., Roth, J. A., & Visher, C. (Eds.). (1986). *Criminal careers and career criminals.* Washington, DC: National Academies Press.

Blyth, D. A., Simmons, R. G., & Carlton-Ford, S. (1983). The adjustment of early adolescents to school transitions. *Journal of Early Adolescence, 31*(1–2), 105–120.

Boardman, J. D. (2009). State-level moderation of genetic tendencies to smoke cigarettes. *American Journal of Public Health, 99*(3), 480–486.

Boardman, J. D., Saint Onge, J. M., Haberstick, B. C., Timberlake, D. S., & Hewitt, J. K. (2008). Do schools moderate the genetic determinants of smoking? *Behavior Genetics, 38*(3), 234–246.

Bolger, N., Davis, A., & Rafaeli, E. (2003). Diary methods: Capturing life as it is lived. *Annual Review of Psychology, 54*, 579–616.

Bolger, N., DeLongis, A., Kessler, R. C., & Schilling, E. (1989). Effects of daily stress on negative mood. *Journal of Personality and Social Psychology, 57*(5), 808–818.

Bowles, S. (1972). Schooling and inequality from generation to generation. *Journal of Political Economy, 80*(3), S219–S251.

Breen, R. (1997). Risk recommodification and the future of the service class. *Sociology, 31*(3), 473–489.

Bride, B. E. (2007). Prevalence of secondary traumatic stress among social workers. *Social Work, 52*(1), 63–70.

Brim, O. G. (1992). *Ambition: How we manage success and failure throughout our lives.* New York: Basic Books.

Brim, O. G., Jr., & Ryff, C. (1980). On the properties of life events. In P. G. Baltes & O. G. Brim (Eds.), *Life-span development and behavior* (Vol. 3, pp. 368–388). New York: Academic Press.

Brines, J. (1994). Economic dependency, gender, and division of labor at home. *American Journal of Sociology, 100*(2), 652–688.

Brines, J., & Joyner, K. (1999). The ties that bind: Principles of cohesion in cohabitation and marriage. *American Sociological Review, 64*(2), 333–355.

Bronfenbrenner, U., & Ceci, S. J. (1994). Nature–nurture reconceptualized in developmental perspective: A bioecological model. *Psychological Review, 101*(4), 568–586.

Bronfenbrenner, U., & Crouter, A. C. (1983). The evolution of environmental models in developmental research. In P. H. Mussen (Ed.), *Handbook of child psychology: Vol. 1. History, theory, and methods* (pp. 357–414). New York: Wiley.

Brown, G., & Harris, T. (1978). *Social origins of depression: A study of psychiatric disorder in women.* New York: Free Press.

Brown, G. W., & Harris, T. O. (1989). *Life events and illness.* New York: Guilford Press.

Brown, L. M., & Gilligan, C. (1992). *Meeting at the crossroads: Women's psychology and girls' development.* Cambridge, MA: Harvard University Press.

Brown, T. H. (2008). *Divergent pathways: Racial/ethnic inequalities in wealth and health trajectories.* PhD dissertation, University of North Carolina at Chapel Hill.

Brückner, E., & Mayer, K. U. (1998). Collecting life history data: Experiences from the German life history study. In J. Z. Giele & G. H. Elder, Jr. (Eds.), *Methods of life course research: Qualitative and quantitative approaches* (pp. 152–181). Thousand Oaks, CA: Sage.

Bryk, A. S., & Raudenbush, S. W. (1992). *Hierarchical linear models: Applications and data analysis methods* (Vol. 1). Newbury Park, CA: Sage.

Buchmann, M. (1989). *The script of life in modern society: Entry into adulthood in a changing world.* Chicago: University of Chicago Press.

Burke, K. (1945). *A grammar of motives.* New York: Prentice-Hall.

Burks, B. S., Jensen, D. W., & Terman, L. M. (1959). *Follow-up studies of a thousand gifted children.* Stanford, CA: Stanford University Press.

Burton, L. M. (1990). Teenage childbearing as an alternative life-course strategy in multigeneration black families. *Human Nature, 1*(2), 123–143.

Burton, L. M. (1996). Age norms, the timing of family role transitions, and intergenerational caregiving among aging African American women. *Gerontologist, 36*(2), 199–208.

Burton, L. M. (1997). Ethnography and the meaning of adolescence in high-risk neighborhoods. *Ethos, 25*(1), 208–217.

Burton, L. M., Cherlin, A., Winn, D. M., Estacion, A., & Holder-Taylor, C. (in press). The role of trust in low-income mothers' intimate unions. *Journal of Marriage and Family.*

Burton, L. M., Obeidallah, D. A., & Allison, K. (1996). Ethnographic insights on social context and adolescent development among inner-city African-American teens. In R. Jessor, A. Colby, & R. Shweder (Eds.), *Ethnography and human development: Context and meaning in social inquiry* (pp. 395–418). Chicago: University of Chicago Press.

Burton, L. M., Skinner, D., & Matthews, S. (2005, August). *"Structuring discovery": A model and method for multi-site team ethnography.* Paper presented at the annual meeting of the American Sociological Association, Philadelphia, PA.

Butler, J., & Burton, L. M. (1990). Rethinking teenage childbearing: Is sexual abuse a missing link? *Family Relations, 39*(1), 73–80.

Button, T. M. M., Corley, R. P., Rhee, S. H., Hewitt, J. K., Young, S. E., & Stallings, M. C. (2007). Delinquent peer affiliation and conduct problems: A twin study. *Journal of Abnormal Psychology, 116*(3), 554–564.

Butz, W. P., & Torrey, B. B. (2006). Some frontiers in social science. *Science, 312*(5782), 1898–1900.

Cadoret, R. J., Yates, W. R., Troughton, E., Woodworth, G., & Stewart, M. (1995). Genetic–environmental interaction in the genesis of aggressivity and conduct disorders. *Archives of General Psychiatry, 52*(11), 916–924.

Cameron, S. J., Armstrong-Stassen, M., Orr, R. R., & Loukas, A. (1991). Stress, coping, and resources in mothers of adults with developmental disabilities. *Counseling Psychology Quarterly, 4*(4), 301–310.

Campbell, R. T., & Henretta, J. C. (1980). Status claims and status attainment: The determinants of financial well-being. *American Journal of Sociology, 86*(3), 618–629.

Carstensen, L. L., Isaacowitz, D. M., & Charles, S. T. (1999). Taking time seriously: A theory of socioemotional selectivity. *American Psychologist, 54*(3), 165–181.

Caspi, A. (2004). Life-course development: The interplay of social selection and social causation within and across generations. In P. L. Chase-Lansdale, K. Kiernan, & R. J. Friedman (Eds.), *Human development across lives and generations: The potential for change.* New York: Cambridge University Press.

Caspi, A., & Moffitt, T. E. (1993). When do individual differences matter?: A paradoxical theory of personality coherence. *Psychological Inquiry, 4*(4), 247–271.

Caspi, A., Moffitt, T. E., Mill, J., Martin, J., Craig, I. W., Taylor, A., et al. (2002). Role of genotype in the cycle of violence in maltreated children. *Science, 297*(5582), 851–854.

Caspi, A., Sugden, K., Moffitt, T. E., Taylor, A., Craig, I. W., Harrington, H., et al. (2003). Influence of life stress on depression: Moderation in the 5-HTT gene. *Science, 301*(5631), 386–389.

Cassell, J., & Wax, M. L. (1980). Toward a moral science of human beings. *Social Problems, 27*(3), 259–264.

Cherlin, A. J., Burton, L. M., Hurt, T. R., & Purvin, D. M. (2004). The influence of physical and sexual abuse on marriage and cohabitation. *American Sociological Review, 69*(6), 768–789.

Chesley, N. (2005). Blurring boundaries?: Linking technology use, spillover, individual distress, and family satisfaction. *Journal of Marriage and the Family, 67*(5), 1237–1248.

Chesley, N., & Moen, P. (2006). When workers care: Dual-earner couples' caregiving strategies benefit use, and psychological well-being. *American Behavioral Scientist, 49*(9), 1–22.

Chiriboga, D. A. (1989). Stress and loss in middle age. In R. A. Kalish (Ed.), *Midlife loss: Coping strategies* (pp. 42–88). Thousand Oaks, CA: Sage.

Chiriboga, D. A. (1997). Crisis, challenge, and stability in the middle years. In M. E. Lachman & J. B. James (Eds.), *Multiple paths of midlife development* (pp. 293–322). Chicago: University of Chicago Press.

Christakis, N. A., & Fowler, J. H. (2007). The spread of obesity in a large social network over 32 years. *New England Journal of Medicine, 357*(4), 370–379.

Chung, I.-J., Hill, K. G., Hawkins, J. D., Gilchrist, L. D., & Nagin, D. S. (2002). Childhood predictors of offense trajectories. *Journal of Research in Crime and Delinquency, 39*(1), 60–90.

Clark, L. A., & Watson, D. (1988). Mood and the mundane: Relations between daily life events and self-reported mood. *Journal of Personality and Social Psychology, 54*(2), 296–308.

Clarkberg, M. (1999). The price of partnering: The role of economic well-being in young adults' first union experiences. *Social Forces, 77*(3), 945–968.

Clarkberg, M., & Moen, P. (2001). Understanding the time-squeeze: Married couples preferred and actual work-hour strategies. *American Behavioral Scientist, 44*(7), 1115–1136.

Clarke, M. (1975). Survival in the field: Implications of personal experience in fieldwork. *Theory and Society, 2*(1), 95–123.

Clark-Plaskie, M., & Lachman, M. E. (1999). The sense of control in midlife. In S. L. Willis & J. D. Reid (Eds.), *Life in the middle: Psychological and social development in middle age* (pp. 181–208). San Diego: Academic Press.

Clarridge, B. R., Sheehy, L. L., & Hauser, T. S. (1977). Tracing members of a panel: A 17-year follow-up. In K. F. Schuessler (Ed.), *Sociological methodology 1978* (pp. 185–203). San Francisco: Jossey-Bass.

Clausen, J. A. (1986). *The life course: A sociological perspective.* Englewood Cliffs, NJ: Prentice-Hall.

Clausen, J. A. (1991). Adolescent competence and the shaping of the life course. *American Journal of Sociology, 96*(4), 805–842.

Clausen, J. A. (1993). *American lives: Looking back at the children of the Great Depression.* New York: Free Press.

Clipp, E. C., Pavalko, E. K., & Elder, G. H., Jr. (1992). Trajectories of health: In concept and empirical pattern. *Behavior, Health, and Aging, 2*(3), 159–179.

Coard, S. J., & Sellers, R. M. (2005). African American families as a context for racial socialization. In V. C. Lloyd, N. E. Hill, & K. A. Dodge (Eds.), *African American family life* (pp. 264–284). New York: Guilford Press.

Cohen, S., Kessler, R. C., & Gordon, L. U. (1997). Strategies for measuring stress in studies of psychiatric and physical disorders. In S. Cohen, R. C. Kessler, & L. U. Gordon (Eds.), *Measuring stress: A guide for health and social scientists* (pp. 3–26). New York: Oxford University Press.

Coleman, J. S., with the assistance of Johnstone, J. W. C., & Jonassohn, K. (1961). *The adolescent society: The social life of the teenager and its impact on education.* New York: Free Press of Glencoe.

Coleman, J. S. (1981). *Longitudinal data analysis.* New York: Basic Books.

Collins, L. M. (2006). Analysis of longitudinal data: The integration of theoretical model, temporal design, and statistical model. *Annual Review of Psychology, 57,* 505–528.

Coltrane, S. (1996). *Family man: Fatherhood, housework, and gender equity.* New York: Oxford University Press.

Coltrane, S., & Adams, M. (2001). Men's family work: Child-centered fathering and the sharing of domestic labor. In R. Hertz & N. L. Marshall (Eds.), *Working families: The transformation of the American home* (pp. 72–99). Berkeley: University of California Press.

Connell, R. W. (1995). *Masculinities.* Berkeley: University of California Press.

Courgeau, D., & Lelièvre, E. (1992). *Event history analysis in demography.* Oxford, England: Clarendon.

Cowan, C. P., & Cowan, P. G. (1999). *When partners become parents: The big life change for couples.* Mahwah, NJ: Erlbaum.

Cross, S., & Markus, H. (1991). Possible selves across the life span. *Human Development, 34*(4), 230–255.

Croudace, T. J., Jarvelin, M.-R., Wadsworth, M. E. J., & Jones, P. B. (2003). Developmental typology of trajectories of nighttime bladder control: Epidemiologic application of longitudinal latent class analysis. *American Journal of Epidemiology, 157*(9), 834–842.

Crowder, K., & South, S. J. (2008). Spatial dynamics of white flight: The effects of local and extralocal racial conditions on neighborhood out-migration. *American Sociological Review, 73*(5), 792–812.

Crystal, S., & Waehrer, K. (1996). Later life economic inequality in longitudinal perspective. *Journals of Gerontology B: Psychological Sciences and Social Sciences, 51*(6), S307–S318.

Csikszentmihalyi, M. (1993). *The evolving self: A psychology for the third millenium.* New York: HarperCollins.

Csikszentmihalyi, M., & Beattie, O. (1979). Life themes: A theoretical and empirical exploration of their origins and effects. *Journal of Humanistic Psychology, 19,* 45–63.

Cudeck, R., & Klebe, K. J. (2002). Multiphase mixed-effects models for repeated measures data. *Psychological Methods, 7*(1), 41–63.

Curran, P. J., & Willoughby, M. T. (2003). Implications of latent trajectory models for the study of developmental psychopathology. *Development and Psychopathology, 15*(3), 581–612.

Dahlin, E., Kelly, E., & Moen, P. (2008). Is work the new neighborhood?: Social ties in the workplace, family, and neighborhood. *Sociological Quarterly, 49*(4), 719–736.

Daly, K. (2003). Family theory versus the theories families live by. *Journal of Marriage and the Family, 65*(4), 771–784.

Dannefer, D. (1987). Aging as intracohort differentiation: Accentuation, the Matthew effect, and the life course. *Sociological Forum, 2*(2), 211–236.

Dannefer, D. (2003). Cumulative advantage/disadvantage and the life course: Cross fertilizing age and social science theory. *Journals of Gerontology B: Psychological Sciences and Social Sciences, 58*(6), S327–S338.

Dannefer, D., & Sell, R. R. (1988). Age structure, the life course, and "aged heterogeneity." *Contemporary Sociology, 2*(1), 1–10.

Davis, J. A., & Smith, T. W. (1992). *The NORC General Social Survey: A user's guide.* Newbury Park, CA: Sage.

Dean, J. P., & Williams, R. M. (1956). *Social and cultural factors affecting role conflict and adjustment among American women: A pilot investigation.* Bethesda, MD: National Institute of Mental Health.

Dempster-McClain, D., & Moen, P. (1997). Finding respondents in a follow-up study. In J. Z. Giele & G. H. Elder, Jr. (Eds.), *Methods of life course research* (pp. 128–151). Thousand Oaks, CA: Sage.

Dentinger, E., & Clarkberg, M. (2002). Informal caregiving and retirement timing among men and women: Gender and caregiving relationships in late midlife. *Journal of Family Issues, 23*(7), 857–879.

Deutscher, I. (1966). Words and deeds: Social science and social policy. *Social Problems, 13*(3), 235–254.

Dick, D. M., Agrawal, A., Schuckit, M. A., Bierut, L., Hinrichs, A., Fox, L., et al. (2006). Marital status, alcohol dependence, and GABRA2: Evidence for gene–environment correlation and interaction. *Journal of Studies on Alcohol, 67*(2), 185–194.

Dillman, D. A. (1991). The design and administration of mail surveys. *Annual Review of Sociology, 17*, 225–249.

Dillman, D. A. (2000). *Mail and Internet surveys: The tailored design method.* New York: Wiley.

Dillon, M., & Wink, P. (2007). *In the course of a lifetime: Tracing religious belief, practice, and change.* Berkeley: University of California Press.

DiPrete, T. A., de Graaf, P. M., Luijkx, R., Tåhlin, M., & Blossfeld, H.-P. (1997). Collectivist versus Individualist Mobility Regimes?: Structural change and job mobility in four countries. *American Journal of Sociology, 103*(2), 318–358.

DiPrete, T. A., & Eirich, G. M. (2006). Cumulative advantage as a mechanism for inequality: A review of theoretical and empirical developments. *Annual Review of Sociology, 32*, 271–297.

Dodson, L. (1998). *Don't call us out of name: The untold lives of women and girls in poor America.* Boston: Beacon Press.

Dodson, L., & Schmalzbauer, L. (2005). Poor mothers and habits of hiding: Participatory methods in poverty research. *Journal of Marriage and Family, 67*(4), 949–959.

Dohrenwend, B. S., & Dohrenwend, B. P. (1974). *Stressful life events: Their nature and effects.* New York: Wiley-Interscience.

D'Onofrio, B. M., Turkheimer, E., Emery, R. E., Slutske, W. S., Heath, A. C., Madden, P. A., et al. (2005). A genetically informed study of marital instability and its association with offspring psychopathology. *Journal of Abnormal Psychology, 114*(4), 570–586.

Drobnic, S., & Blossfeld, H.-P. (2004). Career patterns over the life course:

Gender, class, and linked lives. In A. L. Kalleberg, S. L. Morgan, J. Myles, & R. A. Rosenfeld (Eds.), *Inequality: Structures, dynamics and mechanisms: Essays in honor of Aage B. Sørensen* (Vol. 21, pp. 139–164). Amsterdam: Elsevier.

Dumais, S. A. (2002). *The educational pathways of white working-class students.* Unpublished PhD dissertation, Harvard University, Cambridge, MA.

Duncan, G. J., & Morgan, J. N. (1985). The panel study of income dynamics. In G. H. Elder, Jr. (Ed.), *Life course dynamics: Trajectories and transitions: 1968–1980* (pp. 50–71). Ithaca, NY: Cornell University Press.

Duncan, O. D. (1968). Ability and achievement. *Eugenics Quarterly, 15*(1), 1–11.

Duneier, M. (2007). On the legacy of Elliot Liebow and Carol Stack: Context-driven fieldwork and the need for continuous ethnography. *Focus, 25*(1), 33–38.

D'Unger, A. V., Land, K. C., McCall, P. L., & Nagin, D. S. (1998). How many latent classes of delinquent/criminal careers?: Results from mixed Poisson regression analyses. *American Journal of Sociology, 103*(6), 1593–1630.

Dunn, K. M., Jordan, K., & Croft, P. S. (2006). Characterizing the course of low back pain: A latent class analysis. *American Journal of Epidemiology, 163*(8), 754–761.

Easterlin, R. A. (1987). *Birth and fortune: The impact of numbers on personal welfare* (2nd ed.). Chicago: University of Chicago Press.

Eccles, J. S., & Midgley, C. (1989). Stage–environment fit: Developmentally appropriate classrooms for early adolescents. In R. E. Ames & C. Ames (Eds.), *Research on motivation in education* (Vol. 3, pp. 139–186). New York: Academic Press.

Edin, K. (2000). What do low-income single mothers say about marriage? *Social Problems, 47*(1), 112–133.

Edin, K., & Kefalas, M. (2005). *Promises I can keep: Why poor women put motherhood before marriage.* Berkeley: University of California Press.

Eggleston, E. P., Laub, J. H., & Sampson, R. J. (2004). Methodological sensitivities to latent class analysis of long-term criminal trajectories. *Journal of Quantitative Criminology, 20*(1), 1–26.

Eichorn, D. H., Clausen, J. A., Haan, N., Honzik, M. P., & Mussen, P. H. (1981). *Present and past in middle life.* New York: Academic Press.

Elder, G. H., Jr. (Ed.). (1973). *Linking social structure and personality.* Beverly Hills, CA: Sage.

Elder, G. H., Jr. (1974). *Children of the Great Depression: Social change in life experience.* Chicago: University of Chicago Press.

Elder, G. H., Jr. (1975). Age differentiation and the life course. *Annual Review of Sociology, 1,* 165–190.

Elder, G. H., Jr. (Ed.). (1985a). *Life course dynamics: Trajectories and transitions, 1968–1980.* Ithaca, NY: Cornell University Press.

Elder, G. H., Jr. (1985b). Perspectives on the life course. In *Life course dynamics: Trajectories and transitions, 1968–1980* (pp. 23–49). Ithaca, NY: Cornell University Press.

Elder, G. H., Jr. (1986). Military times and turning points in men's lives. *Developmental Psychology, 22*(2), 233–245.

Elder, G. H., Jr. (1987a). Familes and lives: Some developments in life-course studies. *Journal of Family History, 12,* 179–199.

Elder, G. H., Jr. (1987b). War mobilization and the life course: A cohort of World War II veterans. *Sociological Forum, 2*(3), 449–472.

Elder, G. H., Jr. (1994). Time, human agency, and social change: Perspectives on the life course. *Social Psychology Quarterly, 57*(1), 4–15.

Elder, G. H., Jr. (1998a). The life course as developmental theory. *Child Development, 69*(1), 1–12.

Elder, G. H., Jr. (1998b). The life course and human development. In R. M. Lerner (Ed.), *Handbook of child psychology* (5th ed.): *Vol. 1. Theoretical models of human development* (pp. 939–991). New York: Wiley.

Elder, G. H., Jr. (1999). *Children of the Great Depression: Social change in life experience* (25th anniversary edition). Boulder, CO: Westview Press.

Elder, G. H., Jr. (2000). Life course theory. In A. E. Kazdin (Ed.), *Encyclopedia of psychology* (3rd ed., Vol. 5, pp. 50–52). Washington, DC: American Psychological Association.

Elder, G. H., Jr., & Clipp, E. C. (1988). Wartime losses and social bonding: Influences across 40 years in men's lives. *Psychiatry, 51,* 177–198.

Elder, G. H., Jr., & Conger, R. D. (2000). Legacies of the land. In G. H. Elder, Jr. & R. D. Conger (Eds.), *Children of the land: Adversity and success in rural America* (pp. 221–249). Chicago: University of Chicago Press.

Elder, G. H., Jr., George, L. K., & Shanahan, M. J. (1996). Psychosocial stress over the life course. In H. Kaplan (Ed.), *Psychosocial stress: Perspective on structure, theory, life-course, and methods* (pp. 247–292). San Diego: Academic Press.

Elder, G. H., Jr., Johnson, M. K., & Crosnoe, R. (2003). The emergence and development of the life course. In J. T. Mortimer & M. J. Shanahan (Eds.), *Handbook of the life course.* New York: Plenum Press.

Elder, G. H., Jr., & O'Rand, A. M. (1995). Adult lives in a changing society. In K. S. Cook, G. A. Fine, & J. S. House (Eds.), *Sociological perspectives on social psychology* (pp. 452–475). Boston: Allyn & Bacon.

Elder, G. H., Jr., Pavalko, E. K., & Clipp, E. C. (1993). *Working with archival data: Studying lives* (Vol. 07-088). Newbury Park, CA: Sage.

Elder, G. H., Jr., & Rockwell, R. C. (1979a). Economic depression and postwar opportunity in men's lives: A study of life patterns and health. *Research in Community and Mental Health, 1,* 249–303.

Elder, G. H., Jr., & Rockwell, R. C. (1979b). The life-course and human development: An ecological perspective. *International Journal of Behavioral Development, 2,* 1–21.

Elder, G. H., Jr., & Shanahan, M. J. (2006). The life course and human development. In R. E. Lerner (Ed.), *Handbook of child psychology* (6th ed., Vol. 1, pp. 665–715). Hoboken, NJ: Wiley.

Elder, G. H., Jr., Shanahan, M. J., & Clipp, E. C. (1994). When war comes to men's lives: Life course patterns in family, work, and health. *Psychology and Aging, 9*(1), 5–16.

Elder, G. H., Jr., Shanahan, M. J., & Clipp, E. C. (1997). Linking combat and physical health: The legacy of World War II in men's lives. *American Journal of Psychiatry, 154*(3), 330–336.

Elliott, M. R., Shope, J. T., Raghunathan, T. E., & Waller, P. F. (2006). Gender differences among young drivers in the association between high-risk driving and substance use/environmental influences. *Journal of Studies on Alcohol, 67*(2), 252–260.

Elman, C., & O'Rand, A. M. (1998). Midlife entry into vocational training: A mobility model. *Social Science Research, 27,* 128–158.

Elman, C., & O'Rand, A. M. (2002). Perceived labor market insecurity and entry into work-related education and training among adult workers. *Social Science Research, 31,* 49–76.

Elman, C., & O'Rand, A. M. (2004). The race is to the swift: Socioeconomic origins, adult education, and wage attainment. *American Journal of Sociology, 110*(1), 123–160.

Elman, C., & O'Rand, A. M. (2007). The effects of social origins, life events, and institutional sorting on adults' school transitions. *Social Science Research, 36*(3), 1276–1299.

Elo, I. T., & Preston, S. H. (1996). Educational differentials in mortality: United States, 1979–85. *Social Science and Medicine, 42*(1), 47–57.

Elo, I. T., Turra, C. M., Kestenbaum, B., & Ferguson, B. R. (2004). Mortality among elderly Hispanics in the United States: Past evidence and new results. *Demography, 41*(1), 109–128.

Emerson, R. M., & Pollner, M. (2001). Constructing participant–observation relations. In R. M. Emerson & M. Pollner (Eds.), *Contemporary field research: Perspectives and formulations* (pp. 239–259). Prospect Heights, IL: Waveland Press.

Erikson, E. H. (1963). *Childhood and society* (2nd ed.). New York: Norton.

Erikson, R., & Jonsson, J. O. (1996). *Can education be equalized?: The Swedish case in comparative perspective.* Boulder, CO: Westview Press.

Esping-Andersen, G. (1990). *The three worlds of welfare capitalism.* Cambridge, England: Polity Press.

Etherington, K. (2007). Working with traumatic stories: From transcriber to witness. *International Journal of Social Research Methodology, 10*(2), 85–97.

Featherman, D. L., & Hauser, R. M. (1975). Design for a replicate study of social mobility in the United States. In K. C. Land & S. S. Spilerman (Eds.), *Social indicator models* (pp. 219–251). New York: Russell Sage Foundation.

Featherman, D. L., & Hauser, R. M. (1978). *Opportunity and change.* New York: Academic Press.

Feerick, M. M., & Haugaard, J. J. (1999). Long-term effects of witnessing marital violence for women: The contribution of childhood physical and sexual abuse. *Journal of Family Violence, 14*(4), 377–398.

Feng, D., Silverstein, M., Giarrusso, R., McArdle, J. J., & Bengston, V. L. (2006). Attrition of older adults in longitudinal surveys: Detection and correction of sample selection bias using multigenerational data. *Journals of Gerontology B: Psychological Sciences and Social Sciences, 61*(6), S323–S328.

Fergusson, D. M., Horwood, L. J., & Nagin, D. S. (2000). Offending trajectories in a New Zealand birth cohort. *Criminology, 38*(2), 525–551.

Ferraro, K. F., & Kelley-Moore, J. A. (2003). Cumulative disadvantage and health: Long-term consequences of obesity? *American Sociological Review, 68*(5), 707–729.

Ferri, E., Bynner, J., & Wadsworth, M. (Eds.). (2003). *Changing Britain, changing lives: Three generations at the turn of the century.* London: Institute of Education.

Fine, M., & Weis, L. (1998). *The unknown city: Lives of poor and working class young adults.* Boston: Beacon Press.

Finkelhor, D. (1994). Current information on the scope and nature of child sexual abuse. *The Future of Children, 4*(2), 31–53.

Fish, M., Stifter, C. A., & Belsky, J. (1993). Early patterns of mother–infant dyadic interaction: Infant, mother, and family demographic antecedents. *Infant Behavior & Development, 16*(1), 1–18.

Flanagan, J. C., Cooley, W. W., Lohnes, P. R., Schoenfeldt, L. F., Holdeman, R. W., Combs, J., et al. (1966). *Project TALENT one-year follow-up studies.* Pittsburgh: American Institutes for Research.

Flanagan, J. C., Davis, F. B., Dailey, J. T., Shaycoft, M. F., Orr, D. B., Goldberg, I., et al. (1964). *The American high school student: American Institutes for Research.* Available online at: *www.icpsr.umich.edu/cocoon/ICPSR/STUDY/07823.xml*

Freedman, D. S., & Thornton, A. (1979). The long-term impact of pregnancy at marriage on the family's economic circumstances. *Family Planning Perspectives, 11*(1), 6–21.

Freese, J., Meland, S., & Irwin, W. (2007). Expressions of positive emotion in photographs, personality, and later-life marital and health outcomes. *Journal of Research in Personality, 41*(2), 488–497.

Friedman, H. S., Tucker, J. S., Schwartz, J. E., Tomlinson-Keasey, C., Martin, L. R., Wingard, D. L., et al. (1995). Psychosocial and behavioral predictors of longevity: The aging and death of the "termites." *American Psychologist, 50*(2), 69–78.

Froehlich, G. J. (1941). *The prediction of academic success at the University of Wisconsin, 1909–1941.* Madison: Bureaus of Guidance and Records, University of Wisconsin.

Furstenberg, F. F., Jr., Cook, T. D., Eccles, J., Elder, G. H., Jr., & Sameroff, A. (Eds.). (1999). *Managing to make it: Urban families and adolescent success.* Chicago: University of Chicago Press.

Gager, C. T., & Sanchez, L. (2003). Two as one?: Couples' perception of time spent together, marital quality, and the risk of divorce. *Journal of Family Issues, 24*(1), 21–50.

Gale, J. (1992). When research interviews are more therapeutic than therapy interviews. *The Qualitative Report, 1*(4), 31–38.

Gans, H. J. (1968). The participant–observer as a human being: Observations on the personal aspects of fieldwork. In H. S. Becker, B. Geer, D. Riesman, & R. S. Weiss (Eds.), *Institutions and the person* (pp. 300–374). Chicago: Aldine.

Ge, X., Conger, R. D., Cadoret, R. J., Neiderhiser, J. M., Yates, W. R., Troughton, E., et al. (1996). The developmental interface between nature and nurture: A mutual influence model of child antisocial behavior and parent behaviors. *Developmental Psychology, 32*(4), 574–589.

George, L. K. (1993). Sociological perspectives on life transitions. *Annual Review of Sociology, 19,* 353–373.

George, L. K., Larson, D. B., Koenig, H. G., & McCullough, M. (2000). Spirituality and health: State of the evidence. *Journal of Social and Clinical Psychology, 19,* 102–116.

George, L. K., & Lynch, S. M. (2003). Race differences in depressive symptoms: A dynamic perspective on stress exposure and vulnerability. *Journal of Health and Social Behavior, 44*(3), 353–369.

Geronimus, A. T. (1996). Black/white differences in the relationship of maternal age to birthweight: A population-based test of the weathering hypothesis. *Social Science and Medicine, 42*(4), 589–597.

Gerstel, N. (2000). The third shift: Gender and care work outside the home. *Qualitative Sociology, 23*(4), 467–483.

Giarrusso, R., Feng, D., Silverstein, M., & Bengston, V. L. (2001). Grandparent–adult grandchild affection and consensus: Cross-generational and cross-ethnic comparisons. *Journal of Family Issues, 22*(4), 456–477.

Giele, J. Z. (1987). Coeducation or women's education?: A comparison of findings from two colleges. In C. Lasser (Ed.), *Coeducation: Past, present, and future* (pp. 91–109). Urbana: University of Illinois Press.

Giele, J. Z. (1995). *Two paths to women's equality: Temperance, suffrage, and the origins of modern feminism.* New York: Twayne.

Giele, J. Z. (1998). Innovation in the typical life course. In J. Z. Giele & G. H. Elder, Jr. (Eds.), *Methods of life course research: Qualitative and quantitative approaches* (pp. 231–263). Thousand Oaks, CA: Sage.

Giele, J. Z. (2002a). Life course studies and the theory of action. In R. A. Settersten, Jr. & T. J. Owens (Eds.), *Advances in life-course research: New frontiers in socialization* (Vol. 7, pp. 65–88). London: Elsevier Science.

Giele, J. Z. (2002b). Longitudinal studies and life-course research: Innovations, investigators, and policy ideas. In E. Phelps, F. F. Furstenberg, Jr., & A. Colby (Eds.), *Looking at lives: American longitudinal studies of the twentieth century* (pp. 15–36). New York: Russell Sage Foundation.

Giele, J. Z. (2004). Women and men as agents of change in their own lives. In J. Z. Giele & E. Holst (Eds.), *Advances in life course research: Changing life patterns in Western industrial societies* (Vol. 8, pp. 299–317). Amsterdam: Elsevier Science.

Giele, J. Z. (2008). Homemaker or career woman: Life-course factors and racial influences in the American middle class. *Journal of Comparative Family Studies, 39*(3), 392–411.

Giele, J. Z., & Elder, G. H., Jr. (1998a). Life course research: Development of a field. In *Methods of life course research: Quantitative and qualitative approaches* (pp. 5–27). Thousand Oaks, CA: Sage.

Giele, J. Z., & Elder, G. H., Jr. (Eds.). (1998b). *Methods of life course research: Qualitative and quantitative approaches.* Thousand Oaks, CA: Sage.

Giele, J. Z., & Gilfus, M. (1990). Race and college differences in life patterns of educated women. In J. Antler & S. Biklen (Eds.), *Women and educational change* (pp. 179–197). Albany: State University of New York Press.

Gill, T. M., Allore, H. G., Hardy, S. E., & Guo, Z. C. (2006). The dynamic nature of mobility disability in older persons. *Journal of the American Geriatrics Society, 54*(2), 248–254.

Glenn, N. (1977). *Cohort analysis.* Beverly Hills, CA: Sage.

Glueck, S., & Glueck, E. (1950). *Unraveling juvenile delinquency.* New York: New York Commonwealth Fund.

Glueck, S., & Glueck, E. (1968). *Delinquents and nondelinquents in perspective.* Cambridge, MA: Harvard University Press.

Goffman, E. (1959). *The presentation of self in everyday life.* Garden City, NY: Doubleday.

Goffman, E. (1963). *Stigma: Notes on the preservaton of spoiled identity.* Englewood Cliffs, NJ: Prentice-Hall.

Gold, R. L. (1958). Roles in sociological field observations. *Social Forces, 36*(3), 217–223.

Gottfredson, M. R., & Hirschi, T. (1986). The true value of lambda would appear to be zero: An essay on career criminals, criminal careers, selective incapacitation, cohort studies, and related topics. *Criminology, 24*(2), 213–234.

Gottlieb, G. (2003). On making behavioral genetics truly developmental. *Human Development, 46*(6), 337–355.

Gottman, J. M., & Notarius, C. I. (2000). Decade review: Observing marital interaction. *Journal of Marriage and the Family, 62*(4), 927–947.

Griffin, M. A., Patterson, M. G., & West, M. A. (2001). Job satisfaction and teamwork: The role of supervisor support. *Journal of Organizational Behavior, 22*(5), 537–550.

Griffith, J. (2002). Multilevel analysis of cohesion's relation to stress, well-being, identification, disintegration, and perceived combat readiness. *Military Psychology, 14*(3), 217–239.

Guerrero, T. J., & Naldini, M. (1996). Is the South so different?: Italian and Spanish families in comparative perspective. In M. Rhodes (Ed.), *Southern European welfare states: Between crisis and reform* (Vol. 1, pp. 42–66). London: Frank Cass.

Guo, G., & Zhao, H. (2000). Multilevel modeling for binary data. *Annual Review of Sociology, 26*(1), 441–462.

Gurin, G., Veroff, J., & Feld, S. (1960). *Americans view their mental health: A nationwide interview survey: A report to the staff director, Jack E. Ewalt.* New York: Basic Books.

Guthrie, G. J., & Jenkins, S. (2005). Bertillon Files: An untapped source of nineteenth-century human height data. *Journal of Anthropological Research, 61*(2), 201–215.

Guttmann, M. P., & Fliess, K. H. (1993). The determinants of early fertility decline in Texas. *Demography, 30*(3), 443–457.

Haas, S. (2008). Trajectories of functional health: The "long arm" of childhood health and socioeconomic factors. *Social Science and Medicine, 66*(4), 849–861.

Hall, C. S., & Lindzey, G. (1957). *Theories of personality.* New York: Wiley.

Hallqvist, J., Lynch, J., Bartley, M., Lang, T., & Blane, D. (2004). Can we disentangle life course processes of accumulation, critical period, and social mobility?: An analysis of disadvantaged socio-economic positions and myocardial infarction in the Stockholm Health Epidemiology Program. *Social Science and Medicine, 58*(8), 1555–1562.

Hamil-Luker, J. (2005). Trajectories of public assistance receipt among female high school dropouts. *Population Research and Policy Review, 24*(6), 673–694.

Hamil-Luker, J., & O'Rand, A. M. (2007). Gender differences in the impact of childhood adversity on the risk for heart attack across the life course. *Demography, 44*(1), 137–158.

Hammack, P. L. (2008). Narrative and cultural psychology of identity. *Personality and Social Psychology Review, 12*(3), 222–247.

Han, S.-K., & Moen, P. (1999). Clocking out: Temporal patterning of retirement. *American Journal of Sociology, 105*(1), 191–236.

Han, S.-K., & Moen, P. (2001). Coupled careers: Pathways through work and marriage in the United States. In H.-P. Blossfeld & S. Drobnic (Eds.), *Careers of couples in contemporary societies: From male breadwinner to dual earner families* (pp. 201–232). Oxford, England: Oxford University Press.

Hareven, T. K. (1978). *Transitions: The family and the life course in historical perspective.* New York: Academic Press.

Hareven, T. K. (1982). *Family time and industrial time.* New York: Cambridge University Press.

Harrington, B. (2003). The social psychology of access in ethnographic research. *Journal of Contemporary Ethnography, 32*(5), 592–625.

Hauser, R. M. (1984). Some cross-population comparisons of family bias in the effects of schooling on occupational status. *Social Science Research, 13*(2), 159–187.

Hauser, R. M. (1988). A note on two models of sibling resemblance. *American Journal of Sociology, 93*(6), 1401–1423.

Hauser, R. M. (2005). Survey response in the long run: The Wisconsin Longitudinal Study. *Field Methods, 17,* 3–29.

Hauser, R. M., & Dickinson, P. J. (1974). Inequality on occupational status and income. *American Educational Research Journal, 11,* 161–168.

Hauser, R. M., & Featherman, D. L. (1977). *The process of stratification: Trends and analyses.* New York: Academic Press.

Hauser, R. M., & Mossel, P. A. (1985). Fraternal resemblance in educational attainment and occupational status. *American Journal of Sociology, 91*(3), 650–673.

Hauser, R. M., & Mossel, P. A. (1988). Some structural equation models of sibling resemblance in educational attainment and occupational status. In P. Cuttance & R. Ecob (Eds.), *Structural modeling by example: Applications in educational, sociological, and behavioral research* (pp. 108–137). Cambridge, England: Cambridge University Press.

Hauser, R. M., & Sewell, W. H. (1986). Family effects in simple models of education, occupational status, and earnings: Findings from the Wisconsin and Kalamazoo Studies. *Journal of Labor Economics, 4*(3, Part 2), S83–S115.

Hauser, R. M., Sheridan, J. T., & Warren, J. R. (1999). Socioeconomic achievements of siblings in the life course: New findings from the Wisconsin Longitudinal Study. *Research on Aging, 21*(2), 338–378.

Hauser, R. M., Tsai, S. L., & Sewell, W. H. (1983). A model of stratification with response error in social and psychological variables. *Sociology of Education, 56*(1), 20–46.

Hauser, R. M., Warren, J. R., Huang, M.-H., & Carter, W. Y. (2000). Occupational status, education, and social mobility in the meritocracy. In K. Arrow, S. Bowles, & S. Durlauf (Eds.), *Meritocracy and economic inequality* (pp. 179–229). Princeton, NJ: Princeton University Press.

Hauser, R. M., & Wong, R. S.-K. (1989). Sibling resemblance and inter-sibling effects in educational attainment. *Sociology of Education, 62*(3), 149–171.

Hayward, M. D., & Gorman, B. K. (2004). The long arm of childhood: The influence of early-life social conditions on men's mortality. *Demography, 41*(1), 87–107.

Heckhausen, J. (1999). *Developmental regulation in adulthood: Age-normative and sociostructural constraints as adaptive challenges.* New York: Cambridge University Press.

Heinz, W. R. (1996). Status passages as micro–macro linkages in life course research. In A. Weymann & W. R. Heinz (Eds.), *Society and biography: Interrelationships between social structure, institutions and the life course* (pp. 67–81). Weinheim, Germany: Deutscher Studien Verlag.

Heinz, W. R. (2002). Transition discontinuities and the biographical shaping of early work careers. *Journal of Vocational Behavior, 60*(2), 220–240.

Heise, D. R. (1990). Careers, career trajectories, and the self. In J. Rodin, C. Schooler, & K. W. Schaie (Eds.), *Self-directedness: Cause and effects throughout the life course* (pp. 59–84). Hillsdale, NJ: Erlbaum.

Henmon, V. A. C., & Holt, F. O. (1931). *A report on the administration of scholastic aptitude tests to 34,000 high school seniors in Wisconsin in 1929 and 1930 prepared for the Committee on Cooperation, Wisconsin secondary schools and colleges.* Madison: Bureau of Guidance and Records, University of Wisconsin.

Henmon, V. A. C., & Nelson, M. J. (1946). *Henmon–Nelson Tests of Mental Ability, High School Examination—Grades 7 to 12—Forms A, B, and C: Teacher's manual.* Boston: Houghton-Mifflin.

Henmon, V. A. C., & Nelson, M. J. (1954). *The Henmon–Nelson Tests of Mental Ability: Manual for administration.* Boston: Houghton-Mifflin.

Henretta, J. C., & Campbell, R. T. (1976). Status attainment and status maintenance: A study of stratification in old age. *American Sociological Review, 41*(6), 981–992.

Henry, B., Moffitt, T. E., Caspi, A., Langley, J., & Silva, P. A. (1994). On the "remembrance of things past": A longitudinal evaluation of the retrospective method. *Psychological Assessment, 6*(2), 92–101.

Herd, P., Goesling, B., & House, J. S. (2007). Socioeconomic position and health: The differential effects of education versus income on the onset versus progression of health problems. *Journal of Health and Social Behavior, 48*(3), 223–238.

Hetherington, E. M., & Baltes, P. B. (1988). Child psychology and life-span development. In E. M. Hetherington, R. M. Lerner, & M. Perlmutter (Eds.), *Child development in life-span perspective* (pp. 1–19). Hillsdale, NJ: Erlbaum.

Higginbotham, E. (2001). *Too much to ask: Black women in the era of integration*. Chapel Hill: University of North Carolina Press.

Higuchi, S., Matsushita, S., Imazeki, H., Kinoshita, T., Takagi, S., & Kono, H. (1994). Aldehyde dehydrogenase genotypes in Japanese alcoholics. *Lancet, 343*, 741–742.

Hill, R., & Foote, N. N. (1970). *Family development in three generations: A longitudinal study of changing family patterns of planning and achievement*. Cambridge, MA: Schenkman.

Hirschi, T., & Gottfredson, M. R. (1983). Age and the explanation of crime. *American Journal of Sociology, 89*(2), 552–584.

Hochschild, A. R. (1989). *The second shift: Working parents and the revolution at home*. New York: Penguin Books.

Hogan, D. P. (1981). *Transitions and social change: The early lives of American men*. New York: Academic Press.

Hogan, D. P., & Goldscheider, F. K. (2003). Success and challenge in demographic studies of the life course. In J. T. Mortimer & M. J. Shanahan (Eds.), *Handbook of the life course* (pp. 681–691). New York: Kluwer Academic/Plenum Press.

Hogan, D. P., & Park, J. M. (2000). Family factors and social support in the developmental outcomes of children who were very low birthweight at 32 to 38 months of age. *Seminars in Perinatology, 27*(2), 433–459.

Holahan, C. K., & Sears, R. R. (1995). *The gifted group in later maturity*. Stanford, CA: Stanford University Press.

Holmes, T. H., & Rahe, R. H. (1967). The social readjustment rating scale. *Journal of Psychosomatic Research, 11*, 213–218.

House, J. S., Lantz, P. M., & Herd, P. (2005). Continuity and change in the social stratification of aging and health over the life course: Evidence from a nationally representative Longitudinal Study from 1986 to 2001/2 (Americans' Changing Lives Study). *Journals of Gerontology B: Psychological Sciences and Social Sciences, 60*(Special Issue 2), S15–S26.

Howe, M. J. (1982). Biographical evidence and the development of outstanding individuals. *American Psychologist, 37*(10), 1071–1081.

Hughes, D. C., Blazer, D. G., & George, L. K. (1988). Age differences in life events: A multivariate controlled analysis. *International Journal of Aging and Human Development, 27*(3), 207–220.

Huinink, J. (1989). *Mehrebenenanalyse in den Sozialwissenschaften* [Multi-level analysis in the social sciences]. Wiesbaden: Deutscher Universitäts-Verlag.

Hultsch, D. F., & Plemons, J. K. (1979). Life events and life-span development. In P. B. Baltes & O. G. Brim (Eds.), *Life-span development and behavior* (Vol. 2, pp. 1–36). New York: Academic Press.

Human Capital Initiative Coordinating Committee on Reducing Violence. (1995). Report presented at Reducing Violence: A Research Agenda, Washington, DC.

Hyman, H. H. (1972). *Secondary analysis of sample surveys: Principles, procedures, and potentialities*. New York: Wiley.

Hynes, K., & Clarkberg, M. (2005). Women's employment patterns during early parenthood: A group-based trajectory analysis. *Journal of Marriage and the Family, 67*(1), 222–239.

Jacobs, J. A., & Gerson, K. (2004). *The time divide: Work, family, and gender inequality.* Cambridge, MA: Harvard University Press.

Jaffee, S. R., & Price, T. S. (2007). Gene–environment correlations: A review of the evidence and implications for prevention of mental illness. *Molecular Psychiatry, 12*(5), 432–442.

Jagger, C., Matthews, R., Melzer, D., Matthews, F., Brayne, C., & MRC-CFAS. (2007). Educational differences in the dynamics of disability incidence, recovery, and mortality: Findings from the MRC Cognitive Function and Ageing Study. *International Journal of Epidemiology, 36*(2), 358–365.

Janoski, T., & Hicks, A. M. E. (1994). *The comparative political economy of the welfare state.* Cambridge, England: Cambridge University Press.

Janson, C.-G. (1990). Retrospective data, undesirable behavior, and the longitudinal perspective. In D. Magnusson & L. R. Bergman (Eds.), *Data quality in longitudinal research* (pp. 100–121). Cambridge, England: Cambridge University Press.

Jarvie, I. C. (1969). The problem of ethical integrity in participant observation. *Current Anthropology, 10*(5), 505–508.

Jencks, C., Smith, M., Acland, H., Bane, M. J., Cohen, D., Gintis, H., et al. (1972). *Inequality: A reassessment of the effect of family and schooling in America.* New York: Basic Books.

Johnson, M. K. (2002). Social origins, adolescent experiences, and work value trajectories during the transition to adulthood. *Social Forces, 80*(4), 1307–1341.

Johnson, W. (2007). Genetic and environmental influences on behavior: Capturing all the interplay. *Psychological Review, 114*(2), 423–440.

Johnson, W., & Krueger, R. F. (2004). Genetic and environmental structure of adjectives describing the domains of the Big Five model of personality: A nationwide U.S. twin study. *Journal of Research on Personality, 38*(5), 448–472.

Jones, B. L., Nagin, D. S., & Roeder, K. (2001). A SAS procedure based on mixture models for estimating developmental trajectories. *Sociological Methods and Research, 29*(3), 374–393.

Jordan, N. C., Kaplan, D., Olah, L. N., & Locuniak, M. N. (2006). Number sense growth in kindergarten: A longitudinal investigation of children at risk for mathematical difficulties. *Child Development, 77*(1), 153–175.

Jöreskog, K. G., & Sörbom, D. (1996). *LISREL 8 user's reference guide.* Chicago: Scientific Software International.

Jouriles, E. N., McDonald, R., Norwood, W. D., & Ezell, E. (2001). Issues and controversies in documenting the prevalence of children's exposure to domestic violence. In S. A. Graham-Bermann & J. L. Edleson (Eds.), *Domestic violence in the lives of children: The future of research, intervention, and social policy* (pp. 12–34). Washington, DC: American Psychological Association.

Kahn, R. L., & Antonucci, T. C. (1980). Convoys over the life course: Attachment, roles, and social support. In P. B. Baltes & O. G. Brim, Jr. (Eds.), *Life-span development and behavior* (Vol. 3, pp. 253–286). New York: Academic Press.

Karweit, N., & Kertzer, D. I. (1998). Data organization and conceptualization.

In J. Z. Giele & G. H. Elder, Jr. (Eds.), *Methods of life course research: Qualitative and quantitative approaches* (pp. 81–97). Thousand Oaks, CA: Sage.

Kelley-Moore, J. A., & Ferraro, K. F. (2004). The black/white disability gap: Persistent inequality in later life? *Journal of Gerontology B: Psychological Sciences and Social Sciences, 59*(1), S34–S43.

Kendler, K. S., Neale, M., Kessler, R. C., Heath, A. C., & Eaves, L. (1993). A longitudinal twin study of personality and major depression in women. *Archives of General Psychiatry, 50*(11), 853–862.

Kendler, K. S., Thornton, L. M., & Pedersen, N. L. (2000). Tobacco consumption in Swedish twins reared apart and reared together. *Archives of General Psychiatry, 87*(9), 886–892.

Kerckhoff, A. C. (1976). The status attainment process: Socialization or allocation? *Social Forces, 55*, 368–381.

Kerckhoff, A. C. (1989). On the social psychology of social mobility processes. *Social Forces, 68*(1), 17–25.

Kertzer, D. I., & Hogan, D. P. (1989). *Family, political economy, and demographic change: The transformation of life in Casalecchio, Italy, 1861–1921.* Madison: University of Wisconsin Press.

Kessler, R. C., & Greenberg, D. F. (1981). *Linear panel analysis: Models of quantitative change.* New York: Academic Press.

Kidwell, R. E., Jr., Mossholder, K. W., & Bennett, N. (1997). Cohesiveness and organizational citizenship behavior: A multilevel analysis using work groups and individuals. *Journal of Management, 23*(6), 775–793.

Kiecolt-Glaser, J. K., & Newton, T. L. (2001). Marriage and health: His and hers. *Psychological Bulletin, 127*(4), 472–503.

Kim-Cohen, J., Caspi, A., Taylor, A., Williams, B., Newcombe, R., Craig, I. W., et al. (2006). MAOA, maltreatment, and gene–environment interaction predicting children's mental health: New evidence and a meta-analysis. *Molecular Psychiatry, 11*(10), 903–913.

Kirchler, E., Rodler, C., Holzl, E., & Meier, K. (2001). *Conflict and decision-making in close relationships: Love, money and daily routines.* East Sussex, England: Psychology Press.

Kleinman, S. (1991). Field-workers' feelings: What we feel, who we are, how we analyze. In W. B. Shaffir & R. A. Stebbins (Eds.), *Experiencing fieldwork: An inside view of qualitative research* (pp. 184–195). Newbury Park, CA: Sage.

Kleinman, S., & Copp, M. A. (1993). *Emotions and fieldwork.* Newbury Park, CA: Sage.

Kloos, P. (1969). Role conflicts in social fieldwork. *Current Anthropology, 10*(5), 509–512.

Knaub, P. K., Eversoll, D. B., & Voss, J. H. (1983). Is parenthood a desirable adult role?: An assessment of attitudes held by contemporary women. *Sex Roles, 9*(3), 355–362.

Kohli, M. (1981). Biography: Account, text, method. In D. Bertaux (Ed.), *Biography and society: The life history approach in the social sciences* (pp. 61–75). Beverly Hills, CA: Sage.

Kohn, M. L. (1987). Cross-national research as an analytic strategy. *American Sociological Review, 52*(6), 713–731.

Kohn, M. L., & Schooler, C. (1983). *Work and personality: An inquiry into the impact of social stratification.* Norwood, NJ: Ablex.

Komarovsky, M. (1985). *Women in college: Shaping new feminine identities.* New York: Basic Books.

Komlos, J. (2004). How to (and how not to) analyze deficient height samples. *Historical Methods, 37*(4), 160–173.

Kreuter, F., & Muthén, B. (2008). Analyzing criminal trajectory profiles: Bridging multilevel and group-based approaches using growth mixture modeling. *Journal of Quantitative Criminology, 24*(1), 1–31.

Kuh, D., & Ben-Shlomo, Y. (2004). *A life course approach to chronic disease epidemiology.* New York: Oxford University Press. (Original work published 1997)

Kurtines, W. M., Ferrer-Wreder, L., Berman, S. L., Lorente, C. C., Briones, E., Montgomery, M. J., et al. (2008). Promoting positive youth development: The Miami Youth Development Project (YDP). *Journal of Adolescent Research, 23*(3), 256–267.

Kurz, D. (1996). Separation, divorce, and woman abuse. *Violence Against Women, 2*(1), 63–81.

Lachman, M. E., & Weaver, S. L. (1998). Sociodemographic variations in the sense of control by domain: Findings from the MacArthur studies on midlife. *Psychology and Aging, 13*(4), 553–562.

Land, K. C., McCall, P. L., & Nagin, D. S. (1996). A comparison of Poisson, negative binomial, and semiparametric mixed Poisson regression models with empirical applications to criminal careers data. *Sociological Methods and Research, 24*(4), 387–442.

Larson, R. W., & Almeida, D. M. (1999). Emotional transmission in the daily lives of families: A new paradigm for studying family process. *Journal of Marriage and the Family, 61*(1), 5–20.

Laub, J. H. (2006). Edwin H. Sutherland and the Michael–Adler report: Searching for the soul of criminology 70 years later: The 2005 Sutherland Award address. *Criminology, 44*(2), 235–258.

Laub, J. H., Nagin, D., & Sampson, R. J. (1998). Trajectories of change in criminal offending: Good marriages and the desistance process. *American Sociological Review, 63*, 225–238.

Laub, J. H., & Sampson, R. J. (1993). Turning points in the life course: Why change matters to the study of crime. *Criminology, 31*(3), 301–325.

Laub, J. H., & Sampson, R. J. (2002). Sheldon and Eleanor Gluecks' Unraveling Juvenile Delinquency Study: The lives of 1,000 Boston men in the twentieth century. In E. Phelps, F. F. Furstenberg, Jr., & A. Colby (Eds.), *Looking at lives: American longitudinal studies of the twentieth century* (pp. 87–115). New York: Russell Sage Foundation.

Laub, J. H., & Sampson, R. J. (2003). *Shared beginnings, divergent lives.* Cambridge, MA: Harvard University Press.

Lauderdale, D. S., & Kestenbaum, B. (2002). Mortality rates of elderly Asian American populations based on Medicare and Social Security data. *Demography, 36*(3), 529–540.

Lazarfield, P. F., Berelson, B., & Gaudet, H. (1994). *The people's choice: How the voter makes up his mind in a presidential campaign* (Columbia University Bureau of Applied Research No. B-3). New York: Duell, Sloane, & Pierce.

Lazarus, R. S. (1996). The role of coping in the emotions and how coping changes over the life course. In C. Malatesta-Magai & S. H. McFadden (Eds.), *Handbook of emotion, adult development and aging* (pp. 289–306). New York: Academic Press.

Lazarus, R. S. (1999). *Stress and emotion: A new synthesis.* New York: Springer.

Leone, J. M., Johnson, M. P., Cohan, C. L., & Lloyd, S. E. (2004). Consequences of male partner violence for low-income minority women. *Journal of Marriage and Family, 66*(2), 472–490.

Lieberson, S. (1985). *Making it count: The improvement of social research and theory.* Berkeley: University of California Press.

Link, B. G., & Phelan, J. (1995). Social conditions as fundamental causes of disease. *Journal of Health and Social Behavior, 35*(Extra issue: *Forty Years of Medical Sociology: The State of the Art and Directions for the Future*), 80–94.

Little, J. K. (1958). *A state-wide inquiry into decisions of youth about education beyond high school—follow-up studies.* Madison: University of Wisconsin School of Education.

Little, J. K. (1959). *Explorations into the college plans and experiences of high school graduates: A state-wide inquiry.* Madison: University of Wisconsin School of Education.

Loeber, R., & Hay, D. (1997). Key issues in the development of aggression and violence from childhood to early adulthood. *Annual Review of Psychology, 48*(1), 371–410.

Lorenz, F. O., Wickrama, K. A. S., Conger, R. D., & Elder, G. H., Jr. (2006). The short-term and decade-long effects of divorce on women's midlife health. *Journal of Health and Social Behavior, 47*(2), 111–125.

Lowenthal, M. F., & Chiriboga, D. A. (1972). Transition to the empty nest: Crisis, change, or relief? *Archives of General Psychiatry, 26*(1), 8–14.

Lowenthal, M. F., Thurnher, M., & Chiriboga, D. A. (1975). *Four stages of life: A comparative study of men and women facing transitions.* San Francisco: Jossey-Bass.

Lunney, J. R., Lynn, J., Foley, D. J., Lipson, S., & Guralnik, J. M. (2003). Patterns of functional decline at the end of life. *Journal of the American Medical Association, 289*(18), 2387–2392.

Luo, Y., & Waite, L. J. (2005). The impact of childhood and adult SES on physical, mental, and cognitive well-being in later life. *Journals of Gerontology B: Psychological Sciences and Social Sciences, 60*(2), 93–101.

Luster, T., Small, S. A., & Lower, R. (2002). The correlates of abuse and witnessing abuse among adolescents. *Journal of Interpersonal Violence, 17*(12), 1323–1340.

Lynch, S. M. (2003). Cohort and life-course patterns in the relationship between education and health: A hierarchical approach. *Demography, 40*(2), 309–331.

Lynch, S. M., & George, L. K. (2002). Interlocking trajectories of loss-related events and depressive symptoms among elders. *Journals of Gerontology B: Psychological Sciences and Social Sciences, 57*(2), S117–S125.

Lynn, J. (1997). An 88-year-old woman facing the end of life. *Journal of the American Medical Association, 277*(20), 925–932.

Lynn, J. (2001). Serving patients who may die soon and their families: The role of hospice and other services. *Journal of the American Medical Association, 285*(7), 925–932.

Macmillan, R. (2001). Violence and the life course: The consequences of victimization for personal and social development. *Annual Review of Sociology, 27,* 1–22.

Magnusson, D. (1988). *Individual development from an interactional perspective: A longitudinal study.* Hillsdale, NJ: Erlbaum.

Maguire, M. C. (1999). Treating the dyad as the unit of analysis: A primer on three analytic approaches. *Journal of Marriage and the Family, 61*(1), 213–223.

Manting, D. (1996). The changing meaning of cohabitation and marriage. *European Sociological Review, 12*(1), 53–65.

Marmot, M. G., Smith, G. D., Stansfeld, S., Patel, C., North, F., Head, J., et al. (1991). Health inequalities among British civil servants: The Whitehall II study. *Lancet, 337*(8754), 1387–1393.

Martijn, C., & Sharpe, L. (2006). Pathways to youth homelessness. *Social Science and Medicine, 62*(1), 1–12.

Mason, C. M., & Griffin, M. A. (2003). Group absenteeism and positive affective tone: A longitudinal study. *Journal of Organizational Behavior, 24*(6), 667–687.

Mason, W. M., & Fienberg, S. E. E. (1985). *Cohort analysis in social research.* New York: Springer.

Mayer, K. U. (1990). *Lebensverläufe und sozialer Wandel. Sonderheft 31, Kölner Zeitschrift für Soziologie und Sozialpsychologie* [Life courses and social change. *Kölner Journal of Sociology and Social Psychology.*] Special edition 31. Opladen: Westdeutscher Verlag.

Mayer, K. U. (1997). Notes on a comparative political economy of life courses. *Comparative Social Research, 16,* 203–226.

Mayer, K. U. (2009). New directions in life course research. *Annual Review of Sociology, 35,* 20.1–20.21.

Mayer, K. U., & Huinink, J. (1990). Age, period, and cohort in the study of the life course: A comparison of classical A-P-C analysis with event history analysis or farewell to Lexis? In D. Magnusson & L. R. Bergman (Eds.), *Data quality in longitudinal research* (pp. 211–232). New York: Cambridge University Press.

Mayer, K. U., & Tuma, N. B. (Eds.). (1990). *Event history analysis in life course research.* Madison: University of Wisconsin Press.

McAdams, D. P. (1985). *Power, intimacy, and the life story: Personological inquiries into identity.* Homewood, IL: Dorsey Press.

McAdam, D. (1989). The biographical consequences of activism. *American Sociological Review, 54,* 744–760.

McAdams, D. P. (2001). The psychology of life stories. *Review of General Psychology, 5*(2), 100–122.

McAdams, D. P. (2006). The redemptive self: Generativity and the stories Americans live by. *Research in Human Development, 3*(2 & 3), 81–100.

McClelland, D. C. (1967). *The achieving society.* New York: Free Press.

McClelland, D. C. (1975). *Power: The inner experience.* New York: Irvington.

McDonough, P., & Berglund, P. (2003). Histories of poverty and self-rated health trajectories. *Journal of Health and Social Behavior, 44*(2), 198–214.

McGue, M., & Christensen, K. (2003). The heritability of depression symptoms in elderly Danish twins: Occasion-specific versus general effects. *Behavior Genetics, 33*(2), 83–93.

McLeod, J. D., & Almazan, E. P. (2003). Connections between childhood and adulthood. In J. T. Mortimer & M. J. Shanahan (Eds.), *Handbook of the life course* (pp. 391–412). New York: Kluwer Academic/Plenum Press.

McLeod, J. D., & Fettes, D. L. (2007). Trajectories of failure: The educational careers of children with mental health problems. *American Journal of Sociology, 113*(3), 653–701.

Mead, M. (1963). *Sex and temperament in three primitive societies.* New York: Morrow.

Meland, S. A. (2002). *Objectivity in perceived attractiveness: Development of a new methodology for rating facial physical attractiveness.* Unpublished MA thesis, Department of Sociology, University of Wisconsin–Madison.

Menard, S. (Ed.). (2008). *Handbook of longitudinal research: Design, measurement, and analysis.* Burlington, MA: Elsevier.

Merton, R. K. (1957). Puritanism, pietism, and science. In *Social theory and social structure* (pp. 574–606). Glencoe, IL: Free Press. (Original work published 1949)

Merton, R. K. (1959). Notes on problem finding in sociology. In R. K. Merton, L. Broom, & L. S. Cottrell, Jr. (Eds.), *Sociology today: Problems and prospects* (pp. ix–xxxiv). New York: Basic Books.

Merton, R. K. (1968). The Matthew effect in science. *Science, 159*(3810), 56–63.

Miles, M. B., & Huberman, A. M. (1994). *Qualitative data analysis: An expanded sourcebook* (2nd ed.). Thousand Oaks, CA: Sage.

Minton, H. L. (1988a). Charting life history: Lewis M. Terman's study of the gifted. In J. G. Morawski (Ed.), *The rise of experimentation in American psychology* (pp. 138–162). New Haven, CT: Yale University Press.

Minton, H. L. (1988b). *Lewis M. Terman: Pioneer in psychological testing.* New York: New York University Press.

Mirowsky, J., & Ross, C. E. (2003). *Education, social status, and health.* New York: de Gruyter.

Mishler, E. G. (1996). Missing persons: Recovering developmental stories/histories. In R. Jessor, A. Colby, & R. A. Schweder (Eds.), *Ethnography and human development: Context and meaning in social inquiry* (pp. 73–99). Chicago: University of Chicago Press.

Modell, J. (1989). *Into one's own: From youth to adulthood in the United States 1920–1975.* Berkeley: University of California Press.

Moen, P. (2003). Midcourse: Navigating retirement and a new life stage. In J. T. Mortimer & M. J. Shanahan (Eds.), *Handbook of the life course* (pp. 269–291). New York: Kluwer Academic/Plenum Press.

Moen, P., & Chesley, N. (2008). Toxic job ecologies, time convoys, and work–family conflict: Can families (re)gain control and life course "fit"? In K.

Korabik, D. S. Lero, & D. L. Whitehead (Eds.), *Handbook of work–family integration: Research, theory, and best practices* (pp. 95–122). New York: Elsevier.

Moen, P., Dempster-McClain, D., & Williams, R. M., Jr. (1989). Social integration and longevity: An event history analysis of women's roles and resilience. *American Sociological Review, 54,* 635–647.

Moen, P., Dempster-McClain, D., & Williams, R. M., Jr. (1992). Successful aging: A life-course perspective on women's multiple roles and health. *American Journal of Sociology, 97*(6), 1612–1638.

Moen, P., Erickson, M. A., & Dempster-McClain, D. (1997). Their mothers' daughters?: The intergenerational transmission of gender role orientations in a world of changing roles. *Journal of Marriage and the Family, 59*(2), 281–293.

Moen, P., & Orrange, R. M. (2002). Careers and lives: Socialization, structural lag, and gendered ambivalence. In R. A. Settersten, Jr. & T. J. Owens (Eds.), *Advances in life course research: New frontiers in socialization* (Vol. 7, pp. 231–260). London: Elsevier Science.

Moen, P., & Roehling, P. (2005). *The career mystique: Cracks in the American dream.* Boulder, CO: Rowman & Littlefield.

Moen, P., & Sweet, S. (2002). Two careers, one employer: Couples working for the same corporation. *Journal of Vocational Behavior, 61*(3), 466–483.

Moen, P., & Sweet, S. (2003). Time clocks: Work-hour strategies. In P. Moen (Ed.), *It's about time: Couples and careers* (pp. 17–34). Ithaca, NY: Cornell University Press.

Moen, P., Sweet, S., & Swisher, R. (2005). Embedded career clocks: The case of retirement planning. In R. Macmillan (Ed.), *Advances in life course research: The structure of the life course: Individualized? Standardized? Differentiated?* (Vol. 9, pp. 237–265). New York: Elsevier.

Moffitt, T. E. (1993). Adolescence-limited and life-course-persistent antisocial behavior: A developmental taxonomy. *Psychological Review, 100*(4), 674–701.

Moffitt, T. E., Caspi, A., Harrington, H., & Milne, B. J. (2002). Males on the life-course-persistent and adolescence-limited antisocial pathways: Follow-up at age 26 years. *Development and Psychopathology, 14*(1), 179–207.

Moffitt, T. E., Caspi, A., & Rutter, M. (2005). Strategy for investigating interactions between measured genes and measured environments. *Archives of General Psychiatry, 62*(5), 473–481.

Morrison, D. R., & Ritualo, A. (2000). Routes to children's economy recovery after divorce: Are cohabitation and remarriage equivalent? *American Sociological Review, 65*(4), 560–580.

Mortimer, J. T. (2003). *Working and growing up in America.* Cambridge, MA: Harvard University Press.

Mortimer, J. T., & Shanahan, M. J. (Eds.). (2003). *Handbook on the life course.* New York: Kluwer Academic/Plenum Press.

Mroczek, D. K., & Kolarz, C. M. (1998). The effect of age on positive and negative affect: A developmental perspective on happiness. *Journal of Personality and Social Psychology, 75*(5), 1333–1349.

Murray, H. A. (1938). *Explorations in personality: A clinical and experimental study of fifty men of college age.* New York: Oxford University Press.

Murray, S. A., Kendall, M., Boyd, K., & Sheikh, A. (2005). Illness trajectories and palliative care. *British Medical Journal, 330*(7498), 1007–1008.

Musick, J. S. (1993). *Young, poor, and pregnant: The psychology of teenage motherhood.* New Haven, CT: Yale University Press.

Musick, M. A., House, J. S., & Williams, D. R. (2004). Attendance at religious services and mortality in a national sample. *Journal of Health and Social Behavior, 45*(2), 198–213.

Mustillo, S., Worthman, C., Erkanli, A., Keeler, G., Angold, A., & Costello, E. J. (2003). Obesity and psychiatric disorder: Developmental trajectories. *Pediatrics, 111*(4), 851–859.

Muthén, B. (2001). Latent variable mixture modeling. In G. A. Marcoulides & R. E. Schumacker (Eds.), *New developments and techniques in structural equation modeling* (pp. 1–33). Mahwah, NJ: Erlbaum.

Muthén, B. (2004). Latent variable analysis: Growth mixtures modeling and related techniques for longitudinal data. In D. W. Kaplan (Ed.), *Handbook of quantitative methodology for the social sciences* (pp. 345–368). Newbury Park, CA: Sage.

Muthén, B., & Muthén, L. K. (2000). Integrating person-centered and variable-centered analysis: Growth mixture modeling with latent trajectory classes. *Alcoholism: Clinical and Experimental Research, 24*(6), 882–891.

Nagin, D. S. (1999). Analyzing developmental trajectories: A semiparametric group-based approach. *Psychological Methods, 4*(2), 139–157.

Nagin, D. S. (2005). *Group-based modeling of development over the life course.* Cambridge, MA: Harvard University Press.

Nagin, D. S., Farrington, D. P., & Moffitt, T. E. (1995). Life-course trajectories of different types of offenders. *Criminology, 33*(1), 111–139.

Nagin, D. S., & Land, K. C. (1993). Age, criminal careers and population heterogeneity: Specification and estimation of a nonparametric, mixed poisson model. *Criminology, 31*, 327–362.

Nagin, D. S., & Tremblay, R. E. (1999). Trajectories of boys' physical aggression, opposition, and hyperactivity on the path to physically violent and nonviolent juvenile delinquency. *Child Development, 70*(5), 1181–1196.

Nagin, D., & Tremblay, R. E. (2005a). What has been learned from group-based trajectory modeling?: Examples from physical aggression and other problem behaviors. *Annals of the American Academy of Political and Social Science, 602*, 82–117.

Nagin, D. S., & Tremblay, R. E. (2005b). Developmental trajectory groups: Fact or a useful statistical fiction? *Criminology, 43*(4), 873–904.

Nansel, T. R., Haynie, D. L., & Simons-Morton, B. G. (2003). The association of bullying and victimization with middle school adjustment. In M. J. Elias & J. E. Zins (Eds.), *Bullying, peer harassment, and victimization in the schools: The next generation of prevention* (pp. 45–61). New York: Hawthorn Press.

National Center for Health Statistics. (1994). *National Death Index: General description.* Hyattsville, MD: U.S. Department of Health and Human Services, Public Health Service, Centers for Disease Control and Prevention, National Center for Health Statistics.

National Center for Health Statistics. (1999). *NDI PLUS: Coded causes of death* (rev. July 23, 1999 ed.). Hyattsville, MD: Division of Vital Statistics, National Center for Health Statistics, Centers for Disease Control and Prevention.

National Research Council. (2000). *The aging mind: Opportunities in cognitive research.* Washington, DC: National Academies Press.

National Research Council. (2001). *Cells and surveys: Should biological measures be included in social science research?* Washington, DC: National Academies Press.

National Research Council. (2006a). *Genes, behavior, and the social environment: Moving beyond the nature/nurture debate.* Washington, DC: National Academies Press.

National Research Council. (2006b). *When I'm 64.* Washington, DC: National Academies Press.

National Research Council. (2008). *Biosocial surveys.* Washington, DC: National Academies Press.

Nazio, T., & Blossfeld, H.-P. (2003). The diffusion of cohabitation among young women in West Germany, East Germany and Italy. *European Journal of Population, 19*(1), 47–82.

Nesselroade, J. R., & Baltes, P. B. (1974). Adolescent personality development and historical change: 1970–1972. *Monographs of the Society for Research in Child Development, 39*(1, Serial No. 154), 1–80.

Neugarten, B. L. (1979). Time, age, and the life cycle. *American Journal of Psychiatry, 136*(7), 887–894.

Neugarten, B. L., with a foreword by Dail A. Neugarten. (1996). *The meanings of age: Selected papers of Bernice L. Neugarten.* Chicago: University of Chicago Press.

Neupert, S. D., Almeida, D. M., & Charles, S. T. (2007). Age differences in reactivity to daily stressors: The role of personal control. *Journals of Gerontology B: Psychological Sciences and Social Sciences, 62*(4), 216–225.

Neupert, S. D., Almeida, D. M., Mroczek, D. K., & Spiro, A., III. (2006). The effects of the Columbia shuttle disaster on the daily lives of older adults: Findings from the VA Normative Aging Study. *Aging and Mental Health, 10*(3), 272–281.

Newman, K. S., & Massengill, R. P. (2006). The texture of hardship: Qualitative sociology of poverty. *Annual Review of Sociology, 32,* 423–446.

Nisbet, R. A. (1969). *Social change and history: Aspects of Western theory development.* New York: Oxford University Press.

Northouse, L. L., Mood, D., Templin, T., Mellon, S., & George, T. (2000). Couples' patterns of adjustment to colon cancer. *Social Science and Medicine, 50*(2), 271–284.

Oden, M. H. (1968). The fulfillment of promise: 40-year follow-up of the Terman Gifted Group. *Genetic Psychology Monographs, 77*(1), 3–93.

Ong, A., Bergeman, C. S., & Bisconti, T. L. (2005). Unique effects of daily perceived control on anxiety symptomatology during conjugal bereavement. *Personality and Individual Differences, 38*(3), 1057–1067.

O'Rand, A. M. (1996). The precious and the precocious: Understanding cumulative dis/advantage over the life course. *The Gerontologist, 36*, 230–238.

O'Rand, A. M. (2002). Cumulative advantage theory in life course research. *Annual Review of Gerontology and Geriatrics, 22*, 14–20.

O'Rand, A. M., & Hamil-Luker, J. (2005). Processes of cumulative adversity: Childhood disadvantage and increased risk of heart attack across the life course. *Journals of Gerontology B: Psychological Sciences and Social Sciences, 60*(Special Issue 2), 117–124.

Orbuch, T. L., Thornton, A., & Cancio, J. (2000). The impact of marital quality, divorce, and remarriage on the relationships between parents and their children. *Marriage and Family Review, 29*(4), 221–246.

Orcutt, H. K., Erikson, D. J., & Wolfe, J. (2004). The course of PTSD symptoms among Gulf War veterans: A growth mixture modeling approach. *Journal of Traumatic Stress, 17*(3), 195–202.

Ortiz, S. M. (2004). Leaving the private world of wives of professional athletes: A male sociologist's reflections. *Journal of Contemporary Ethnography, 33*(4), 466–487.

Osgood, D. W. (2005). Making sense of crime and the life course. *Annals of the American Academy of Political and Social Science, 602*, 196–211.

Palloni, A. (2006). Reproducing inequalities: Luck, wallets and the enduring effects of childhood health. *Demography, 43*(4), 587–616.

Pampel, F. C., & Rogers, R. G. (2004). Socioeconomic status, smoking and health: A test of competing theories of cumulative advantage. *Journal of Health and Social Behavior, 45*(3), 306–321.

Park, J. M., Hogan, D. P., & Goldscheider, F. K. (2003). Child disability and mothers' tubal sterilization. *Perspectives on Sexual and Reproductive Health, 35*(3), 138–143.

Parsons, T. (1966). *Societies: Evolutionary and comparative perspectives*. Englewood Cliffs, NJ: Prentice-Hall.

Parsons, T., Bales, R. F., & Shils, E. A. (1953). *Working papers in the theory of action*. Glencoe, IL: Free Press.

Patterson, G. R., & Yoerger, K. (1993). Developmental models for delinquent behavior. In S. Hodgins (Ed.), *Mental disorder and crime* (pp. 140–172). Newbury Park, CA: Sage.

Pavalko, E. K., & Elder, G. H., Jr. (1993). Women behind the men: Variations in wives' support of husbands' careers. *Gender and Society, 7*(4), 548–567.

Pavalko, E. K., & Smith, B. (1999). The rhythm of work: Health effects of women's work dynamics. *Social Forces, 77*(3), 1141–1162.

Pavalko, E. K., & Woodbury, S. (2000). Social roles as process: Caregiving careers and women's health. *Journal of Health and Social Behavior, 41*(1), 91–105.

Pearlin, L. I. (1999). The stress process revisited: Reflections on concepts and their interrelationships. In C. S. Aneshensel & J. C. Phelan (Eds.), *Handbook of the sociobiology of mental health* (pp. 395–415). New York: Kluwer.

Pearlin, L. I., Menaghan, E. G., Lieberman, M. A., & Mullan, J. T. (1981). The stress process. *Journal of Health and Social Behavior, 22*, 337–356.

Pearlin, L. I., Schieman, S., Fazio, E. M., & Meersman, S. C. (2005). Stress, health, and the life course: Some conceptual perspectives. *Journal of Health and Social Behavior, 46*(2), 205–219.

Pearlin, L. I., & Schooler, C. (1978). The structure of coping. *Journal of Health and Social Behavior, 19*(1), 2–21.

Pearlin, L. I., & Skaff, M. M. (1996). Stress and the life course: A paradigmatic alliance. *Gerontologist, 36*(2), 239–247.

Pearlman, L. A., & Saakvitne, K. W. (1995). *Trauma and the therapist: Countertransference and vicarious traumatization in psychotherapy with incest survivors.* New York: Norton.

Pedersen, N. L., & Reynolds, C. A. (1998). Stability and change in adult personality: Genetic and environmental components. *European Journal of Personality, 12*(5), 365–386.

Pellegrini, A. D. (2002). Bullying and victimization in middle school: A dominance relations perspective. *Educational Psychologist, 37*(3), 151–163.

Peterson, C., Seligman, M. E. P., Yurko, K. H., Martin, L. R., & Friedman, H. S. (1998). Catastrophizing and untimely death. *Psychological Science, 9*(2), 127–130.

Peterson, R. R. (1996). A re-evaluation of the economic consequences of divorce. *American Sociological Review, 61*(2), 528–536.

Pettigrew, T. F. (1998). Intergroup conflict theory. *Annual Review of Psychology, 49*, 65–85.

Phelan, J. C., Link, B. G., Diez-Roux, A., Kawachi, I., & Levin, B. (2004). "Fundamental causes" of social inequalities in mortality: A test of the theory. *Journal of Health and Social Behavior, 45*(3), 265–285.

Phelps, E., Furstenberg, F. F., Jr., & Colby, A. (Eds.). (2002). *Looking at lives: American longitudinal studies of the twentieth century.* New York: Russell Sage Foundation.

Piquero, A. R. (2008). Taking stock of developmental trajectories of criminal activity over the life course. In A. Liberman (Ed.), *The long view of crime: A synthesis of longitudinal research* (pp. 23–78). New York: Springer.

Pixley, J. E. (2008). Life course patterns of career-prioritizing decisions and occupational attainment in dual-earner couples. *Work and Occupations, 35*(2), 127–163.

Plomin, R., DeFries, J. C., & Loehlin, J. C. (1977). Genotype–environment interaction and correlation in the analysis of human behavior. *Psychological Bulletin, 84*(2), 309–322.

Plomin, R., Pedersen, N. L., Lichtenstein, P., & McClearn, G. E. (1994). Variability and stability in cognitive abilities are largely genetic later in life. *Behavior Genetics, 24*(3), 207–215.

Pollner, M., & Emerson, R. M. (1983). The dynamics of inclusion and distance in fieldwork relations. In R. M. Emerson (Ed.), *Contemporary field research: A collection of readings* (pp. 235–252). Boston: Little, Brown.

Porter, J. N. (1974). Race, socialization and occupational mobility in educational and early occupational attainment. *American Sociological Review, 39*(3), 303–316.

Portes, A., & Wilson, K. (1976). Black–white differences in educational attainment. *American Sociological Review, 41*(3), 414–431.

Purvin, D. M. (2003). Weaving a tangled safety net—the intergenerational legacy of domestic violence and poverty. *Violence Against Women, 9*(10), 1263–1277.

Purvin, D. M. (2007). At the crossroads and in the crosshairs: Social welfare policy and low-income women's vulnerability to domestic violence. *Social Problems, 54*(2), 188–210.

Quick, H. E., & Moen, P. (1998). Gender, employment, and retirement quality: A life course approach to the differential experiences of men and women. *Journal of Occupational Health Psychology, 3*(1), 44–64.

Ragin, C. C. (1987). *The comparative method: Moving beyond qualitative and quantitative strategies.* Berkeley: University of California Press.

Ragin, C. C. (2000). *Fuzzy-set social science.* Chicago: University of Chicago Press.

Raley, S. B., Mattingly, M. J., & Bianchi, S. M. (2006). How dual are dual-income couples?: Documenting change from 1970 to 2001. *Journal of Marriage and the Family, 68*(1), 11–28.

Raudenbush, S. W. (2001). Comparing personal trajectories and drawing causal inferences from longitudinal data. *Annual Review of Psychology, 52*(1), 501–525.

Raudenbush, S. W. (2005). How do we study "what happens next"? *Annals of the American Academy of Political and Social Science, 602*(1), 131–144.

Reichart, E., Chesley, N., & Moen, P. (2007). Beyond the career mystique?: Policies structuring gendered paths in the United States and Germany. *Journal of Family Research, 3,* 336–369.

Reiss, A. J., Jr. (1989). *Ending criminal careers.* Washington, DC: MacArthur Foundation and National Institute of Justice.

Reiss, A. J., Jr., & Rhodes, A. L. (1961). The distribution of juvenile delinquency in the social class structure. *American Sociological Review, 26*(5), 720–732.

Reiss, A. J., Jr., & Roth, J. A. E. (1994). *Consequences and control* (Vol. 4). Washington, DC: National Academies Press.

Reither, E. N., Hauser, R. M., & Swallen, K. E. (2009). Predicting adult health and mortality from adolescent facial characteristics in yearbook photographs. *Demography, 46*(1), 27–41.

Rhodes, A. L., Reiss, A. J., Jr., & Duncan, O. D. (1965). Occupational segregation in a metropolitan school system. *American Journal of Sociology, 70*(6), 682–694.

Riley, M. W. (1973). Aging and cohort succession: Interpretations and misinterpretations. *Public Opinion Quarterly, 37*(1), 35–49.

Riley, M. W., Johnson, M. E., & Foner, A. (1972). *Aging and society: Vol. 3. A sociology of age stratification.* New York: Russell Sage Foundation.

Rimer, S. (2008, October 10). Math skills suffer in U.S., study finds. *New York Times,* pp. 15, 19.

Rindfuss, R. R., Swicegood, C. G., & Rosenfeld, R. A. (1987). Disorder in the life course: How common and does it matter? *American Sociological Review,* *52,* 785–801.

Rodgers, J. L., St. John, C. A., & Coleman, R. (2005). Did fertility go up after the Oklahoma City bombing?: An analysis of births in metropolitan counties in Oklahoma, 1990–1999. *Demography, 42*(4), 675–692.

Rodgers, W. L. (1982). Estimable functions of age, period, and cohort effects. *American Sociological Review, 47*(6), 774–787.

Rossi, A. S., & Rossi, P. H. (1990). *Of human bonding: Parent–child relations across the life course.* New York: Aldine.

Rowe, D. C., Jacobson, K. C., & Van den Oord, E. J. C. G. (1999). Genetic and environmental influences on vocabulary IQ: Parental education level as moderator. *Child Development, 70*(5), 1151–1162.

Rowlison, R. T., & Felner, R. D. (1988). Major life events, hassles, and adaptation in adolescence: Confounding in the conceptualization and measurement of life stress and adjustment revisited. *Journal of Personality and Social Psychology, 55*(3), 432–444.

Ruggles, S. (2002). *Integrated public use microdata series.* Retrieved December 2, 2003, from *www.ipums.unm.edu.*

Ryder, N. B. (1965). The cohort as a concept in the study of social change. *American Sociological Review, 30*(6), 843–861.

Rylander-Rudqvist, T., Hakansson, N., Tybring, G., & Wolk, A. (2006). Quality and quantity of saliva DNA obtained from the self-administrated oragene method—a pilot study on the cohort of Swedish men. *Cancer Epidemiology Biomarkers and Prevention, 15*(9), 1742–1745.

Sampson, R. J., & Laub, J. H. (1993). *Crime in the making: Pathways and turning points through life.* Cambridge, MA: Harvard University Press.

Sampson, R. J., & Laub, J. H. (1996). Socioeconomic achievement in the life course of disadvantaged men: Military service as a turning point, circa 1940–1965. *American Sociological Review, 61*(3), 347–367.

Sampson, R. J., & Laub, J. H. (2003). Life-course desisters?: Trajectories of crime among delinquent boys followed to age 70. *Criminology, 41*(3), 555–592.

Sampson, R. J., & Laub, J. H. (2005a). A life course view of the development of crime. *Annals of the American Academy of Political and Social Science, 602*(1), 12–45.

Sampson, R. J., & Laub, J. H. (2005b). Seductions of method: Rejoinder to Nagin and Tremblay's "Developmental trajectory groups: Fact or fiction?" *Criminology, 43*(4), 905–914.

Sampson, R. J., Laub, J. H., & Eggleston, E. P. (2004a). *The aftermath of incarceration in the lives of disadvantaged men: A 50-year follow-up study: Final Report prepared for "The 'Mass' Incarceration Working Group."* New York: Russell Sage Foundation.

Sampson, R. J., Laub, J. H., & Eggleston, E. P. (2004b). On the robustness and validity of groups. *Journal of Quantitative Criminology, 20*(1), 37–42.

Sampson, R. J., Morenoff, J. D., & Earls, F. (1999). Beyond social capital: Spatial dynamics of collective efficacy for children. *American Sociological Review, 64*(5), 633–660.

Savla, J., Almeida, D. M., Davey, A., & Zarit, S. H. (2008). Routine assistance to parents: Effects on daily mood and other stressors. *Journals of Gerontology B: Psychological Sciences and Social Sciences, 63*(3), S154–S161.

Schaeffer, C. M., Petras, H., Ialongo, N., Masyn, K. E., Hubbard, S., Poduska, J., et al. (2006). A comparison of girls' and boys' aggressive–disruptive behavior trajectories across elementary school: Prediction to young adult antisocial outcomes. *Journal of Consulting and Clinical Psychology, 74*(3), 500–510.

Schauben, L. J., & Frazier, P. A. (1995). Vicarious trauma: The effects on female counselors of working with sexual violence survivors. *Psychology of Women Quarterly, 19*(1), 49–64.

Schoen, R., Rogers, S. J., & Amato, P. R. (2006). Wives' employment and spouses' marital happiness: Assessing the direction of influence using longitudinal couple data. *Journal of Family Issues, 27*(4), 506–528.

Schwalbe, M. L. (1987). On practical and discursive self-knowledge. *Humanity and Society, 11*, 366–384.

Scott, E. K., London, A. S., & Myers, N. A. (2002). Dangerous dependencies: The intersection of welfare reform and domestic violence. *Gender and Society, 16*(6), 878–897.

Scott, J., & Alwin, D. (1998). Retrospective versus prospective measurement of life histories in longitudinal research. In J. Z. Giele & G. H. Elder, Jr. (Eds.), *Methods of life course research: Qualitative and quantitative approaches* (pp. 98–127). Thousand Oaks, CA: Sage.

Segal, D. R., & Segal, M. W. (2004). America's military population. *Population Bulletin, 59*(4), 3–40.

Sewell, W. H. (1988). The changing institutional structure of sociology and my career. In M. W. Riley (Ed.), *Sociological lives* (pp. 119–143). Newbury Park, CA: Sage.

Sewell, W. H., & Armer, J. M. (1966a). Neighborhood context and college plans. *American Sociological Review, 31*(2), 159–168.

Sewell, W. H., & Armer, J. M. (1966b). Reply to Turner, Michael, and Boyle (On neighborhood context and college plans [I], [II], [III]). *American Sociological Review, 31*(5), 698–712.

Sewell, W. H., & Armer, J. M. (1972). High school context and college plans: A comment. *American Sociological Review, 37*(5), 637–639.

Sewell, W. H., Haller, A. O., & Ohlendorf, G. W. (1970). The educational and early occupational status attainment process: Replication and revision. *American Sociological Review, 35*(6), 1014–1027.

Sewell, W. H., Haller, A. O., & Portes, A. (1969). The educational and early occupational attainment process. *American Sociological Review, 34*(1), 82–92.

Sewell, W. H., & Hauser, R. M. (1972). Causes and consequences of higher education: Models of the status attainment process. *American Journal of Agricultural Economics, 54*(6), 851–861.

Sewell, W. H., & Hauser, R. M. (1975). *Education, occupation, and earnings: Achievement in the early career.* New York: Academic Press.

Sewell, W. H., & Hauser, R. M. (1992). The influence of the American occupational structure on the Wisconsin Model. *Contemporary Sociology, 21*(5), 598–603.

Sewell, W. H., Hauser, R. M., Springer, K. W., & Hauser, T. S. (2004). As we age:

The Wisconsin Longitudinal Study, 1957–2001. In K. Leicht (Ed.), *Research in social stratification and mobility* (Vol. 20, pp. 3–111). London: Elsevier.

Sewell, W. H., Hauser, R. M., & Wolf, W. C. (1980). Sex, schooling and occupational status. *American Journal of Sociology, 86*(3), 551–583.

Shanahan, M. J., & Elder, G. H., Jr. (2002). History, agency, and the life course. In L. J. Crockett (Ed.), *Agency, motivation, and the life course* (pp. 145–185). Lincoln, NE: University of Nebraska Press.

Shanahan, M. J., Erickson, L. D., Vaisey, S., & Smolen, A. (2007). Helping relationships and genetic propensities: A combinatoric study of DRD2, mentoring, and educational continuation. *Twin Research and Human Genetics, 10*(2), 285–298.

Shanahan, M. J., & Hofer, S. M. (2005). Social context in gene–environment interactions: Retrospect and prospect. *Journals of Gerontology B: Psychological Sciences and Social Sciences, 60*, 65–76.

Shanahan, M. J., Hofer, S. M., & Shanahan, L. (2003). Biological models of behavior and the life course. In J. T. Mortimer & M. J. Shanahan (Eds.), *Handbook of the life course* (pp. 597–622). New York: Kluwer Academic/Plenum Press.

Shanahan, M. J., & Macmillan, R. (2007). *Biography and the sociological imagination: Contexts and contingencies.* New York: Norton.

Shanahan, M. J., Vaisey, S., Erickson, L. D., & Smolen, A. (2008). Environmental contingencies and genetic propensities: Social capital, educational continuation, and a dopamine receptor polymorphism. *American Journal of Sociology, 114*(S1), S260–S286.

Shavit, Y., & Blossfeld, H.-P. E. (1993). *Persistent inequality: Changing educational attainment in thirteen countries.* Boulder, CO: Westview Press.

Shuey, K. M., & Willson, A. E. (2008). Cumulative disadvantage and black/white disparities in life-course heath trajectories. *Research on Aging, 60*(2), 169–199.

Silverstein, M., Bengston, V. L., & Lawton, L. (1997). Intergenerational solidarity and the structure of adult child–parent relationships in American families. *American Journal of Sociology, 103*(2), 429–460.

Silverstein, M., & Long, J. D. (1998). Trajectories of grandparents' perceived solidarity with adult grandchildren: A growth curve analysis over 23 years. *Journal of Marriage and the Family, 60*(3), 912–923.

Simmons, R. G., Rosenberg, F., & Rosenberg, M. (1973). Disturbance in the self image of adolescence. *American Sociological Review, 38*(4), 553–568.

Singer, B., & Ryff, C. D. (2001). Person-centered methods for understanding aging: The integration of numbers and narratives. In R. H. Binstock & L. K. George (Eds.), *Handbook of aging and the social sciences* (5th ed., pp. 44–65). San Diego: Academic Press.

Singer, J. A. (2004). Narrative identity and meaning making across the adult lifespan: An introduction. *Journal of Personality, 72*(3), 437–460.

Singer, J. D., & Willett, J. B. (2003). *Applied longitudinal data analysis: Modeling change and event occurrence.* New York: Oxford University Press.

Singer, M., Hertas, E., & Scott, G. (2000). Am I my brother's keeper?: A case study of the responsibilities of research. *Human Organization, 59*(4), 389–400.

Singley, S. G., & Hynes, K. (2005). Transitions to parenthood. *Gender and Society, 19*(3), 376–397.

Slevin, K. F., & Wingrove, C. R. (1998). *From stumbling blocks to stepping stones: The life experiences of fifty professional African American women.* New York: New York University Press.

Smith, P. H., Tessaro, I., & Earp, J. A. L. (1995). Women's experiences with battering: A conceptualization from qualitative research. *Women's Health Issues, 5*(4), 173–182.

Sokoloff, N. J., & Dupont, I. (2005). Domestic violence at the intersections of race, class, and gender: Challenges and contributions to understanding violence against marginalized women in diverse communities. *Violence Against Women, 11,* 38–64.

Soskice, D. (1991). The institutional infrastructure for international competitiveness: A comparative analysis of the U.K. and Germany. In A. B. Atkinson & R. Brunetta (Eds.), *Economics for the New Europe: Proceedings of a conference held by the International Economic Association in Venice, Italy, November, 1990* (pp. 45–66). New York: New York University Press.

Spradley, J. P. (1980). *Participant observation.* New York: Holt, Rinehart & Winston.

Stebbins, R. A. (1972). The unstructured interview as incipient interpersonal relationship. *Sociology and Social Research, 56*(2), 164–179.

Stolzenberg, R. M. (2001). It's about time and gender: Spousal employment and health. *American Journal of Sociology, 107*(1), 61–100.

Stone, P. (2007). *Opting out?: Why women really quit careers and head home.* Berkeley: University of California Press.

Stouffer, S. A., Lumsdaine, A. A., Lumsdaine, M. H., Williams, R. M., Jr., Smith, M. B., Janis, I. L., et al. (1949). *The American soldier: Vol. II. Combat and its aftermath.* Princeton, NJ: Princeton University Press.

Stouffer, S. A., Suchman, E. A., DeVinney, L. C., Star, S. A., & Williams, R. M., Jr. (1949). *The American soldier: Vol. I. Adjustment during army life.* Princeton, NJ: Princeton University Press.

Straits, B. C. (1996). Ego-net diversity: Same- and cross-sex coworker ties. *Social Networks, 18*(1), 29–45.

Straus, M. A. (1992). Children as witnesses to marital violence: A risk factor of lifelong problems among a nationally representative sample of American men and women. In D. F. Schwartz (Ed.), *Children and violence: Report of the 23rd Ross Roundtable on Critical Approaches to Common Pediatric Problems* (pp. 98–109). Columbus, OH: Ross Laboratories.

Strauss, A. L., & Corbin, J. (1990). *Basics of qualitative research: Grounded theory procedures and techniques.* Newbury Park, CA: Sage.

Strober, M. H., & Chan, A. M. K. (1999). *The road winds uphill all the way: Gender, work, and family in the United States and Japan.* Cambridge, MA: MIT Press.

Strohschein, L. (2005). Parental divorce and child mental health trajectories. *Journal of Marriage and the Family, 67*(5), 1286–1300.

Sweet, S., & Moen, P. (2007). Integrating educational careers in work and family. *Community, Work and Family, 10*(2), 231–250.

Taylor, M. G. (2005). *Disaggregating disability trajectories: Exploring differences in the disability experience of older adults in the United States*. Unpublished dissertation, Duke University, Durham, NC.

Taylor, M. G. (2008). Timing, accumulation and the black/white disability gap in later life: A test of weathering. *Research on Aging, 30*(2), 226–250.

Taylor, M. G., & Lynch, S. M. (2004). Trajectories of impairment, social support, and depressive symptoms in later life. *Journals of Gerontology B: Psychological Sciences and Social Sciences, 59*(4), S238–S246.

Terman, L. M. (1925). *Mental and physical traits of a thousand gifted children*. Stanford, CA: Stanford University Press.

Terman, L. M., & Oden, M. H. (1959a). *Genetic studies of genius: Vol. 5. The gifted group at mid-life: Thirty-five years of follow-up of the superior child*. Stanford, CA: Stanford University Press.

Terman, L. M., & Oden, M. H. (1959b). *Genetic studies of genius: Vol. 4. The gifted child grows up: Twenty-five years' follow-up of a superior group*. Stanford, CA: Stanford University Press.

Thernstrom, S. (1964). *Poverty and progress: Social mobility in a 19th-century city*. Cambridge, MA: Harvard University Press.

Thomas, W. I., & Znaniecki, F. (1918–1920). *The Polish peasant in Europe and America: Monograph of an immigrant group* (Vol. 1–5). Chicago: University of Chicago Press; Boston: Badger Press.

Thompson, L., & Walker, A. J. (1982). The dyad as the unit of analysis: Conceptual and methodological issues. *Journal of Marriage and Family, 44*(3), 889–900.

Titma, M., & Tuma, N. B. (Eds.). (1995). *Paths of a generation: A comparative longitudinal study of young adults in the former Soviet Union*. Stanford, CA: Stanford University Press.

Tremblay, R. E., Japel, C., Perusse, D., Mcduff, P., Boivin, M., Zoccolillo, M., et al. (1999). The search for age of "onset" of physical aggression: Rousseau and Bandura revisited. *Criminal Behavior and Mental Health, 9*(1), 8–23.

Turnbull, J. E., George, L. K., Landerman, R., Swartz, M. S., & Blazer, D. G. (1990). Social outcomes related to age of onset among psychiatric disorders. *Journal of Consulting and Clinical Psychology, 58*(6), 832–839.

Turner, R. H. (1960). Sponsored and contest mobility and the school system. *American Sociological Review, 25*(6), 855–867.

Turner, R. H. (1964). *The social context of ambition*. San Francisco: Chandler.

U.S. Department of Health and Human Services, Centers for Disease Control and Prevention. (1988). National Maternal and Infant Health Survey. Retrieved August 14, 2008, from *www.cdc.gov/nchs/about/major/nmihs/abnmihs.htm*

U.S. Department of Health and Human Services. (1999). Annual update of the Health and Human Services poverty guidelines. *Federal Register, 64*, 13428–13430.

U.S. Public Health Service. (1980). *International classification of diseases, 9th revision, clinical modification*. Washington, DC: Author.

van de Rijt, A., & Buskens, V. (2006). Trust in intimate relationships: The increased importance of embeddedness for marriage in the United States. *Rationality and Society, 18*(2), 123–156.

Verbrugge, L. M., Gruber-Baldini, A. L., & Fozard, J. L. (1996). Age differences and age changes in activities: Baltimore Longitudinal Study of Aging. *Journals of Gerontology B: Psychological Sciences and Social Sciences, 51*(1), S30–S41.

Vidich, A. J. (1955). Participant observation and the collection and interpretation of data. *American Journal of Sociology, 60*(4), 354–360.

Volkart, E. H. (1951). *Social behavior and personality: Contributions of W. I. Thomas to theory and social research.* New York: Social Science Research Council.

von Eye, A., & Bogat, G. A. (2006). Person-oriented and variable-oriented research: Concepts, results, and development. *Merrill–Palmer Quarterly Journal of Developmental Psychology, 52*(3), 390–420.

Wadsworth, M. E. J. (1991). *The imprint of time: Childhood, history, and adult life.* Oxford, England: Clarendon Press.

Wagmiller, R. L., Jr., Lennon, M. C., Kuang, L., Alberti, P., & Aber, J. L. (2006). The dynamics of economic disadvantage and children's life chances. *American Sociological Review, 71*(5), 847–866.

Wang, M. (2007). Profiling retirees in the retirement transition and adjustment process: Examining the longitudinal change patterns of retirees' psychological well-being. *Journal of Applied Psychology, 92*(2), 455–474.

Warren, J. R., & Halpern-Manners, A. (2007). Is the glass emptying or filling up?: Reconciling divergent trends in high school completion and droput. *Educational Researcher, 36*(6), 335–343.

Warren, J. R., Sheridan, J. T., & Hauser, R. M. (2002). Occupational stratification across the life course: Evidence from the Wisconsin Longitudinal Study. *American Sociological Review, 67*(3, June), 432–455.

Wax, R. (1956). Reciprocity as a field technique. *Human Organization, 11*(3), 34–41.

Weber, M. (1930). *The Protestant ethic and the spirit of capitalism* (T. Parsons, Trans.). New York: Scribner.

Weinstein, E. A., & Deutschberger, P. (1963). Some dimensions of altercasting. *Sociometry, 26*(4), 454–466.

Wellman, B., Wong, R. Y.-L., Tindall, D., & Nazer, N. (1997). A decade of network change: Turnover, persistence and stability in personal communities. *Social Networks, 19*, 27–50.

Wells, T., Sandefur, G. D., & Hogan, D. P. (2004). What happens after the high school years among young persons with disabilities? *Social Forces, 82*(2), 803–832.

West, C., & Zimmerman, D. H. (1987). Doing gender. *Gender and Society, 1*(2), 125–151.

Weyman, A., Heinz, W. R., & Alheit, P. (1996). *Society and biography.* Paper presented at the Third International Symposium of the Sonderforschungsbereich 186.

Wheaton, B. (1990). Life transitions, role histories, and mental health. *American Sociological Review, 55*(2), 209–223.

Wheaton, B. (1999). The nature of stressors. In A. V. Horowitz & T. L. Scheid (Eds.), *A handbook for the study of mental health: Social contexts, theories, and systems* (pp. 176–197). New York: Cambridge University Press.

Wheaton, B., & Clarke, P. (2003). Space meets time: Integrating temporal and contextual influences on mental health in early adulthood. *American Sociological Review, 68,* 680–706.

White, R. W. (1966). *Lives in progress: A study of the natural growth of personality* (2nd ed.). New York: Holt, Rinehart & Winston. (Original work published 1952)

Williams, D. R., Lavizzo-Mourney, R., & Warren, R. C. (1994). The concept of race and health status in America. *Public Health Reports, 109*(1), 26–41.

Williams, L. A. (2003). Understanding child abuse and violence against women: A life course perspective. *Journal of Interpersonal Violence, 18*(4), 441–451.

Willie, C. V. (1988). Commentary on *Sociological Lives.* In M. W. Riley (Ed.), *Sociological lives* (Vol. 2, pp. 163–176). Newbury Park, CA: Sage.

Willson, A. E., Shuey, K. M., & Elder, G. H., Jr. (2007). Cumulative advantage processes as mechanisms of inequality in life course health. *American Journal of Sociology, 112*(6), 1886–1924.

Winship, C., & Morgan, S. L. (1999). The estimation of causal effects from observational data. *Annual Review of Sociology, 25,* 659–706.

Winston, P., with Angel, R. J., Burton, L. M., Chase-Lansdale, P. L., Cherlin, A. J., Moffitt, R. A., & Wilson, W. J. (1999). *Welfare, children, and families: A three-city study.* Overview and design. Available online at *web.jhu.edu/three-citystudy/images/overviewanddesign.pdf.*

Yates, M. E., Tennstedt, S., & Chang, B. H. (1999). Contributors to and mediators of psychological well-being for informal caregivers. *Journals of Gerontology B: Psychological Sciences and Social Sciences, 54*(1), P12–P22.

Yorgason, J. B., Almeida, D. M., Neupert, S. D., Spiro, A., III, & Hoffman, L. (2006). A dyadic examination of daily health symptoms and emotional well-being in late-life couples. *Family Relations, 55*(5), 613–624.

Zarit, S. H., & Eggebeen, D. J. (2002). Parent–child relationships in adulthood and later years. In M. H. Bornstein (Ed.), *Handbook of parenting* (2nd ed., Vol. 1, pp. 135–161). Mahwah, NJ: Erlbaum.

Zautra, A. J. (2003). *Emotions, stress, and health.* New York: Oxford University Press.

Zautra, A. J., Finch, J. F., Reich, J. W., & Guarnaccia, C. A. (1991). Predicting the everyday life events of older adults. *Journal of Personality, 59*(3), 507–538.

Zimmer, Z., & House, J. S. (2003). Education, income and functional limitation transitions among American adults: Contrasting onset and progression. *International Journal of Epidemiology, 32*(6), 1089–1097.

Author Index

Subject Index

About the Editors

Glen H. Elder, Jr. (PhD, University of North Carolina at Chapel Hill) is Research Professor of Sociology and Psychology at the University of North Carolina at Chapel Hill. He was formerly the Howard W. Odum Distinguished Professor of Sociology and Psychology. He is a pioneering figure in the development of life course theory and methods through longitudinal studies of children and adults who were influenced by the hard times of the Great Depression and World War II. Other major longitudinal projects include a multigenerational study of families and children under economic stress in the Midwest, and an inner-city longitudinal study of white and minority young people in Philadelphia. His books include *Children of the Great Depression: Social Change in Life Experience* (1974), which has been reissued in a 25th anniversary expanded edition (1999). He is a member of the American Academy of Arts and Sciences and has served as vice president of the American Sociological Association as well as president of the Society for Research on Child Development.

Janet Z. Giele (PhD, Harvard University) is Professor Emerita of Sociology, Social Policy, and Women's Studies at the Heller School for Social Policy and Management of Brandeis University. Her research focuses on the changing life course of women and the emergence of American family policy. Her work has been supported by the Ford and Rockefeller Foundations, German Marshall Fund, Lilly Endowment, National Institute on Aging, and National Science Foundation. She is the author, editor, or coeditor of *Women: Roles and Status in Eight Countries* (1977), *Women and the Future* (1978), *Women in the Middle Years* (1982), *Women and Work: The Continuing Struggle Worldwide* (1992), *Two Paths to Women's Equality* (1995), *Methods of Life Course Research* (1998), *Women and Equality in the Workplace* (2003), and *Changing Life Patterns in Western Industrial Societies* (2004).

Contributors

David M. Almeida (PhD, University of Victoria) is Professor of Human Development and Family Studies at The Pennsylvania State University. His current work involves linking naturally occurring daily stressors to physiological indicators of well-being, including endocrine and immune functioning. Dr. Almeida is the Principal Investigator of the National Study of Daily Experiences, an in-depth study of the National Survey of Midlife in the United States, and a Principal Investigator of Workplace Practices and Daily Family Well-Being Project. He currently serves on the editorial board of *Psychology and Aging*.

Hans-Peter Blossfeld (Dr. rer. pol., University of Mannheim) is Chair of Sociology I at the University of Bamberg, Director of the University's Institute of Longitudinal Studies in Education and State Institute for Family Research, and Principal Investigator of the National Educational Panel Study. He has published books and articles on social inequality, youth, family, and educational sociology, labor market research, demography, social stratification and mobility, the modern methods of quantitative social research, and statistical methods for longitudinal data analysis. Currently, he is interested in the flexibility trends for work in modern societies, the division of domestic work in the family, partner choice via the Internet, and the development of individual competences and educational careers over the life course. He is Editor-in-Chief of the *European Sociological Review*, as well as coeditor of *International Sociology*.

Jason D. Boardman (PhD, University of Texas at Austin) is Associate Professor of Sociology and Research Associate with the Population Program of the Institute of Behavioral Science at the University of Colorado at Boulder. His work examines health disparities with recent focus on the interplay between genetic and social factors as determinants of physical and psychological well-being. He has served on advisory councils with the National Institutes of Health, and he is currently on the editorial board of the *Journal of Health and Social Behavior*.

Linda M. Burton (PhD, University of Southern California) is the James B. Duke Professor of Sociology at Duke University. She directed the ethnographic component of Welfare, Children, and Families: A Three-City Study and is currently Principal Investigator of a multisite team ethnographic study (Family Life Project) of poverty, family processes, and child development in six rural communities. Her research integrates ethnographic and demographic approaches and examines the roles that poverty and intergenerational family dynamics play in accelerating the life course transitions of children and adults. She is a recipient of the Family Research Consortium IV Legacy Award and the American Family Therapy Academy Award for Innovative Contributions to Family Research. Dr. Burton is currently a member of the Board on Children, Youth, and Families, National Academy of Sciences, and is coeditor of the *Journal of Research on Adolescence*.

Elaine Eggleston Doherty (PhD, University of Maryland, College Park) is a research associate in the Department of Health, Behavior and Society at the Johns Hopkins Bloomberg School of Public Health. Her primary interests include crime and deviance over the life course, longitudinal data analysis and methodology, and the intersection of criminology and public health. Dr. Doherty is currently investigating a variety of research topics related to crime and drug use over the life course using the Woodlawn study, which is a prospective and longitudinal study of an urban community population of African Americans followed from age 6 to age 42.

Glen H. Elder, Jr. (*see* "About the Editors").

Raymond Garrett-Peters (MS, North Carolina State University) is a doctoral student in sociology at North Carolina State University and a data manager and analyst for Welfare, Children, and Families: A Three-City Study and Family Life Project team ethnographies at the Duke Population Research Institute. He has done previous ethnographic research on displaced professional-managerial workers' coping with unemployment. His current dissertation research uses ethnographic data from the Family Life Project to look at the dynamics of social support and coping among low-income rural mothers.

Linda K. George (PhD, Duke University) is Professor of Sociology and Associate Director of the Center for the Study of Aging and Human Development at Duke University. She is the author or editor of seven books, as well as the past president of the Gerontological Society and former editor of the *Journal of Gerontology: Social Sciences*. Her major research interests include social factors and depression; the effects of stress and coping, especially the stress of caring for an impaired family member; the relationship between religion and health; and the effects of medical technology on population health. She is a recipient of the Mentorship Award of the Behavioral and Social Sciences Section of the Gerontological Society of America and the 2004 Matilda White Riley Award of the American Sociological Association for distinguished scholarship on aging and the life course.

Janet Z. Giele (see "About the Editors").

Robert M. Hauser (PhD, University of Michigan) is Vilas Research Professor of Sociology at the University of Wisconsin–Madison, where he directs the Center for Demography of Health and Aging. He has worked on the Wisconsin Longitudinal Study since 1969 and been Principal Investigator since 1980. His current research interests include trends in educational progression and achievement among American racial and ethnic groups, the uses of educational assessment as a policy tool, and changes in socioeconomic standing, cognition, personality, health, and well-being across the life course. Recent publications include a report of the National Research Council, *Measuring Literacy: Performance Levels for Adults*, and analyses of trends and differentials in grade retention. He is a member of the National Academy of Sciences, the National Academy of Education, and the American Philosophical Society.

Elaine Hernandez (MPH, University of Minnesota) is currently a PhD candidate in the Department of Sociology at the University of Minnesota. She received a predoctoral National Research Service Award fellowship from the National Institute of Mental Health. Her research focuses broadly on health inequalities and integrates medical sociology and life course perspectives. For her dissertation, she is investigating the role of health knowledge and social networks in the reproduction of health inequalities.

Dennis P. Hogan (PhD, University of Wisconsin–Madison) is Chair of the Department of Sociology and Robert E. Turner Distinguished Professor of Sociology at Brown University. He does social demographic research on the life course of children, adolescents, and young adults. His research has included historical studies of the effects of changing social structures on the life course of American men born in the first half of the 20th century in the United States. His books *Transitions and Social Change: The Early Lives of American Men* and *Family, Political Economy*, and *Demographic Change: The Transformation of Life in Casalecchio, Italy 1861–1921*, with David I. Kertzer, illustrate the use of archival records. He is currently involved in a longitudinal study of adolescents living in rural Western Ethiopia and is beginning work on the impact of the Israeli occupation on the life course of Palestinians in the West Bank. He is also completing the book *Exceptional Children, Challenged Families: Raising Children with Disabilities* on the life course of children with disabilities and the linked life courses of their family members.

John H. Laub (PhD, State University of New York at Albany) is Distinguished University Professor in the Department of Criminology and Criminal Justice at the University of Maryland, College Park, as well as a Visiting Scholar at the Institute for Quantitative Social Science at Harvard University. His research interests include crime and the life course, juvenile delinquency and juvenile justice, and the history of criminology. He has published widely, including the award-winning *Crime in the Making: Pathways and Turning Points through Life* and *Shared Beginnings, Divergent Lives: Delinquent Boys to Age 70*, both with Robert Sampson. In 1996, he was named a fellow of the American Society of Criminology; in 2002–2003, he served as the President of the American Society of

Criminology, and in 2005, he received the Edwin H. Sutherland Award from the American Society of Criminology. He is past Editor of the *Journal of Quantitative Criminology* and is currently Associate Editor of *Criminology*.

Phyllis Moen (PhD, University of Minnesota) holds the McKnight Presidential Endowed Chair and is Professor of Sociology at the University of Minnesota. She served as president of the Eastern Sociological Society and is Emerita Professor of Sociology and of Human Development at Cornell University. Dr. Moen codirects (with Erin Kelly) the Flexible Work and Well-Being Center, part of a larger National Institutes of Health-funded network initiative, investigating ways to promote work redesign around employees' work–time control, as a means to reduce or prevent work–family conflict and to enhance individual and family health and life quality. She studies occupational careers, retirement, health, gender, policy, and families, as they intersect and play out over the life course. Her two most recent books are *It's About Time: Couples and Careers* (2003) and the award-winning *Career Mystique: Cracks in the American Dream* (2005, with Patricia Roehling).

Angela M. O'Rand (PhD, Temple University) is currently Professor and Chair of the Department of Sociology at Duke University. Prior to Duke, she was on the faculty of the University of Florida, where she helped to found the gerontology program at that institution. Her publications have focused on stratification processes in economic security and health over the life course. She has been active in the American Sociological Association's Section on Aging and the Life Course, from which she recently received the Matilda White Riley Award for exceptional contributions to the sociology of aging and the life course. She has been Editor of the journal *Research on Aging* since 1997 and Deputy Editor of *Demography* since 2007. In 2008, she was elected President of the Southern Sociological Society for 2009–2010.

Diane Purvin (PhD, Brandeis University) is a senior research associate at Casey Family Services, the Direct Service Agency of the Annie E. Casey Foundation. She was a data manager and family ethnographer for the Boston site of Welfare, Children, and Families: A Three-City Study, and her postdoctoral research used longitudinal ethnographic data from the Three-City Study to examine the impact of domestic abuse on low-income women and children through life course, developmental, and social policy perspectives. Prior to embarking on a research career, Dr. Purvin served as an advocate and program coordinator for children affected by domestic violence in a community-based shelter and service agency.

Robert J. Sampson (PhD, State University of New York at Albany) is Chair of the Department of Sociology and the Henry Ford II Professor of the Social Sciences at Harvard University. He also serves as Senior Advisor in the Social Sciences at the Radcliffe Institute for Advanced Study. He was elected a Fellow of the American Academy of Arts and Sciences in 2005 and a member of the National Academy of Sciences in 2006, and was a Fellow at the Center for Advanced

Study in the Behavioral Sciences in Stanford, California. Professor Sampson's research interests include crime, the life course, neighborhood effects, and the social organization of cities. With John Laub, he is coauthor of *Crime in the Making: Pathways and Turning Points through Life* and *Shared Beginnings, Divergent Lives: Delinquent Boys to Age 70.*

Michael J. Shanahan (PhD, University of Minnesota) is Professor of Sociology at the University of North Carolina at Chapel Hill. His interests include life course theory and research and the intersection of sociology and behavioral genetics. He is coeditor (with Jeylan Mortimer) of the *Handbook of the Life Course* (2003) and coauthor (with Ross Macmillan) of *Biography and the Sociological Imagination* (2008). He is a former Fellow of the Center for Advanced Study in the Behavioral Sciences (Stanford) and served as a Visiting Professor of Developmental Psychology at Friedrich Schiller University (Germany).

Carrie E. Spearin (PhD, Brown University) is Visiting Assistant Professor of Sociology and an affiliate of the Population Studies and Training Center at Brown University. Understanding family change from a life course perspective is a unifying theme of her research. Her most current research examines how the presence of children affects the relationship choices mothers and fathers make over time. This research is innovative as it combines family sociology and demography to explore the family lives of men, in comparison to women, using a life course perspective. Additional research interests include how families cope and adapt to the often unanticipated experience of having a child with a disability, the dynamic family lives of men, fatherhood, and divorce and remarriage and their impacts on children.

Miles G. Taylor (PhD, Duke University) is Assistant Professor of Sociology and Research Associate at the Pepper Institute for Aging and Public Policy at Florida State University. Funded by a National Institute on Aging Career Development Award, her current research examines the disparity between black and white older adults in functional limitations and mortality. She focuses on individual and structural mechanisms, including health insurance and neighborhood factors, while utilizing advanced trajectory methods to disentangle the timing of disparities, the mediating and moderating influences of individual socioeconomic and health factors, and cohort differences. She recently received a dissertation award from the Gerontological Association of America and currently serves on the editorial board of *Demography.*

Jen D. Wong (MS, The Pennsylvania State University) is a doctoral candidate in the Human Development and Family Studies Program at The Pennsylvania State University. She received her undergraduate degree from Hampshire College in Amherst, Massachusetts. Her research interests focus on daily stress, health, and employment transitions, with an emphasis on retirees and older workers. She is a past recipient of a grant for Research Training in Mental Health and Aging from the National Institute of Mental Health.